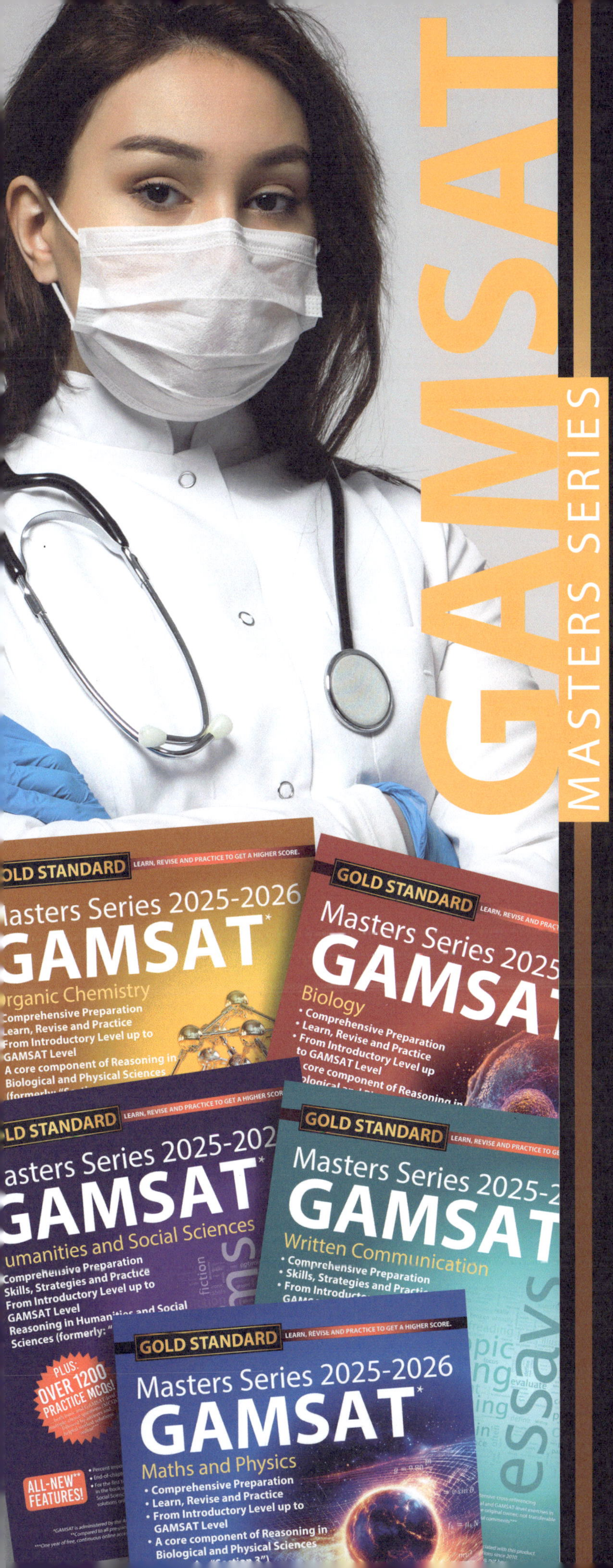

GOLD STANDARD

PERMISSION GRANTED

If you wish to share your study experience in social media (e.g. Instagram, TikTok, YouTube, etc.), Gold Standard GAMSAT gives you the permission to include any of our books (cover and/or interior pages, though never all pages from a chapter), and/or short segments of our videos, in your content. Share your study journey and inspire others!

01 **Editor and Author**
Brett Ferdinand BSc MD-CM

02 **Contributors**
Lisa Ferdinand BA MA
Sean Pierre BSc MD
Kristin Finkenzeller BSc MD
Ibrahima Diouf BSc MSc PhD
Charles Haccoun BSc MD-CM
Timothy Ruger BA MA
Jeanne Tan Te

03 **Illustrators**
Harvie W. Gallatiera BS CompE
Gilbert Rafanan BSc

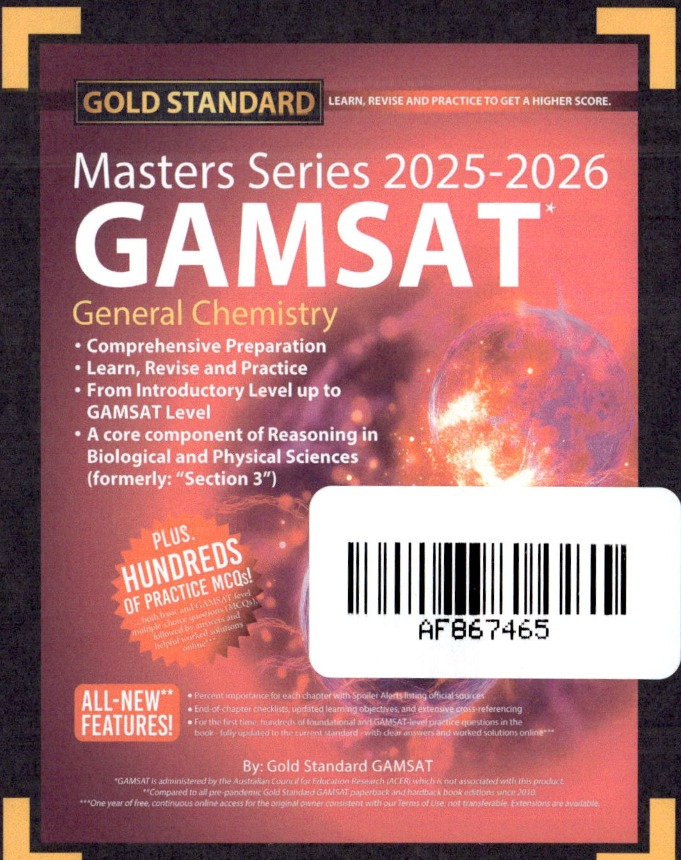

Register your book!

Free Online Access*

Answers and detailed worked solutions for hundreds of end-of-chapter practice questions, as well as the full-length practice test GS-Free which has the new digital GAMSAT format and cross-references to this Masters Series book.

*One year of continuous access for the original owner of this textbook upon online registration at www.gamsat-prep.com/gamsat-general-chemistry
If you purchased this textbook or the eBook directly from www.gamsat-prep.com, then your online access is automated.

Please note: Benefits last for one year from the date of online registration, for the original book owner only, and are not transferable; unauthorized access and use outside the Terms of Use posted on GAMSAT-prep.com may result in account deletion; if you are not the original owner, or if you are seeking an extension, you can purchase your virtual access card separately at GAMSAT-prep.com.

Online access: reduces digital piracy; allows the addition of relevant multimedia including videos; permits the updating of strategies and content to reflect the evolving GAMSAT; permits more detailed worked solutions; reduces the retail price; and ultimately, saves trees!

ISBN 978-1-927338-85-8

Address all inquiries, comments, or suggestions to the publisher. For Terms of Use go to: www.GAMSAT-prep.com

Gold Standard GAMSAT Product Contact Information

Distribution in Australia, NZ, Asia

Woodslane Pty Ltd 10 Apollo Street
Warriewood NSW 2102 Australia
ABN: 76 003 677 549
learn@gamsat-prep.com

Distribution in Europe

Central Books 99 Wallis
Road LONDON,
E9 5LN, United Kingdom
orders@centralbooks.com

Distribution in North America

RuveneCo Publishing
334 Cornelia Street #559
Plattsburgh, New York 12901, USA
buy@gamsatbooks.com

GAMSAT (Graduate Medical School Admissions Test)

Computer-based exam held at test centres internationally for graduate-entry medicine

Written Communication (Writing Tasks A & B)

- formerly "Section 2"

2 essays responding to 2 different themes using sound reasoning and competent English-writing skills (essays must be typed)

Writing Task A: sociocultural theme (e.g., free speech, justice, social media)
Writing Task B: personal-social themes (e.g., humour, love, happiness)

Reasoning in Humanities and Social Sciences

- formerly "Section 1"

multiple-choice section with stimulus materials requiring comprehension and analysis of non-science content

poetry • proverbs cartoons • novels or play excerpts • travel and/or medical journal entries • social science graphs

Reasoning in Biological and Physical Sciences

- formerly "Section 3"

multiple-choice section with questions mostly based on science passages that require problem-solving and graph analysis

first-year undergraduate level Biology (40%), General Chemistry (20%) & Organic Chemistry (20%) • A-level/Leaving Certificate/ Year 12 level Physics (20%)

Top GAMSAT Score: 100
Average GAMSAT Score: 57

Summary of the new Digital-format GAMSAT Exam Day

	KEY POINTS	EVENT	DURATION
Written Communication	Produce ideas in writing with clarity and soundness; essays are typed with no copy/paste function	2 essays typed on a computer (for all sections including the essays: no longer is there a formal, dedicated reading time)	65 minutes
Arrival and Sitting of Exam	Bring only the acceptable ID documents and permitted items to the test centre as specified in ACER's GAMSAT Information Booklet	Security, identification, health protocols	15-45 minutes
Reasoning in Humanities and Social Sciences	Key skills are reading speed and comprehension of information within socio-cultural contexts	62 MCQs* (the test centre will provide you with 2 sheets of A4 scratch paper; *option*: whiteboard)	100 minutes
Break	Consider packing your own lunch to avoid queues with nervous chatter	–	20 minutes
Reasoning in Biological and Physical Sciences	Analyse and solve problems: 40% Biology, 40% Chemistry (equally split between General and Organic); 20% Physics	75 MCQs* (the test centre will provide you with 2 new sheets of A4 scratch paper; *option*: whiteboard)	150 minutes
Total Test Time	Success requires stamina; stamina improves with practice.	–	5 hours, 15 minutes

*MCQs: multiple-choice questions, 4 options per question with only 1 best answer. Note that the 'old' GAMSAT had a dedicated 'reading time' of 10 minutes for each of Section 1 and 3, and 5 minutes for Section 2. During that reading time, students were not permitted to write or mark their exam paper in any way. The new digital GAMSAT has added time for each of the 3 exam sections as a legacy to 'reading time'; however, in practice, you can use your exam time in any way that you see fit.

**It might be a good idea to allocate a whole day to sit the GAMSAT test to allow for any contingencies and/or technical issues that you might encounter. Safety measures and health protocols should be carefully anticipated when making travel arrangements and accommodations to and from the testing centre.

Common formula for acceptance:

GPA + GAMSAT score + Interview = Medical School Admissions

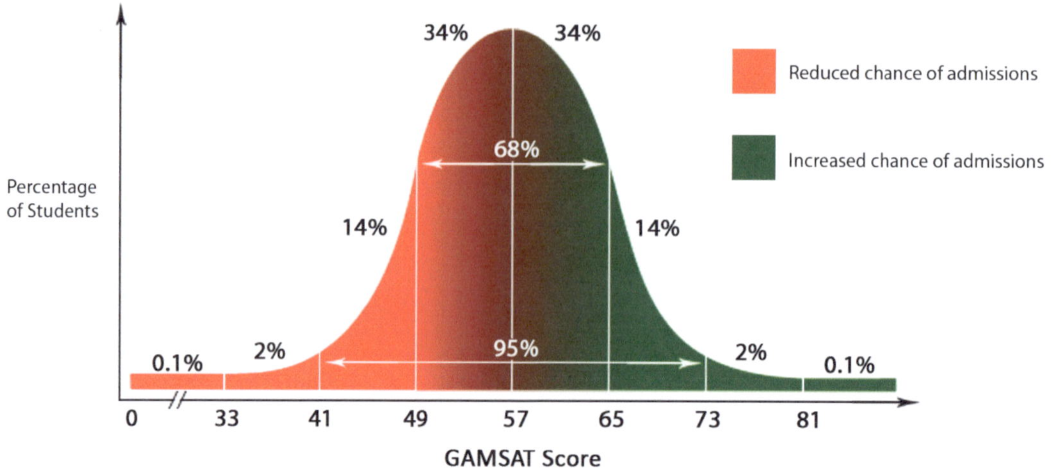

Typical Overall GAMSAT Score Distribution (Approx)

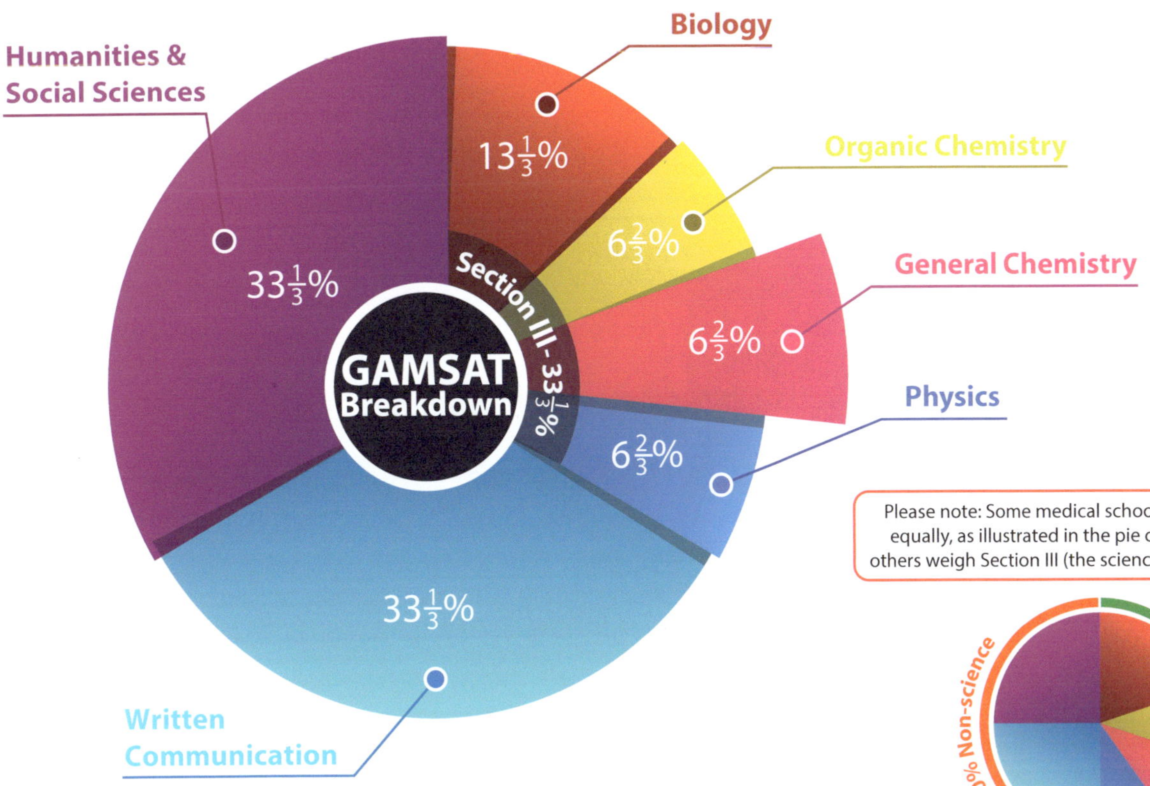

Please note: Some medical schools weigh all 3 sections equally, as illustrated in the pie chart to the left, while others weigh Section III (the sciences) twice as seen below.

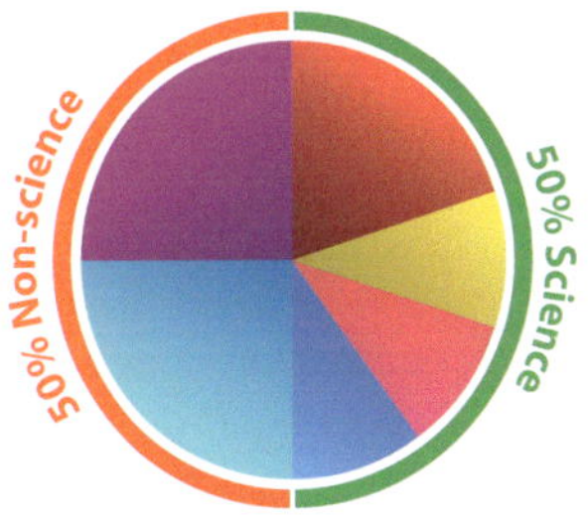

GAMSAT is challenging, get organised.

gamsat-prep.com/free-GAMSAT-study-schedule

1. How to study

- Learn, revise and practice using the GAMSAT Masters Series book(s) and/or videos.
- Complete all exercises and multiple-choice practice questions in this book.
- Consolidate: create and study from your personal summaries (= Gold Notes) daily. Create study cards or audio files from your Gold Notes to increase your study efficiency.

2. Once you have completed your studies

- Sit a full-length GAMSAT practice test.
- Analyse mistakes and all worked solutions.
- Consolidate: Revise all your Gold Notes and create more.

3. Sit multiple mock exams

- ACER GAMSAT practice exams with free Gold Standard worked solutions on YouTube
- Free full-length Gold Standard (GS) mock exam GS-Free with helpful, detailed worked solutions
- HEAPS: 15 full-length exams, 5 in the book and 10 online with the new, digital GAMSAT format

4. How much time do you need to study?

- On average, 3-6 hours per day for 3-6 months, depending on life experiences, 2 weeks may be enough and 8 months could be insufficient.
- Try to study full on for 1-2 weeks and then adjust your expectations for your personal, ideal study time.

5. Recommended GAMSAT Communities

- All countries (mainly Australia): pagingdr.net
- Mainly the UK: thestudentroom.co.uk (Medicine Community Discussion)
- Mainly Ireland: boards.ie (GAMSAT and GEM forum)

Is there something in the Masters Series that you did not understand? Don't get frustrated, get online:

gamsat-prep.com/forum

Table of Contents

Note that: H = High-level Importance; M = Medium-level Importance; L = Low-level Importance.

Note that: H = High-level Importance; M = Medium-level Importance; L = Low-level Importance.

Table of Contents

Note that: H = High-level Importance; M = Medium-level Importance; L = Low-level Importance.

Note that: H = High-level Importance; M = Medium-level Importance; L = Low-level Importance.

INTRODUCTION

GAMSAT Reasoning in Biological and Physical Sciences (i.e. GAMSAT Sciences, previously called: Section 3) is the final and longest of the 3 GAMSAT subtests. 'Biological Sciences' refers to Organic Chemistry and Biology. 'Physical Sciences' refers to Physics and General (Inorganic, not Organic) Chemistry. In our experience, most students with a non-science background (NSB) can successfully learn the assumed knowledge for GAMSAT independently, while a smaller number may need to enrol in a short tertiary-level science course, or use a video series to supplement their learning.

Essentially, 20% of GAMSAT Sciences is General Chemistry. The level of assumed knowledge is first year university Chemistry.

For a typical secondary or tertiary-level exam, you could read all the chapters in the relevant book, commit as much to memory as possible, walk into the exam room, match the questions with your knowledge, and reply. Your training: study anytime, even the night before the exam since you might encounter something that is word-for-word on exam day, replicate what you read, and you can ace the exam, in fact, you are brilliant!

The GAMSAT: study all you want even the night before, extremely unlikely to be able to identify something word-for-word on exam day, no feeling of being brilliant (this is true even for many students who actually 'ace' the exam). The actual exam includes 2 atypical sensations: **1)** you must learn a lot of new information *during* the exam; **2)** the topics and questions almost seem random. In some ways, these atypical sensations emulate life as a doctor!

In summary, you have been trained to focus on 'knowledge' as a priority to succeed in university studies. Frankly, for some exams, 'understanding' is secondary. If you had both knowledge and understanding, you would likely ace any exam – except GAMSAT. We will continually try to adjust the way you study while you read chapters herein.

What is General Chemistry?

General Chemistry is principally concerned with atoms and molecules, how they interact, and how they transform into other atoms and molecules. The one basic force that underlies virtually all GAMSAT General Chemistry, *electrostatics*, boils down to the one catch phrase that almost everyone has heard before: 'opposites attract' and thus like charges repel. The latter is not an oversimplification, it is one of the founding principles of Chemistry.

General Chemistry includes stoichiometry (the quantitative relationship between reactants and products), the infamous periodic table, the different phases of matter (gas, liquid, solid), acids & bases, heat changes in reactions (thermodynamics), how quickly reactions occur (rate processes), and the production of electricity from chemicals (electrochemistry).

You have always been a chemist. As a child, you likely experimented by mixing water with some solid or crystals (dirt, salt, sugar, whatever!) and observed solubility and precipitation (= 2 common GAMSAT topics; the latter relates to the inability to dissolve any more). As an adult, you took it much further: brewing coffee or tea; dissolving sugar (easier at high temperature rather than low temperature); noting the separation of oil and water; observing the phase changes of water – ice (solid), 'water' (liquid), steam (gas); acids (pH < 7) with their sour taste as opposed to bases (pH > 7); the in-house chemistry lab: the kitchen (adding energy to *denature* or change certain bonding patterns); the curious energy stored in batteries (electrochemistry) – just to name a few.

How do I study GAMSAT General Chemistry?

We do not believe that it would be an efficient use of your time to plan to read all chapters in this textbook multiple times, nor to attempt to read straight through from the beginning to the end in one go. Ideally, you would plan to read each chapter once while taking very brief notes (less than 1 page per chapter). Either before or after reading a chapter – where applicable – you may choose to watch some online videos relevant to that chapter while also taking very brief notes. Revise your notes often according to your GAMSAT study schedule which you can modify from the one we created (gamsat-prep.com/free-GAMSAT-study-schedule).

Practice questions

We have 3 levels of multiple-choice practice questions, the first two are at the back of each chapter:

1) Foundational practice questions: Basic, understanding questions to ensure that you have read the chapter; if you have a non-science background (NSB), if you do not know the answer, it would be better to treat these questions as 'open-book' questions rather than just looking at the worked solutions in your online account;

2) GAMSAT-level practice questions: Reasoning, application questions with the normal GAMSAT dosage of graphs, tables, diagrams and algebraic manipulations;

3) Full-length practice tests which span the depth and breadth of a simulation of the real exam. Be warned: We do not replicate real-exam questions, we replicate real-exam reasoning. You can start with GS-Free which is a full-length GAMSAT mock exam with the new digital format, with free answers and worked solutions at gamsat-prep.com. There are also 15 GS/HEAPS full-length mock exams.

For GAMSAT Sciences, "Study, practice, then full-length testing" should be your mantra for success!

Note for NSB students: If you read poems for months, you will increase your comfort reading poems. Reading science chapters is quite similar. It will feel bewildering at times, but less so as you progress. The real GAMSAT will have some articles that even the best science students do not fully grasp during the exam. However, they can still manage to obtain top GAMSAT scores by focusing on the minimum required in order to answer the questions correctly. This is a skill you can develop but it will not always feel comfortable.

The Importance of GAMSAT Maths

Gold Standard GAMSAT has completed an extensive analysis of ACER's official GAMSAT practice materials. We can lay the data in your lap to hopefully guide you towards more efficient studies.

We placed the step-by-step worked solutions to all of the over 400 multiple-choice Sciences official ACER GAMSAT practice questions on YouTube for free access in the Gold Standard GAMSAT Channel. Then we re-examined all of ACER's practice materials multiple times and compared the data generated with students' experiences as publicly reported in online forums. If we have erred, it is on the side of conservative estimates.

We can confirm that most students will experience more than 50% of GAMSAT Sciences questions as intimately related to maths: in other words, either based on graphs, calculations, equation manipulation with little or no background, etc. As a consequence, maths is a more important component to GAMSAT Sciences success than any other standard science subject. As a reminder, GAMSAT Sciences is: 40% Biology, 20% Physics, 20% General Chemistry and 20% Organic Chemistry; the "more than 50%" GAMSAT Maths primarily overlaps with the GAMSAT Biology, Physics and General Chemistry.

Despite being a digital exam, GAMSAT will have many numerical calculations and equation manipulations requiring the use of scratch paper which will be provided to you by an attendant at your exam centre (two A4 sheets for the entirety of GAMSAT Sciences; *whiteboard* optional). No calculator is permitted, just old-fashioned longhand calculations. Keeping your scratch paper organised using lines separating the work from different questions, and neat so that all work remains crystal clear to you, is paramount. Feel free to use A4 scratch paper for the multiple-choice questions at the end of chapters in this book to become accustomed to the experience.

Note that we have added a GAMSAT Maths primer which precedes GAMSAT General Chemistry Chapter 1.

What is so *new* about the new GAMSAT Masters Series?

The trifecta: We have introduced 3 new tools to increase your study efficiency comprising of Percent Importance, Spoiler Alerts and Chapter Checklists.

Percent Importance

'Importance' deals with the classic-student conundrum: How much effort should I invest in studying this or that chapter? How relevant is it to the GAMSAT?

After an exhaustive analysis of ACER's materials, we converted our previous Importance boxes to reveal percentages so students are better informed as to what they should emphasise when studying.

Here is the summary of Importance for the 10 GAMSAT General Chemistry chapters in this book:

Chapter	1	2	3	4	5	6	7	8	9	10
Percent Importance	5%	0%	2%	15%	18%	22%	0%	6%	26%	6%
Relative Importance	M	L	L	H	H	H	L	M	H	M

HIGH H (> 10%) MEDIUM M (3% to 10%) LOW L (< 3%)

The data is clear. The labels representing 'relative importance' is, of course, subjective. We will always remind you of the percentages on the first page of each chapter so that you do not have to accept our judgement as to the level of importance, you can decide for yourself. Note that 80% of GAMSAT General Chemistry lies within just 4 of the 10 chapters: 4, 5, 6 and 9.

Spoiler Alert!

And for those who only believe if they can see for themselves: Spoiler Alert! This feature is at the end of each chapter and provides specific cross-references to ACER official practice materials. This way, you may choose to either check our work through specific examples from official ACER GAMSAT content or continue your studies for that particular chapter. Please note: 1-2% of official ACER practice questions either change or are moved every year.

Chapter Checklists

Part 3 of the trifecta to improve your study efficiency: At the end of each chapter, we encourage you to participate in a reassessment of your understanding based on the learning objectives for that chapter, to take appropriate notes, to engage in multimedia learning, and more.

More changes?

In addition to the trifecta, for the first time as compared to all pre-pandemic paperback and hardback editions since 2010, this book contains many other features with the sole aim of increasing your study efficiency and understanding. As examples: A Maths Primer before the first General Chemistry chapter; *Need for Speed* exercises at the beginning of most chapters; improved quality and quantity of practice questions; detailed worked solutions; re-editing of each and every page; GAMSAT General Chemistry Key Points summary at the back of the book; and finally, more online discussion boards to ensure that you have access to resolve any question you may have regarding the content in this book.

A word about your online access . . .

The GS Online Access has saved thousands of trees and have reduced the cost of this book to you. It is not just the hundreds of online answers and worked solutions that you get access to with your gamsat-prep.com account, it is the fact that we do not have to limit the length of our worked solutions because of printing cost restrictions. It permits this textbook to sell for less than most with the same production value, while at the same time, providing you with more detailed worked solutions than any other GAMSAT publication, ever. You will also find that many of the solutions include videos.

Cross-references!

Wherever possible, we will identify another chapter, section or subsection of the book where you can find more information regarding a particular topic. For the most part, each book is self-contained but there are some exceptional cases where we cross-reference between different Masters Series books. The following table contains a summary of the abbreviations used throughout the Masters Series.

Cross-references to the Masters Series books, videos, apps, etc.

Abbreviation	Subject	Theme, Book
RHSS	Reasoning in Humanities & Social Sciences	Book 1
WC	Written Communication	Book 2
GM	GAMSAT Maths	Physical Sciences, Book 3
PHY	Physics	Physical Sciences, Book 3
CHM	General Chemistry	Physical Sciences, Book 4
ORG	Organic Chemistry	Biological Sciences, Book 5
BIO	Biology	Biological Sciences, Book 6

For example, CHM 2.4 means that you will find more information by looking at the Masters Series textbook, Chapter 2 General Chemistry, in the section 2.4. After a few chapters, you will find the system to be quite straightforward and, often, helpful.

Note: Despite the many new additions throughout this textbook, including over 100 pages of brand-new content, it remains 99% error-free. Should you have any doubts, join us at gamsat-prep.com/forum.

Good luck!

- BF, MD

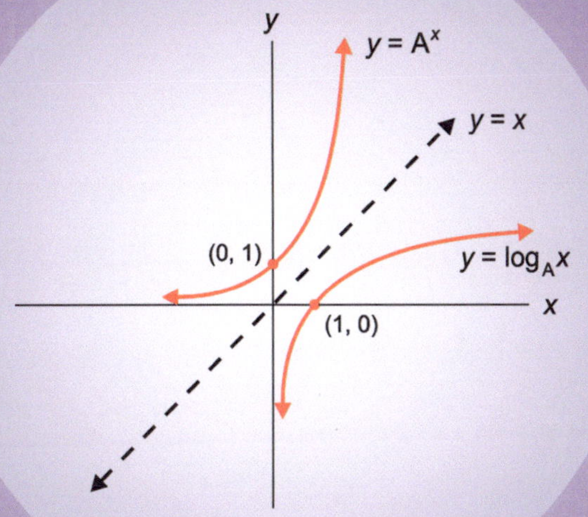

GAMSAT-Prep.com

GAMSAT MATHS

Maths for GAMSAT

General Chemistry: A Primer

PROLOGUE: A GAMSAT MATHS PRIMER

We cannot replicate all 6 chapters, over 150 pages, of the GAMSAT Maths section from the Masters Series Maths and Physics book. We must assume that you have read those chapters or that you have a basic understanding of algebra, including SI units, dimensional analysis, logs and graph analysis. Either way, this small GAMSAT Maths section can serve either as a primer or as revision of the fundamentals.

Here by section and subsection are some highlights which are most relevant to GAMSAT General Chemistry.

1.4 Fractions, Decimals, and Percentages

1.4.2 Manipulating Fractions

G. Fractions: Summary

Multiplying $$\left(\frac{a}{b}\right)\left(\frac{c}{d}\right) = \frac{ac}{bd}$$

Addition $$\frac{a}{b}+\frac{c}{d} = \frac{ad+bc}{bd}$$

Dividing $$\frac{\left({}^{a}\!/_{b}\right)}{\left({}^{c}\!/_{d}\right)} = \frac{ad}{bc}$$

Subtraction $$\frac{a}{b}-\frac{c}{d} = \frac{ad-bc}{bd}$$

1.4.3 Decimals and Percentages

Fraction-Decimal Conversions to Know:
Having these common conversions between fractions and decimals memorised will help you save valuable time on the test.

Fraction	Decimal
1/2	.5
1/3	~ .33
1/4	.25
1/5	.2
1/6	~.167
1/8	.125
1/10	.1

1.5 Roots and Exponents

1.5.5 Summary of the Rules for Exponents

$a^0 = 1$ $\qquad$ $a^1 = a$

$a^n a^m = a^{n+m}$ $\qquad$ $a^n/a^m = a^{n-m}$

$(a^n)^m = a^{nm}$ $\qquad$ $a^{\frac{1}{n}} = \sqrt[n]{a}$ {note that $a^{\frac{1}{2}}$ is simply $\sqrt{a}$}

1.5.6 Recognising Number Patterns

x	1	2	3	4	5	6	7	8	9	10	11	12	13	14	15	20
x^2	1	4	9	16	25	36	49	64	81	100	121	144	169	196	225	400
x^3	1	8	27	64	125	-	-	-	-	1000	-	-	-	-	-	-

Table 1: Common squares and cubes that are helpful to know. Applying the rules of exponents (GM 1.5.3, 1.5.5), $5^2 = 25$, $5^3 = 125$; square root of 121 = $(121)^{1/2} = \sqrt[2]{121} = \sqrt{121} = 11$; cube (= 3rd) root of 64 = $(64)^{1/3} = \sqrt[3]{64} = 4$. These basic manipulations are commonly required for the real exam.

2.1 Systems of Measurement

2.1.3 SI Units

Table 1: SI Base Units

Base quantity	SI base unit: Name	SI base unit: Symbol
length	metre	m
mass	kilogram	kg
time	second	s
electric current	ampere	A
thermodynamic temperature	kelvin	K
amount of substance	mole	mol

Table 2: Examples of SI Derived Units

	SI derived unit	
area	square metre	m^2
volume	cubic metre	m^3
speed, velocity	metre per second	m/s
acceleration	metre per second squared	m/s^2

Table 3: SI Derived Units with Special Names and Symbols

			SI base unit	
frequency	hertz	Hz	-	s^{-1}
force	newton	N	-	$m \cdot kg \cdot s^{-2}$
pressure, stress	pascal	Pa	N/m^2	$m^{-1} \cdot kg \cdot s^{-2}$
energy, work, quantity of heat	joule	J	N·m	$m^2 \cdot kg \cdot s^{-2}$
power	watt	W	J/s	$m^2 \cdot kg \cdot s^{-3}$
electric charge, quantity of electricity	coulomb	C	-	s·A
electric potential difference, electromotive force	volt	V	W/A	$m^2 \cdot kg \cdot s^{-3} \cdot A^{-1}$

NOTE

We will see all the units from these 3 tables in the GAMSAT Physics and General Chemistry chapters.

Do not try to memorise the last 2 columns in Table 3. However, if this is your second time studying from this page, you should be able to derive all the units displayed in the last 2 columns of Table 3. In fact, the derivation of units through dimensional analysis is a regular type of GAMSAT question. You will be tested on this point with the GAMSAT-level practice questions in this book (and also in GAMSAT Physics and Biology).

Table 4: Important SI prefixes for GAMSAT, A closer look

Prefix		Base 10	Decimal	English Word
Name	Symbol			
tera	T	10^{12}	1 000 000 000 000	trillion
giga	G	10^{9}	1 000 000 000	billion
mega	M	10^{6}	1 000 000	million
kilo	k	10^{3}	1000	thousand
hecto	h	10^{2}	100	hundred
deca	da	10^{1}	10	ten
BASE UNIT	-	10^{0}	1	one
deci	d	10^{-1}	0.1	tenth
centi	c	10^{-2}	0.01	hundredth
milli	m	10^{-3}	0.001	thousandth
micro	μ	10^{-6}	0.000001	millionth
nano	n	10^{-9}	0.000000001	billionth
pico	p	10^{-12}	0.000000000001	trillionth

2.2 Mathematics of Conversions (Dimensional Analysis)

2.2.1 Dimensional Analysis with Numeric Calculations

Dimensional analysis (also called 'factor-label method' or the 'unit-factor method') permits the solving of problems across the sciences simply by carefully analysing and manipulating units. Equations developed during the process of dimensional analysis require you to focus on numbers and units. **Dimensional analysis uses the fact that any number or expression can be multiplied by one without changing its value.** For example, you can choose to multiply (*conversion of units*) using any of the following, depending on what units you wish to cancel, because:

$$1 = \frac{1\text{ hour}}{60\text{ minutes}} = \frac{60\text{ minutes}}{1\text{ hour}}$$

Chapter 3: Algebra and Graph Analysis

Need for Speed **GM Chapter 3**

Circle the correct response: On the axis of a graph using a log scale, halfway between the numbers 100 and 1000 would yield a number most consistent with which of the following?

A. Between 300 and 400 **B.** Between 400 and 500 **C.** 500 **D.** Above 500

Note: The answer is coming in section 3.8.

3.5 Basic Graphs

3.5.1 The Graph of a Linear Equation

$$y = mx + b$$

$$m = (y_2 - y_1)/(x_2 - x_1)$$
$$= \Delta y/\Delta x = \text{rise/run}$$

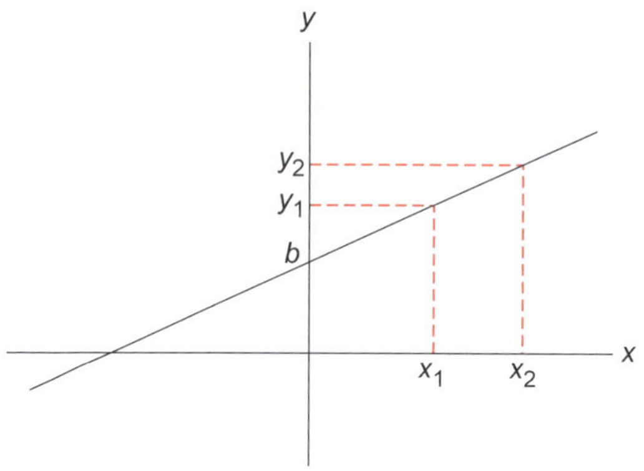

3.7 Logarithms

3.7.1 Log Rules and Logarithmic Scales

Table 1: Common values for the log base 10 (note the trends)

x	Exponential form	$\log_{10}(x)$
0.0001	10^{-4}	-4
0.001	10^{-3}	-3
0.01	10^{-2}	-2
0.1	10^{-1}	-1
1	10^{0}	0
10	10^{1}	1
100	10^{2}	2
1000	10^{3}	3
10 000	10^{4}	4

Here are the log rules you must know:

1) $\log_a a = 1$
2) $\log_a M^k = k \log_a M$
3) $\log_a(MN) = \log_a M + \log_a N$
4) $\log_a(M/N) = \log_a M - \log_a N$
5) $10^{\log 10 M} = M$
6) $\log_a(1) = 0$, given "a" is greater than zero.

EXAMPLE 1

Given:

$$pH = -\log_{10}[H^+]$$

Let us calculate the pH of 0.001 H^+ (for now, ignore the chemistry, focus only on the maths):

$[H^+] = 0.001$
using the #1 Rule of Algebra (GM 3.1.1):
$-\log[H^+] = -\log(0.001)$
$pH = -\log(10^{-3})$
$pH = 3 \log 10$ (log rule #2)
$pH = 3$ (rule #1, a = 10)

EXAMPLE 2

What is log (1 000 000)?
log (1 000 000) = log 10^6 = 6

EXAMPLE 3

What is log (1/100)?
log (1/100) = log 10^{-2} = -2

EXAMPLE 4

Given that $\ln 2 = 0.69$, what is $\ln 2e^3$?

Try to solve the problem while keeping in mind: (1) ln is the natural logarithm, meaning that it is log to the base e; (2) our 3rd rule of logarithms permits you separate factors.

$$\ln 2e^3 = \ln 2 + \ln e^3 = 0.69 + 3 = 3.69$$

Notice that if you have the base of the log and the base of the number with the exponent the same, then the answer is simply the exponent. Thus

$$\text{Log}(1000) = \log 10^3 = \ln e^3 = 3.$$

EXAMPLE 5

Approximate log(200).

Because the number 200 is between 100 and 1000 (but clearly closer to 100), and since log(100) = 2 and log(1000) = 3, log(200) must be a number between 2 and 3 but closer to the number 2. Such an approximation is sufficient for a multiple choice exam. {Incidentally, log(200) happens to be approximately 2.3.}

3.8 Exponential and Logarithmic Curves

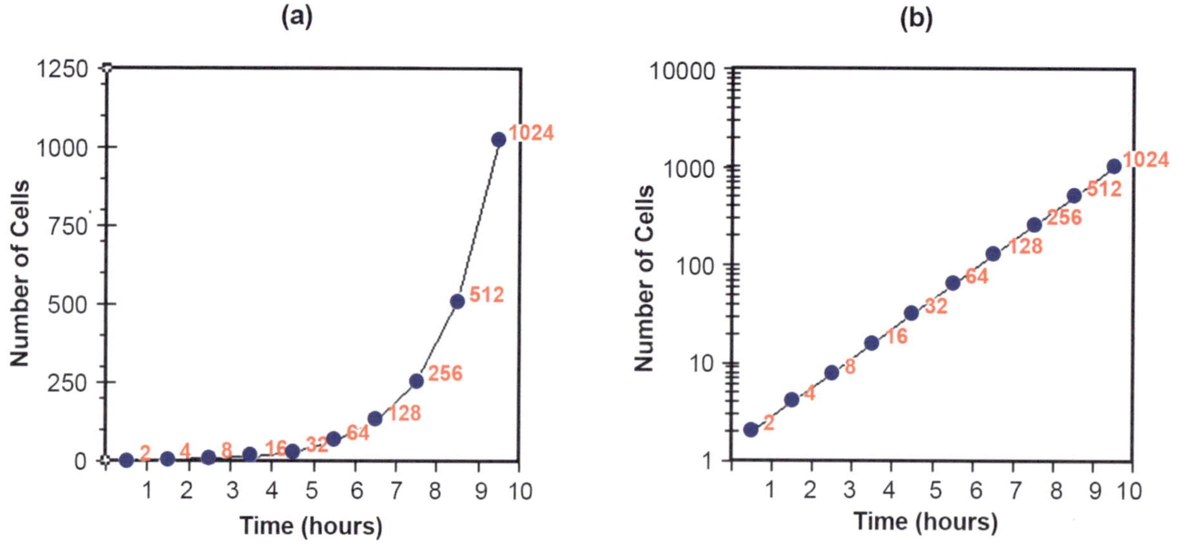

Figure IV.3.4: Growth curves of cells dividing mitotically. (a) An exponential curve with a linear scale for the x and y-axis. (b) A logarithmic scale on the y-axis converts the data rising exponentially into a linear graph. This is referred to as a semi-log graph or semi-log plot (GM 3.7.1). Notice that it is observation or analysis that leads to the conclusion as to what type of graph is being assessed as neither graph is labelled "exponential" nor "logarithm" anywhere. Also, carefully count the notches along the y-axis of the log scale (b), and notice that halfway between 1 and 10, is a number between 3 and 4, halfway between 10 and 100 is 30-40, halfway between 100 and 1000 is 300-400 (answer A in GM 3.0 *Need for Speed*), and so on.

3.9 Nomograms: The Art of Unusual Graphs

EXAMPLE 3

Ternary (AKA trilinear, triangular) graphs or plots, tephigrams (commonly used in weather analysis and forecasting), and some thermodynamic diagrams can be loosely defined as nomograms. The ternary graph is encountered the most frequently.

The following is the most widely-used scale for a ternary graph. From time to time, return to this common scale to confirm your understanding.

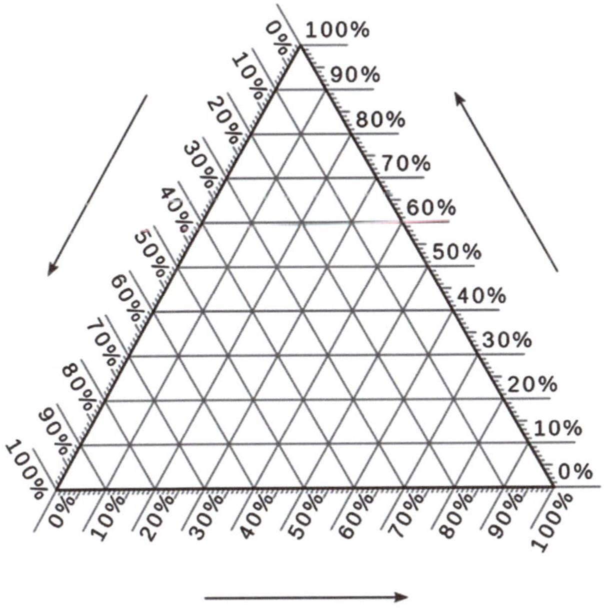

Now we will learn how to read a ternary graph with the following 3 variables: organic matter, clay and sand.

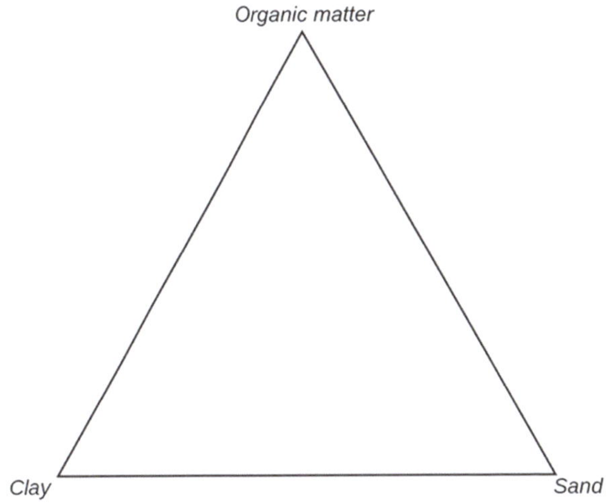

As a general rule, the percentage of one component is given by a line that is parallel with the line between the other 2 components. For example, consider the diagram below. Notice that the percentage of 'Organic matter' is represented by a line that is parallel to the Clay-Sand line.

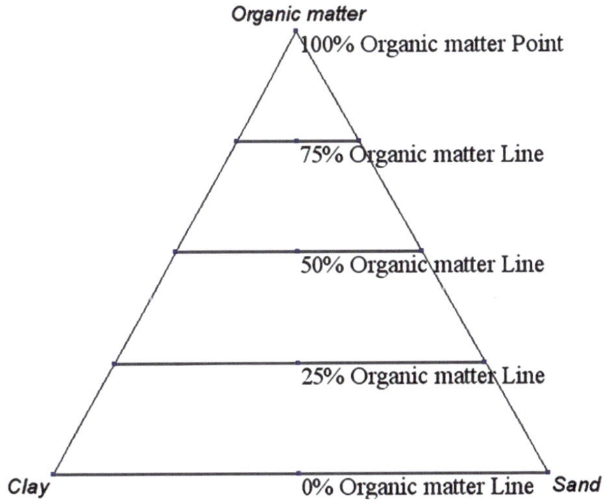

Notice that the percentage of 'Clay' in the following diagram is represented by a line that is parallel to the Organic matter-Sand line. The caption in the diagram reads: "One coordinate only tells us the one proportion: at any point along these lines, the proportion of Clay is the percentage given, but we don't know the proportions of Organic matter or Sand."

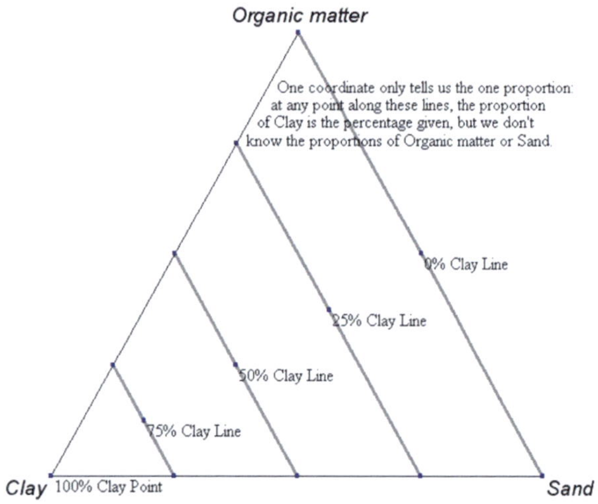

Notice in the following diagram that the percentage of 'Sand' is represented by a line that is parallel to the Clay-Organic matter line.

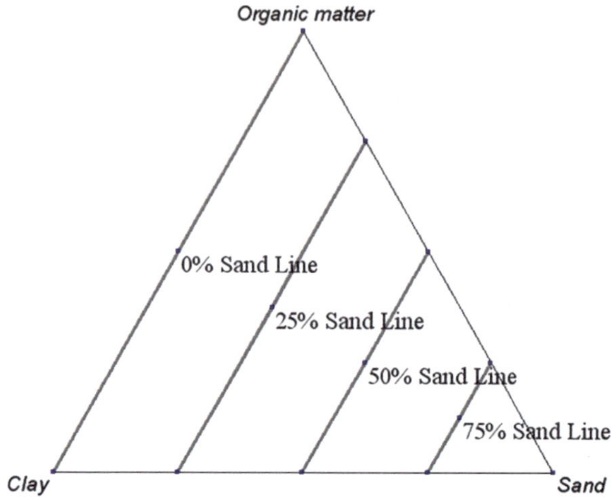

4.2 2D Figures

4.2.2 Types of Triangles

A. Right Triangles

A **right triangle** is a triangle that contains a right angle. The other two angles in a right triangle add up to 90°.

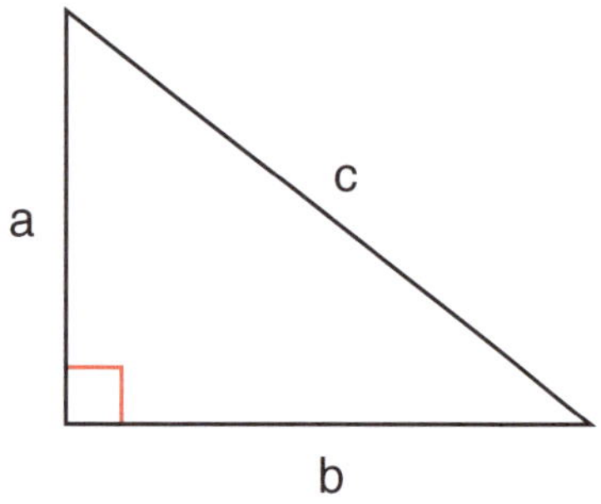

The two short legs of a right triangle (the legs that come together to form the right angle) and the hypotenuse (the side opposite the right angle) are related by the Pythagorean Theorem:

$$a^2 + b^2 = c^2$$

$$\text{Area} = \frac{1}{2}(a \times b)$$

GAMSAT GENERAL CHEMISTRY

5 Sections • 10 Chapters

01
Atoms: Shapes, Classifications, Bonds to Make Molecules, and Balance

Chapter 1: Stoichiometry
Chapter 2: Electronic Structure and the Periodic Table
Chapter 3: Bonding

02
Solids, Liquids and Gases

Chapter 4: Phases and Phase Equilibria
Chapter 5: Solution Chemistry

03
Special Case: Protons in Water

Chapter 6: Acids and Bases

04
Chemical Reactions: Heat, Spontaneity, and Speed

Chapter 7: Thermodynamics
Chapter 8: Enthalpy and Thermochemistry
Chapter 9: Rate Processes in Chemical Reactions

05
Electricity from Chemicals: Redox Reactions

Chapter 10: Electrochemistry

GAMSAT-prep.com

STOICHIOMETRY

Chapter 1

Memorise

* Define: molecular weight
* Define: empirical/molecular formula

Understand

* Composition by % mass
* Mole concept, limiting reactants
* Avogadro's number
* Calculate theoretical yield
* Basic types of reactions

Importance

Medium level: 4% of GAMSAT General Chemistry

questions released by ACER are related to content in this chapter (in our estimation).

* Note that approximately 80% of the questions in GAMSAT General Chemistry are related to just 4 chapters: 4, 5, 6, and 9.

GAMSAT-Prep.com

Introduction

An atom is the smallest unit of matter that forms a chemical element. Every solid, liquid, gas, and living thing in the known universe is composed of neutral or ionised atoms. Atoms are tiny! Sprinkle a few grams of salt (NaCl) in the palm of your hand and imagine how many atoms of sodium (Na) and chloride (Cl) might be there. Thousands? Millions? Billions of billions? Not even close! The number is shockingly huge. That number, which shall be revealed in this chapter, can be related to some 'simplifications': the mole concept and Avogadro's number.

From a GAMSAT perspective, the total number of atoms on each side of an equation remains the same. Atoms may change partners, or go off on their own, but none are created or destroyed. Stoichiometry exists to ensure that there is truly a balance of atoms on both sides of a chemical reaction (AKA, *chemical equation*). Typically, stoichiometry is the rather simple maths behind the chemistry.

Multimedia Resources at GAMSAT-Prep.com

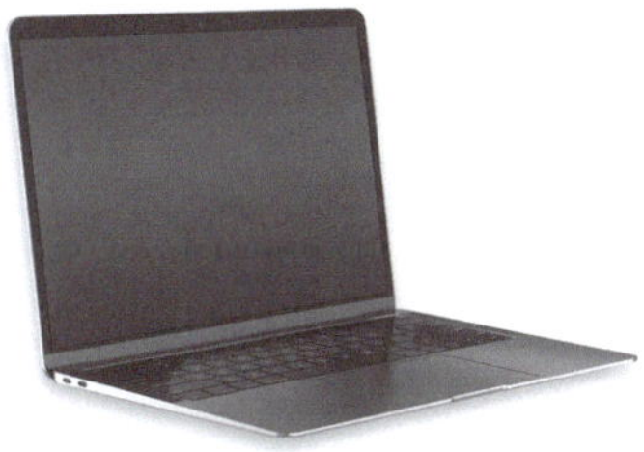

Open Discussion Boards
(*gamsat-prep.com/forum*)

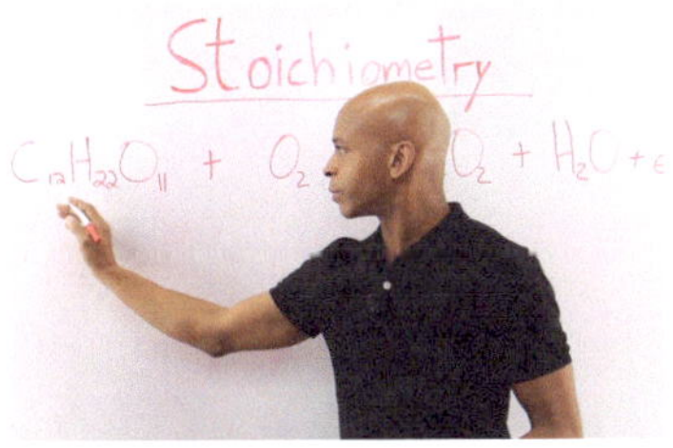

Science Preparation Videos

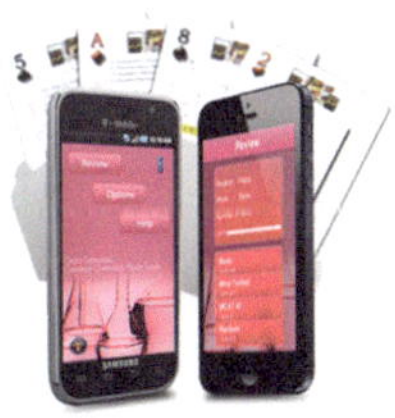

Flashcards

* The real GAMSAT may have advanced-level information presented (i.e. in a passage) but previous knowledge of said information is not required to answer the questions that would follow. Practice questions at the end of this chapter, as well as ACER and GS (HEAPS) practice GAMSATs can help you clarify this point.

1.0 GAMSAT has a *Need for Speed*!

If you are a NSB student, first read through the chapter content while taking brief notes then return to this section to complete the *Need for Speed* exercises. Otherwise, complete the straightforward exercises in the table below as warm up, read through the chapter while taking brief notes, and then: All candidates should attack the GAMSAT practice questions at the end of the chapter. Find the answers by going to the section number marked in the first column below, and then looking for the use of a pink highlighter.

<table>
<tr><th>Section</th><th>GAMSAT General Chemistry Need for Speed Exercises</th></tr>
<tr><td rowspan="3">1.1</td><td>Name any 3 of the most common atoms in your body.</td></tr>
<tr><td>If two or more atoms are held together by chemical bonds, what do they form?</td></tr>
<tr><td>Is the air we breathe an atom, a molecule or a mixture?</td></tr>
<tr><td>1.2
Complete the missing entries for the empirical formulas in the table on the right.</td><td>
<table>
<tr><th>Compound</th><th>Molecular Formula</th><th>Empirical Formula</th></tr>
<tr><td>Water</td><td>H_2O</td><td></td></tr>
<tr><td>Hydrogen peroxide</td><td>H_2O_2</td><td></td></tr>
<tr><td>Glucose</td><td>$C_6H_{12}O_6$</td><td></td></tr>
<tr><td>Benzene</td><td>C_6H_6</td><td></td></tr>
<tr><td>Caffeine</td><td>$C_8H_{10}N_4O_2$</td><td></td></tr>
</table>
</td></tr>
<tr><td>1.3</td><td>Can you calculate the number of moles of a compound from the number of grams and the molecular weight? If so, how?</td></tr>
<tr><td>1.5</td><td>Balancing a chemical equation requires that there are the same number of atoms on the left side and the right side of the arrow. Balance the following chemical equations using the smallest, whole-number coefficients.

$CH_4 + O_2 \rightarrow CO_2 + H_2O$

$BiCl_3 + H_2O \rightarrow Bi_2O_3 + HCl$</td></tr>
<tr><td>1.5.1
Balance the equations.</td><td>$CaCl_2(aq) + Na_2CO_3(aq) \rightarrow CaCO_3(s) + NaCl(aq)$

$HCl(l) + Ba(OH)_2(aq) \rightarrow H_2O(l) + BaCl_2(aq)$

$H_2(g) + O_2(g) \rightarrow H_2O(l)$ | $NaCl(s) \rightarrow Na(l) + Cl_2(g)$</td></tr>
</table>

Medium-level Importance

1.1 Atoms, Stuff, and Things that Matter

Matter is stuff. Matter is things. Matter is simply anything that has mass and occupies space. Chemistry is concerned with matter, but leans towards pure substances like elements and compounds. In fact, to summarise the 10 chapters of this textbook: Chemistry deals with the properties, composition, and structure of elements and compounds, how they can change, and the energy that is released or absorbed when they change.

There are more than 100 elements in the periodic table of the elements (CHM 2.4.1), but only 94 occur naturally on Earth. Every person, every rock, the sky, the soda, every shape and colour that you have ever seen: 94 elements. In fact, almost 99% of the mass of your body is stunningly composed of only six elements: oxygen, carbon, hydrogen, nitrogen, calcium, and phosphorus. These elements are, of course, atoms.

An element is a pure substance which cannot be broken down by chemical means, and consists of atoms which have identical numbers of protons in their nuclei (GAMSAT Physics Chapter 12). When two or more atoms are held together by chemical bonds,

Medium-level Importance

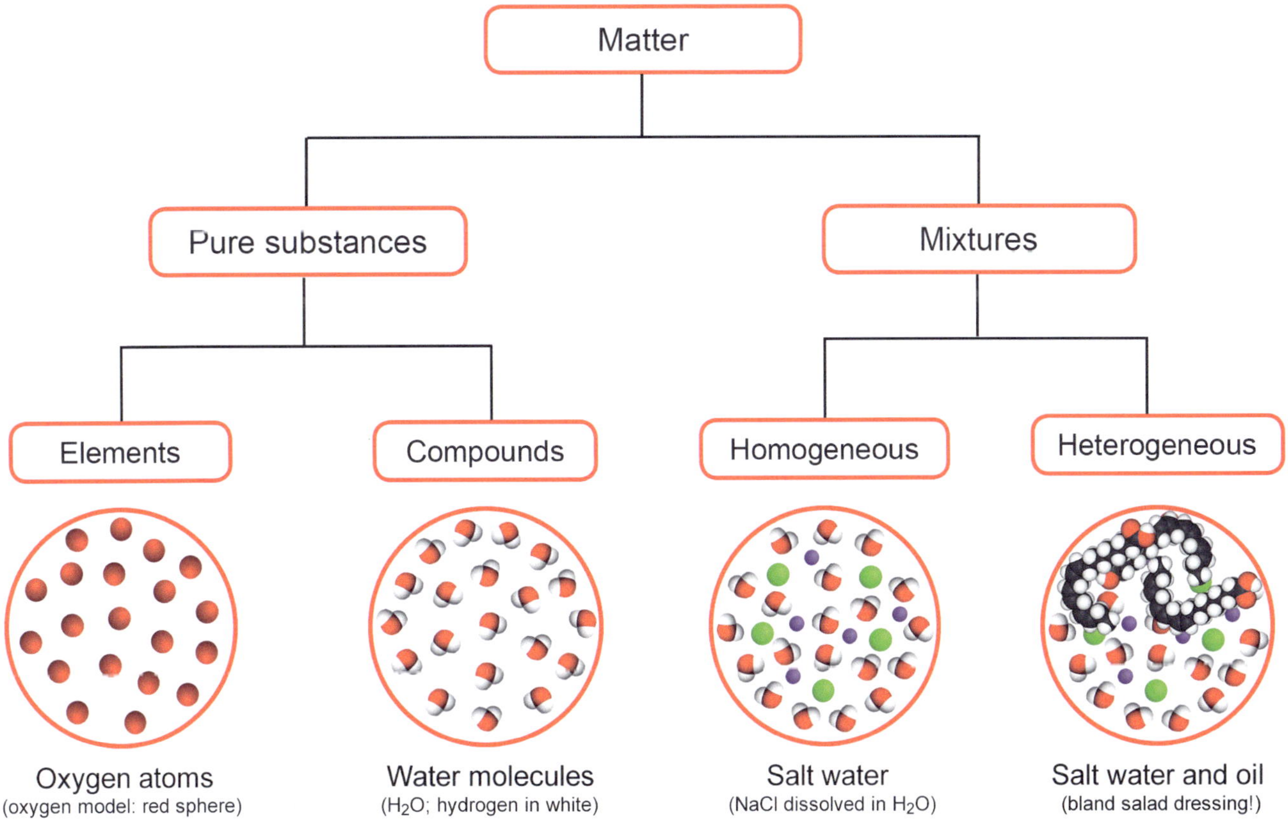

Figure III.A.1.1: Your world. Everything that you have ever seen, touched, inhaled, etc., falls into four simple categories of things (*matter*). It does not matter if it is solid, liquid or gas, it's matter.

they form a *molecule*. When the molecule, like water (2 hydrogen atoms + 1 oxygen atom: H_2O), is composed of atoms from more than one element, then it is a *compound*.

In our daily lives, we interact with mixtures far more than pure substances (i.e. elements and compounds). It is unlikely that you have ever experienced pure H_2O since it is usually a mixture which includes many different minerals, and sometimes additives like fluoride. The air that we breathe is a mixture of the pure compounds: nitrogen (~78%), oxygen (~21%), water vapor and many other gases (~1%). The exact compositional ratio of air, or any other mixture, may vary from one location to another. {*Solid mixtures and an awesome ternary graph await you in GAMSAT-level Practice Questions at the end of this chapter, not to be missed!*}

A mixture can be *homogeneous* (uniform in composition) or *heterogeneous* (lacks uniformity). A homogeneous mixture means that when dividing the volume in half, the same amount of material is suspended in both halves of the substance, like air, or salt water.

1.2 Empirical Formula vs. Molecular Formula

The molecules of oxygen (O_2) are made up of two atoms of the same element. Water molecules on the other hand are composed of two different elements: hydrogen and oxygen in the specific ratio 2:1. Note that water is not a mixture of hydrogen and oxygen since this ratio is specific and does not vary with the location or the experimental conditions.

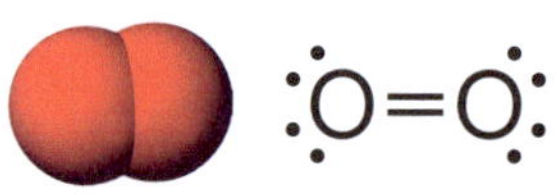

Oxygen

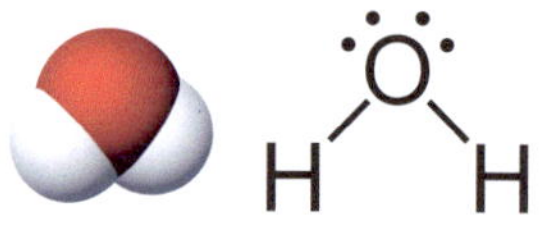

Water

The *empirical formula* of a pure compound is the simplest whole number ratio between the numbers of atoms of the

Compound	Molecular Formula	Empirical Formula
Water	H_2O	H_2O
Hydrogen peroxide	H_2O_2	HO
Glucose	$C_6H_{12}O_6$	CH_2O*
Benzene	C_6H_6	CH
Caffeine	$C_8H_{10}N_4O_2$	$C_4H_5N_2O$

*Notice that the empirical formula of glucose (a simple sugar), CH_2O, shows carbon (C) bonded to water (H_2O). Consider that you hydrate when you drink water, thus glucose is a "carbon-hydrate" or a *carbohydrate*!

different elements making up the compound. For instance, the empirical formula of water is H_2O (2:1 ratio) while the empirical formula of hydrogen peroxide is HO (1:1 ratio).

The *molecular formula* of a given molecule states the exact number of the different atoms that make up this molecule. The empirical formula of water is identical to its molecular formula, i.e. H_2O; however, the molecular formula of hydrogen peroxide, H_2O_2, is different from its empirical formula (both correspond to a 1:1 ratio).

1.3 Mole - Atomic and Molecular Weights

Because of the small size of atoms and molecules chemists have to consider collections of a large number of these particles to bring chemical problems to our human, macroscopic scale. Collections of tens or dozens of atoms are still too small to achieve this practical purpose. For various reasons, the number 6.02×10^{23} (Avogadro's number: N_A) was chosen. It is the number of atoms in 12 grams of the most abundant *isotope* of carbon (isotopes are elements which are identical chemically since the number of protons are the same; their masses differ slightly since the number of neutrons differ; PHY 12.2).

The number 6 followed by 23 zeroes is a shocking number. If you had 6.02×10^{23} dollars, and spent that money at a rate of one billion dollars every second, it would take you about 20 million years to run out of money! One billion dollars every second.

Diamonds and graphite are composed of carbon. If you sprinkle exactly 12 grams of pure graphite in the palm of your hand (or diamonds – the way you've been spending lately!), you would be holding precisely 6.02×10^{23} atoms of carbon. That number is too big to continue repeating, so there is a word for it: *mole*. You know how the word 'dozen' represents the number 12? But a dozen roses, a dozen people and a dozen buses do not weigh the same! Well, the word 'mole' represents 6.02×10^{23} things (usually small things like atoms and molecules), and a mole of carbon, a mole of water, and a mole of caffeine do not weigh the same!

And so, a mole of atoms or molecules (or in fact any particles in general) contains an Avogadro number of these particles. The weight in grams of a mole of atoms of a given element is the gram-atomic weight, GAW, of that element (sometimes weight is measured in atomic mass units - *see* PHY 12.2, 12.3). Along the same lines, the weight in grams of a mole of molecules of a given compound is its gram-molecular weight, GMW. Here are some equations relating these concepts:

For an element:

$$\text{moles} = \frac{\text{weight of sample in grams}}{\text{GAW}}$$

For a compound:

$$\text{moles} = \frac{\text{weight of sample in grams}}{\text{GMW}}$$

Medium-level Importance

For either elements or compounds, the dimensional analysis (GM 2.2) is quite simple:

$$\text{moles} = \frac{\text{grams}}{\left(\frac{\text{grams}}{\text{mole}}\right)}$$

{Note that some students like to simplify to: $n = m/M$, which means that the number of moles n is equal to mass/molar mass.}

Note that on the right side of the equation, grams cancel and the denominator in the denominator (mole) becomes the numerator.

The GAW of a given element is not to be confused with the mass of a single atom of this element. For instance, the mass of a single atom of carbon-12 (GAW = 12 g) is $12/N_A = 1.993 \times 10^{-23}$ grams.

Atomic weights are dimensionless numbers based on carbon-12 as the reference standard isotope and are defined as follows:

$$\frac{\text{mass of an atom of X}}{\text{mass of an atom of Y}} = \frac{\text{atomic weight of element X}}{\text{atomic weight of element Y}}$$

Clearly if the reference element Y is chosen to be carbon-12 (which is the case in standard periodic tables) the GAW of any element X is numerically equal to its atomic weight. In the table of atomic weights, all the elements then have values in which are relative to the carbon-12 isotope.

The molecular weight of a given molecule is equal to the sum of the atomic weights of the atoms that make up the molecule. For example, the molecular weight of H_2O is equal to 18.0 amu/molecule (H = 1.008 and O = 16.00). The molar weight (or molar mass) of H_2O is numerically equal to the molecular weight (18.0); however, the units are in grams/mol as the molar weight is based on a mole amount of substance. Thus, molecular weight and molar weight are numerically equivalent; however, molecular weight is the weight (amu) per molecule and molar weight is based on the weight (grams) per mole (1 mol = 6.02×10^{23} molecules).

Medium-level Importance

1.4 Composition of a Compound by Percent Mass

The percentage composition of a compound is the percent of the total mass of a given element in that compound. For instance, the chemical analysis of a 100 g sample of pure vitamin C demonstrates that there are 40.9 g of carbon, 4.58 g of hydrogen and 54.5 g of oxygen. The percentage composition of pure vitamin C is:

%C = 40.9; %H = 4.58; %O = 54.5

The composition of a compound by percent mass is closely related to its empirical formula. For instance, in the case of vitamin C, the determination of the number of moles of atoms of C, H or O in a 100 g of vitamin C is rather straightforward (note that in each case, the numerator is in grams, and the denominator is in grams/mole, thus the answer is in moles):

moles of atoms of C in a 100 g of vitamin C = 40.9/12.0 = 3.41

moles of atoms of H in a 100 g of vitamin C = 4.58/1.01= 4.53

moles of atoms of O in a 100 g of vitamin C = 54.5/16.0 = 3.41

[GAW can be determined from the periodic table in Chapter 2]

To deduce the smallest ratio between the numbers above, one follows the simple procedure:

(i) divide each one of the previously obtained numbers of moles by the smallest one of them (3.41 in our case):

for C: 3.41 mol/3.41 mol = 1.00
for H: 4.53 mol/3.41 mol = 1.33
for O: 3.41 mol/ 3.41 mol = 1.00

(ii) multiply the numbers obtained in the previous step by a small number to obtain a whole number ratio. In our case we need to multiply by 3 (in most cases this factor is between 1 and 5) so that:

for C: 1.00 × 3 = 3
for H: 1.33 × 3 = 4
for O: 1.00 × 3 = 3

Therefore, in this example, the simplest whole number ratio is 3C:4H:3O and we conclude that the empirical formula for vitamin C is: $C_3H_4O_3$.

In the previous example, instead of giving the composition of vitamin C by percent weight we could have provided the raw chemical analysis data and asked for the determination of that composition.

For instance, this data would be that the burning of a 4.00 mg sample of pure vitamin C yields 6.00 mg of CO_2 and 1.632 mg of H_2O. Since there are 12.0 g of carbon in 44.0 g of CO_2, the number of milligrams of carbon in 6.00 mg of CO_2 (which corresponds to the number of mg of carbon in 4.00 mg of vitamin C) is simply:

6.00 mg × (12.0 g C/44.0 g CO_2) = 1.636 mg of C in 6.00 mg of CO_2 or 4.00 mg of vitamin C for further clarification.

To convert this number into a percent mass is then trivial (GM 1.4.3). Similarly, the percent mass of hydrogen is obtained from the previous data and bearing in mind that there are 2.02 g of hydrogen (and not 1.01 g) in 18.0 g of water.

Incidentally, "burning" means combustion (CHM 1.5.1, ORG 3.2.1) which takes place in the presence of excess oxygen and results in the production of heat (*exothermic*, CHM 8.2), the conversion of the chemical species (new products), and light can be produced (glowing or a flame).

> The real GAMSAT does not usually provide a periodic table so the atomic weights (amu) will be given when required. Also, since calculators are not permitted, you should practice performing all calculations that you see in this textbook.

Medium-level Importance

1.5 Description of Reactions by Chemical Equations

Medium-level Importance

We have seen that atoms combine in very specific ratios to form molecules (e.g., 2 hydrogen atoms + 1 oxygen atom = 1 water molecule, H_2O). During a chemical reaction, molecules may break down into individual atoms which then recombine to form new compounds. Stoichiometry establishes relationships between the specific ratios within and between molecules in a chemical equation.

The convention for writing chemical equations is as follows: compounds which initially combine or react in a chemical reaction are called *reactants*; they are always written on the left-hand side of the chemical equation. The compounds which are produced during the same process are referred to as the *products* of the chemical reaction; they always appear on the right-hand side of the chemical equation.

Consider the combustion of methane gas (CH_4) producing carbon dioxide and water. Here is a model of the atoms and the chemical equation:

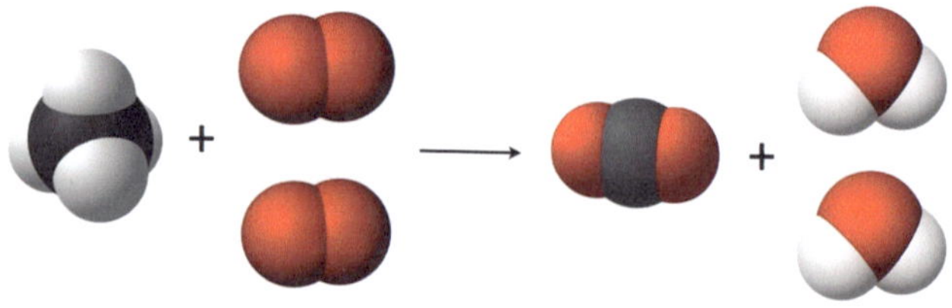

$$CH_4 + 2O_2 \longrightarrow CO_2 + 2H_2O$$

Notice that the atoms change partners but no atom is created or destroyed. For the chemical equation to have the same number of each atom on each side, note the coefficients representing the relative number of moles of reactants (1 methane + 2 oxygen) that combine to form the corresponding relative number of moles of products (1 carbon dioxide + 2 water): they are the stoichiometric coefficients of the balanced chemical equation with the ratio 1:2:1:2. The law of conservation of mass requires that the number of atoms of a given element remains constant during the process of a chemical reaction.

Balancing a chemical equation is putting conservation of mass into practice. Many equations are balanced by trial and error; however, caution must be practiced when balancing a chemical equation. It is always easier to balance elements that appear only in one compound on each side of the equation; therefore, as a general rule, always balance those elements first and then deal with those which appear in more than one compound last. Consider the following unbalanced chemical equation.

$$BiCl_3 + H_2O \rightarrow Bi_2O_3 + HCl$$

Let us consider a systematic approach to balancing chemical equations: **(1)** count and compare the atoms on both sides of the chemical equation; **(2)** balance each element one at a time by placing whole number coefficients in front of the formulas resulting in the same number of atoms of each element on each side of the equation. Remember that a coefficient in front of a formula multiplies every atom in the formula (i.e., $2BiCl_3 = 2Bi + 6Cl$). It is best to leave pure elements or metals until the end. **(3)** Balance hydrogens, if any, in both the reactant and products; and **(4)** finally, check if all elements are balanced with the smallest possible set of whole number coefficients.

Consider the balanced equation:

$2\ BiCl_3 + 3\ H_2O \rightarrow Bi_2O_3 + 6\ HCl$

Given the preceding chemical reaction, if H_2O is present in excessive quantity, then $BiCl_3$ would be considered the **limiting reactant.** In other words, since the amount of $BiCl_3$ is relatively small, it is the $BiCl_3$ which determines how much product will be formed. Thus if you were given 316 grams of $BiCl_3$ in *excess* H_2O and you needed to determine the quantity of HCl produced (theoretical yield), you would proceed as follows:

- Determine the number of moles of $BiCl_3$ (*see* CHM 1.3) given Bi = 209 g/mol and Cl = 35.5 g/mol, thus $BiCl_3 = (1 \times 209) + (3 \times 35.5) = 315.5$ or approximately 316 g/mol:

$$\#\text{ moles } BiCl_3 = (316\text{ g})/(316\text{ g/mol}) = 1.0\text{ mole of } BiCl_3.$$

- From the stoichiometric coefficients of the balanced equation:

  2 moles of $BiCl_3$: 6 moles of HCl; therefore,
  1 mole of $BiCl_3$: 3 moles of HCl

- Given H = 1.00 g/mol, thus HCl = 36.5 g/mol, we get:

$3\text{ moles} \times 36.5\text{ g/mol} = 110\text{ g}$ of HCl (approx.).

Please note: The theoretical yield is the calculated amount of product that can be predicted from a balanced chemical reaction and is seldom obtained in the laboratory. The actual yield is the actual amount of product produced and recovered in the laboratory. The Percentage yield = Actual yield/ Theoretical Yield × 100%.

Medium-level Importance

1.5.0.1 Hydrates

A **hydrate** is a substance that contains water or its constituent elements. In General Chemistry, hydrates are typically inorganic salts containing water molecules combined in a definite ratio as an integral part of the crystal. A colorful example is cobalt(II) chloride, which turns from blue to red upon hydration, and can thus be used as a water indicator.

The notation "*hydrated compound*·$\boldsymbol{n}$$\mathbf{H_2O}$", where n is the number of water molecules per formula unit of the salt, is commonly used to show that a salt is hydrated. The n is usually a low integer, though it is possible for fractional values to occur. For example, in a **monohydrate** n = 1, and in a **hexahydrate** n = 6. Thus, here is the notation for cobalt(II) chloride hexahydrate: $CoCl_2 \cdot 6H_2O$.

Numerical prefixes of Greek origin are: Hemi – ½; Mono – 1; Di – 2; Tri – 3; Tetra – 4; Penta – 5; Hexa – 6; Hepta – 7; Octa – 8; Nona – 9; Deca – 10.

A hydrate that has lost water is referred to as an *anhydride*; the remaining water, if any exists, can only be removed with very strong heating. A substance that does not contain any water is *anhydrous*. Some anhydrous compounds are hydrated so easily that they are deemed to be *hygroscopic* and are used as drying agents or *desiccants*.

1.5.1 Categories of Chemical Reactions

Throughout the chapters in General Chemistry we will explore many different types of chemicals and some of their associated reactions. The various chemical reactions may be classified generally as either a *redox* type or as a *non-redox* type reaction. We will explore redox (i.e. reduction-oxidation) reactions in detail in Chapter 10.

The following chart is an overview of major chemical reaction classifications (categories) followed by examples (please confirm that all reactions are balanced). Note that compounds in the chart are identified as solid (s), liquid (l), gas (g), or solubilised in water which is an *aqueous* (aq) solution. Follow the chart like a story that you should revisit but do not memorise.

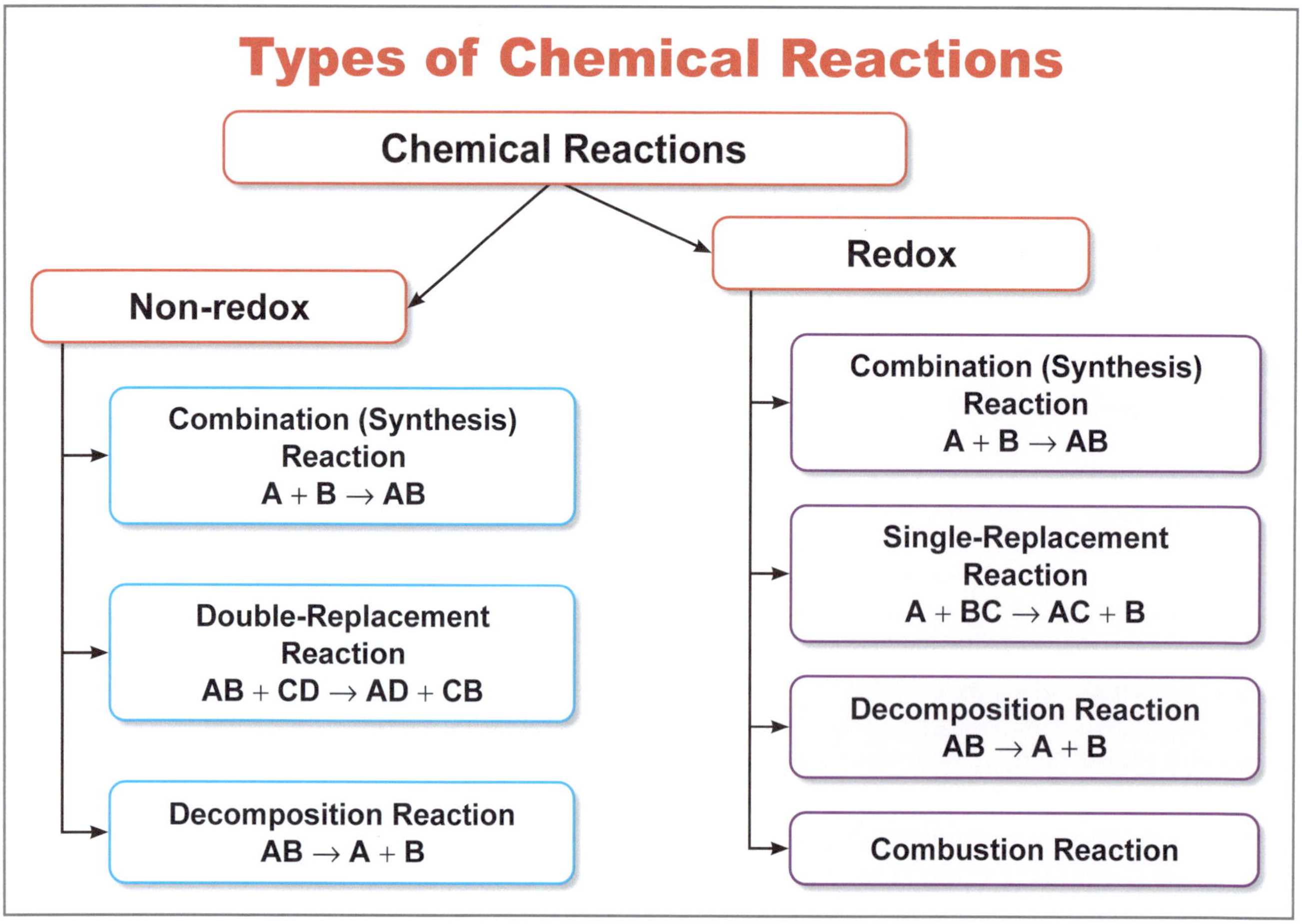

Medium-level Importance

Non-redox

Combination (Synthesis) Reaction

General equation: $A + B \rightarrow AB$

Example: $SO_2(g) + H_2O(l) \rightarrow H_2SO_3\,(aq)$

Double-Replacement Reaction (or Metathesis Reaction)

(a) Precipitation Type

General equation: $AB + CD \rightarrow AD + CB$

Example: $CaCl_2(aq) + Na_2CO_3(aq) \rightarrow CaCO_3(s) + 2NaCl(aq)$

(b) Acid-Base Neutralisation Type

General equation: $HA + BOH \rightarrow H_2O + BA$
(HA = any H^+ acid & BOH = any OH^- base)

Example:
$2HCl(l) + Ba(OH)_2(aq) \rightarrow 2H_2O(l) + BaCl_2(aq)$

(c) Gas Evolution Type Reaction

General equation: $HA + B \rightarrow H_2O + BA$
(HA = H^+ acid & B = special base salt $NaHCO_3$)

Example: $HCl(aq) + NaHCO_3(aq) \rightarrow H_2CO_3(aq)^* + NaCl(aq) \rightarrow H_2O(l) + CO_2(g) + NaCl(aq)$
(*H_2CO_3 is carbonic acid, the "fizz" in sodas, which degrades to $CO_2(g)$ and $H_2O(l)$)

Decomposition Reaction (CHM 4.3.1)

General equation: $AB \rightarrow A + B$

Example: $H_2CO_3(aq) \rightarrow H_2O(l) + CO_2(g)$

Redox

Combination (Synthesis) Reaction

General equation: $A + B \rightarrow AB$

Example: $2H_2(g) + O_2(g) \rightarrow 2H_2O(l)$

Single-Replacement Reaction

General equation: $A + BC \rightarrow AC + B$

Example:
$Zn(s) + CuSO_4(aq) \rightarrow Cu(s) + ZnSO_4(aq)$

Decomposition Reaction

General equation: $AB \rightarrow A + B$

Example: $2NaCl(s) \rightarrow 2Na(l) + Cl_2(g)$
(electrolysis reaction, CHM 10.4)

Combustion Reaction

Example: $CH_4(g) + 2O_2(g) \rightarrow CO_2(g) + 2H_2O(g)$

Medium-level Importance

1.6 Oxidation Numbers

This is a legacy section previously entitled: 1.6 Oxidation Numbers, Redox Reactions, Oxidising vs. Reducing Agents. This section has been moved in its entirety to General Chemistry Chapter 10, CHM 10.0.1.

CHAPTER 1: Stoichiometry

GOLD STANDARD FOUNDATIONAL GAMSAT PRACTICE QUESTIONS

Foundational practice questions are meant to underline some basic assumed knowledge. Students with little or no background in this subject can treat the questions as open-book practice questions. Expect mistakes! Remember: This is not a traditional exam. Practice is a process.

And finally, our Foundational GAMSAT Practice Questions are followed by GAMSAT-level Practice Questions. Only students with a solid background in the sciences should consider using a timer when completing any multiple-choice questions (*maximum average of 2 minutes per question according to the new digital GAMSAT timing*). For others, take your time and try your best before consulting the online answers and worked solutions. Good luck!

Medium-level Importance

1) Consider the following chemical reaction:

$$CH_4 + 2O_2 \rightarrow CO_2 + 2H_2O$$

What amount of oxygen is needed to completely react with 1 mole of CH_4?

A. 2 molecules
B. 2 grams
C. 2 atoms
D. 2 moles

2) What is the total number of atoms represented in the formula $CuSO_4 \cdot 5H_2O$?

A. 6
B. 13
C. 21
D. 29

3) What is the molecular weight of K_2CO_3?

- Note that: K = 39 g/mol, C = 12 g/mol, O = 16 g/mol

A. 138 g
B. 106 g
C. 99 g
D. 67 g

4) What is the molecular weight of $(NH_4)_3PO_4$?

- Note that: H = 1.0 g/mol, N = 14 g/mol, O = 16 g/mol, P = 31 g/mol

A. 113 g
B. 121 g
C. 149 g
D. 404 g

5) When the following equation is balanced, how many moles of water will be produced for each mole of calcium phosphate?

$$\_Ca(OH)_2 + \_H_3PO_4 \rightarrow \_H_2O + \_Ca_3(PO_4)_2$$

A. 2
B. 3
C. 4
D. 6

6) Approximately what is the percent, by mass, of nitrogen in NH_4NO_2?

- Note that: H = 1.0 g/mol, N = 14 g/mol, O = 16 g/mol

A. 38%
B. 44%
C. 48%
D. 54%

7) Molecule A contains only carbon and chlorine, and has a molecular weight of 285 g mol^{-1}. What is the molecular formula for this compound? (C = 12 amu; Cl = 35.5 amu)

A. C_2Cl_2
B. C_4Cl_4
C. C_5Cl_5
D. C_6Cl_6

8) Balance the following chemical equation:

$$MnO_2 + Al \rightarrow Al_2O_3 + Mn$$

If the preceding reaction runs to completion, how many moles of Al_2O_3 would be produced from reacting 1 mole of MnO_2 with an excess of Al?

A. 3
B. 2/3
C. 1/4
D. 1/2

9) Two moles of a diatomic gas P_2 were mixed with four moles of another diatomic gas Q_2 in a closed vessel. All of the P_2 and Q_2 molecules reacted to yield one triatomic product. Which of the following shows the net reaction between P and Q?

A. $2P_2 + 4Q_2 \rightarrow P_4Q_8$
B. $P_2 + 2Q_2 \rightarrow 2PQ_2$
C. $2P + 4Q \rightarrow P_2Q_4$
D. $P_2 + Q_4 \rightarrow P_2Q_4$

10) Assume that the composition by volume of air is 80% N_2 and 20% O_2. Which of the following gases are denser than air assuming they are at the same temperature and pressure?

$$CH_4, Cl_2, CO_2, NH_3, NO_2, O_3, SO_2$$

Note that:

- H = 1.0 g/mol, C = 12 g/mol, N = 14 g/mol, O = 16 g/mol, S = 32 g/mol, Cl = 35.5 g/mol
- Assume that density of a gas is directly related to its weight.

A. CH_4, CO_2, Cl_2, SO_2
B. CO_2, Cl_2, SO_2, NH_3, O_3
C. Cl_2, CO_2, NH_3, NO_2, O_3, SO_2
D. Cl_2, CO_2, NO_2, O_3, SO_2

GOLD STANDARD GAMSAT-LEVEL PRACTICE QUESTIONS

Questions 11–14

A ternary plot graphically depicts the ratios of three variables as positions in an equilateral triangle. Every point on a ternary plot represents a different composition of the three components. The concentration of each component is 100% (pure phase) in each corner of the triangle and 0% at the line opposite it.

(*continue au verso*)

The percentage of a specific component decreases linearly with increasing distance from its corner. By drawing parallel lines at regular intervals between the zero line and the corner, divisions can be established for estimation of the content of a component. Using Figure 1 as an example: Sample RX-68, a soil sample containing a mixture of three components, was determined to have a composition of 10% clay, 20% silt and 70% sand, which represents a point in sandy loam.

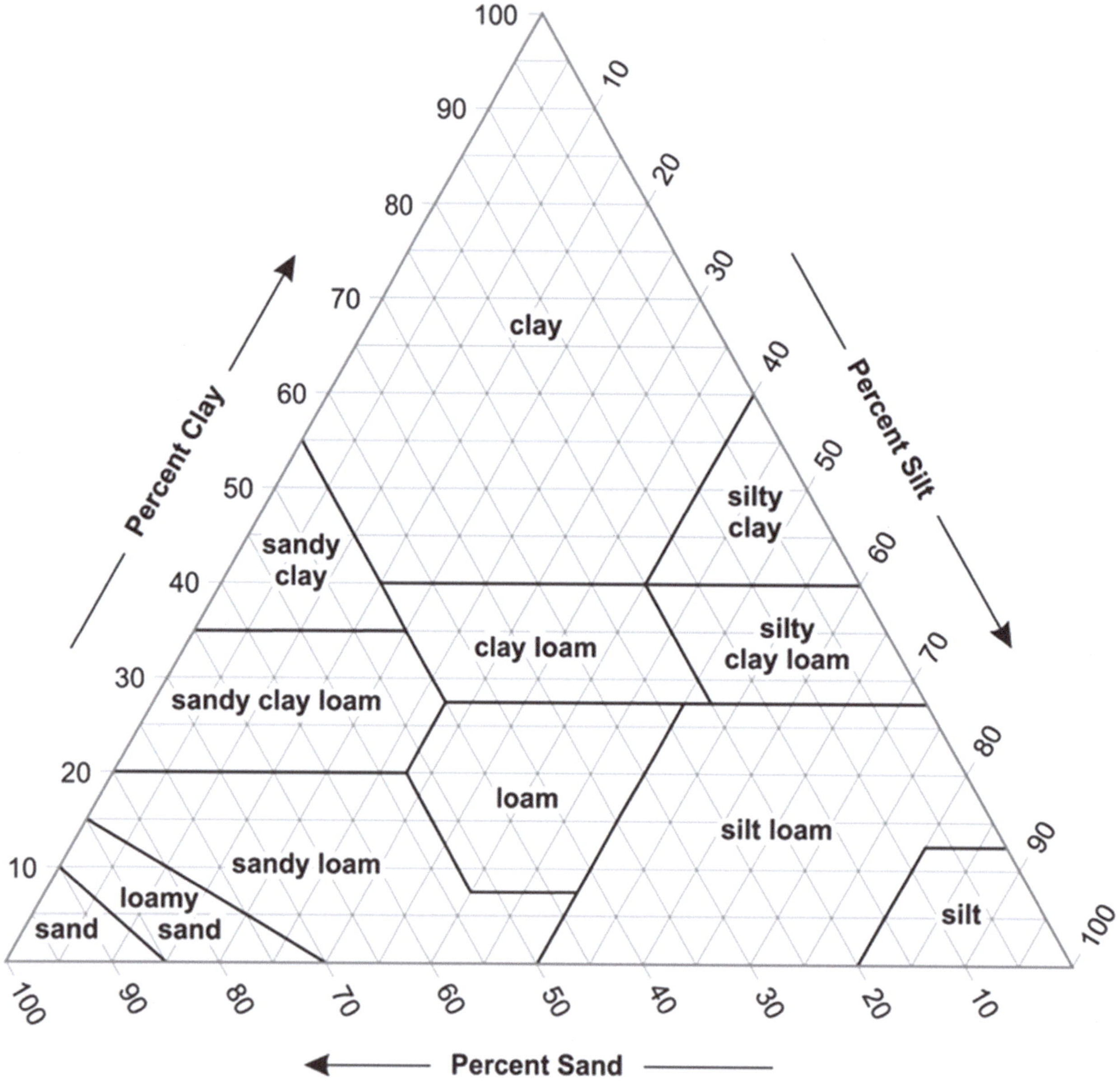

Figure 1: Soil composition mixture. (USDA; 2020)

11) According to Figure 1, which of the following would NOT be considered possible for a specimen labelled "clay"?

A. Less than 50% clay
B. Less than 80% sand
C. More than 80% silt
D. More than 50% clay

12) Sample RX-68 is mixed with an equal volume of pure silt. According to Figure 1, which of the following would be the accurate label for this new mixture?

A. Silt loam
B. Silty clay
C. Silty clay loam
D. Silt

13) If all of the sand was removed from the original Sample RX-68, what would be the resultant mixture?

A. Silt loam
B. Silty clay
C. Silty clay loam
D. Silt

14) At any given point in the ternary graph, the percentage of sand could be given by which of the following? (let a = percentage of clay; let b = percentage of silt)

A. $(a + b)/100$
B. $(2a + 2b)/100$
C. $100 - 2a - 2b$
D. $100 - a - b$

Questions 15–19

One proposal made to NASA for the robotic exploration of the surface of Mars involved the use of a "fuel factory" in which NASA would land a wheeled, robotic vehicle (*rover*) that would operate in conjunction with a robotic chemical lab. The lab would land with a supply of liquefied hydrogen gas aboard. The lightest of elements, the stored hydrogen would not add appreciably to the overall mass of the vehicle. Once landed upon the surface of Mars, the lab would begin to create the fuel for the rover from the hydrogen gas.

CO_2 from the atmosphere would be converted into its component carbon and oxygen molecules, while hematite (Fe_2O_3 or rust) incorporated into the Martian soil would be processed in order to liberate oxygen molecules. The carbon would be then converted into methane with hydrogen from the lab's stores. The Martian rover could then use oxygen and methane to power its engine; the waste products would be stored by the rover, and reconverted into fuel by the lab.

The fuel creation and conversion processes are as follows:

(i) Liberation of oxygen from hematite; heating hematite to a high degree yields:

$$2Fe_2O_3 \rightarrow 4FeO + O_2$$

(ii) Decomposition of CO_2:

$$CO_2 + E \text{ (energy)} \rightarrow C + O_2$$

(iii) Creation of methane:

$$2H_2 + C \rightarrow CH_4$$

The rover's engine burns methane with pure oxygen generated by steps **(i)** and **(ii)**.

The waste products from combustion can be stored by the rover, and reused by the lab. Waste water, for example, can be decomposed through hydrolysis:

(iv) $$2H_2O + E \rightarrow O_2 + 2H_2$$

Note that the following atomic mass units (amu) may be of use for calculations: H = 1.0, C = 12, O = 16, Fe = 56.

15) The limiting reagent is the reactant that is completely used up in a reaction, and thus determines when the reaction stops. Which of the following represents the limiting reagent in the fuel production process described in the passage?

A. Fe_2O_3
B. CO_2
C. CH_4
D. H_2

16) How much methane can be generated if the lab processes 12 kg H_2 with 79.8 kg Fe_2O_3 and 132 kg CO_2?

A. 3 kg
B. 18 kg
C. 36 kg
D. 48 kg

17) Given only 9 kg of H_2O, what is the maximum amount of methane that the lab can produce from the rover's waste products?

A. 1 kg
B. 2 kg
C. 4 kg
D. 8 kg

18) Which of the following represents the combustion of methane?

A. $O_2 + CH_4 \rightarrow CO_2 + 2H_2$
B. $O_2 + CH_4 \rightarrow CO + H_2O + H_2$
C. $3O_2 + CH_4 \rightarrow 2CO_2 + 2H_2O$
D. $2O_2 + CH_4 \rightarrow CO_2 + 2H_2O$

19) One of the potential problems that NASA engineers foresaw with the lab/rover concept was the possibility that some of the rover's waste products might irretrievably become lost into the atmosphere (due to leaks, for example). If the system burns 1 kg CH_4 per day, and 5% of the methane gas cannot be regenerated by the lab due to waste loss, how many mole(s) of H_2 will be lost after 1 week of continuous operation?

A. 43.8 moles
B. 2.1×10^{-3} moles
C. 3.6×10^{-2} moles
D. 1.05 moles

20) What would be the approximate ratio between the mass of manganese (Mn) and the mass of chlorine gas (Cl_2) produced?

$$2MnO_4^- + 16H^+ + 10Cl^- \rightarrow 2Mn^{2+} + 5Cl_2(g) + 8H_2O$$

Note that the following approximate atomic mass units (amu) may be of use: H = 1.0, O = 16, Cl = 35.5, Mn = 55.

A. 2:5
B. 3:2
C. 3:4
D. 1:3

How many moles are in guacamole?
Avocado's number. :)

High-level Importance

SPOILER ALERT

Gold Standard has cross-referenced the content in this chapter to examples from ACER's official GAMSAT practice materials (note that only ACER sells their eBooks brand new). It is for you to decide when you want to explore these questions since you may want to preserve some of ACER's materials for timed mock-exam practice.

Number	1	2	3	4	5
Title	GAMSAT Practice Questions	GAMSAT Sample Questions	GAMSAT Practice Test 1	GAMSAT Practice Test 2	GAMSAT Practice Test 3

Examples – Empirical formulas (the definition is not given thus it is assumed knowledge): Q37 and Q39 of 1; ternary graph for a mixture of medications: Q14-17 of 5 (these questions were not counted as being dependent on any assumed knowledge for Chapter 1); straight stoichiometry though the reaction is atomic physics: Q28 and Q30 of 5, or biochemistry: Q36 of 5. Note that "Q" is followed by the question number, and, for example, "of 1" refers to booklet number 1 in the table above. Also note that your gamsat-prep.com Masters Series online account has direct links to the step-by-step worked solutions for all of ACER's GAMSAT Sciences practice questions (the solutions can also be found in the Gold Standard GAMSAT YouTube Channel). The 15 full-length GAMSAT practice tests by Gold Standard, HEAPS-1 through HEAPS-15, contain specific cross-references to this chapter within the worked solutions. Note that there are ½ dozen units with ternary graphs among the HEAPS exams including one that is in GS-Free. The NASA unit is from HEAPS-8. Also note that your account has the worked solution for ACER's ternary-graph unit (Q14-17 of 5) in which we discuss the step-by-step approach to deconstruct ternary graphs.

Chapter Checklist

- ☐ Access your free online account at www.gamsat-prep.com/gamsat-general-chemistry to view answers, worked solutions and discussion boards for chapter-ending practice questions.
- ☐ Reassess your 'learning objectives' for this chapter: Go back to the first page of this chapter and re-evaluate the top 3 boxes and the Introduction.
  - ☐ Please be sure that you have completed the *Need for Speed* exercises at the beginning of this chapter.
- ☐ Complete a maximum of 1 page of notes using symbols/abbreviations to represent the entire chapter based on your learning objectives. These are your Gold Notes.
- ☐ Consider your multimedia options based on your optimal way of learning:
  - ☐ Download the free Gold Standard GAMSAT app for your Android device or iPhone.
  - ☐ Create your own, tangible study cards or try the free app: Anki.
  - ☐ Record your voice reading your Gold Notes onto your smartphone (audio files, e.g., *memo* or MP3s) and listen during exercise, transportation, etc.
  - ☐ Try out the Gold Standard GAMSAT online videos at gamsat-prep.com, or you can try other options on YouTube like Khan Academy or Crash Course Chemistry.
- ☐ Schedule your full-length GAMSAT practice tests: ACER and/or HEAPS exams. Schedule one full day to complete a practice test and 1-2 days for a thorough assessment of worked solutions while adding to your abbreviated Gold Notes.
- ☐ Schedule and/or evaluate stress reduction techniques such as regular exercise (sports), yoga, meditation and/or mindfulness exercises (*see* YouTube for suggestions).

High-level Importance

ELECTRONIC STRUCTURE AND THE PERIODIC TABLE
Chapter 2

Memorise

* Nothing**

Understand
(a little bit!)

* Conventional notation, Pauli, Hund's
* Box diagrams, ionisation potential, electronegativity
* Valence, electron affinity
* Variation in shells, atomic size
* Trends in the periodic table

Importance

Low level: 0% of GAMSAT General Chemistry
questions released by ACER are related to content in this chapter (in our estimation).
* Note that approximately 80% of the questions in GAMSAT General Chemistry are related to just 4 chapters: 4, 5, 6, and 9.

Introduction

The periodic table of the elements provides data and abbreviations for the names of elements in a tabular layout. The purpose of the table is to illustrate recurring (*periodic*) trends and to classify and compare the different types of chemical behavior. To do so, we must first better understand the atom.

Please note: 'Importance Level' does not apply to the GAMSAT-level, multiple-choice questions (MCQs) at the end of the chapter, since they will help you practice reasoning skills that apply to all of GAMSAT Sciences. However, this chapter contains a lot of content with a negligible GAMSAT assumed-knowledge footprint. The next chapter (Chapter 3: Bonding) is similar in that respect. Alas, a conundrum. Most chemistry professors would say: "If you have not studied the periodic table, nor chemical bonding, then you have not studied chemistry!" However, our purpose is not to teach you chemistry, but rather to teach you GAMSAT Chemistry.

We suggest 3 options depending on your objectives: **1)** If you are a science student who wants a perfect GAMSAT Sciences score: Read these 2 chapters like any textbook and then attack the GAMSAT-level MCQs; **2)** If you have a non-science background and Chapter 1 was traumatic: Read these 2 chapters like a comic book, glance at all highlighted text, images and captions, then take your time with the GAMSAT-level MCQs and worked solutions; **3)** If you are somewhere in between: Read like it's a novel, identify main characters and themes with the confidence that the GAMSAT-level MCQs will make sure that you are exam-ready.

**ACER does not typically provide a periodic table for the GAMSAT. The following would be normal to commit to memory for introductory-level chemistry: the location of the first 20 elements in the periodic table; the names of common elements and their symbols; and the trends (especially electronegativity, which will be revisited in context in the ORG Masters Series). However, none of ACER's practice materials have any such assumed knowledge for GAMSAT General Chemistry, thus we cannot advise content for you to commit to memory for this chapter.

Multimedia Resources at GAMSAT-Prep.com

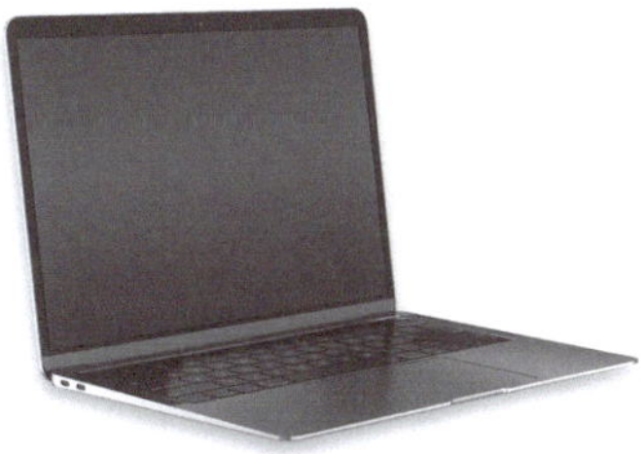

Open Discussion Boards
(*gamsat-prep.com/forum*)

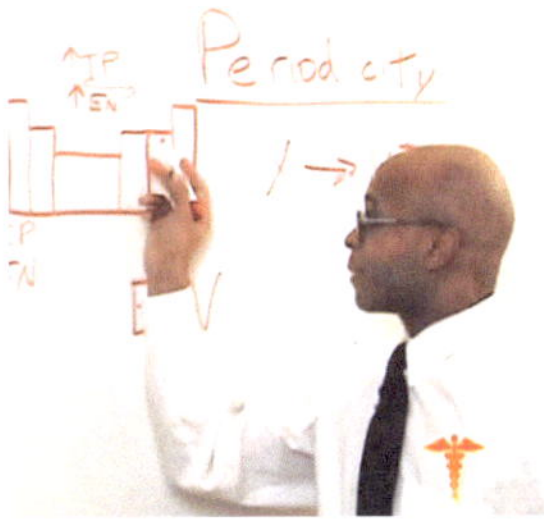

Science Preparation Videos

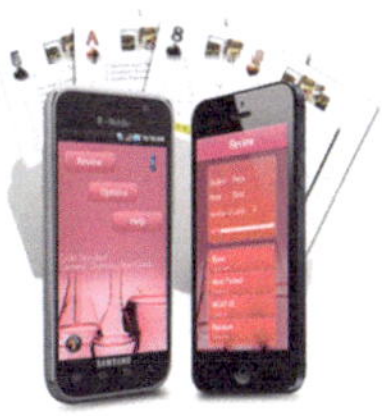

Flashcards

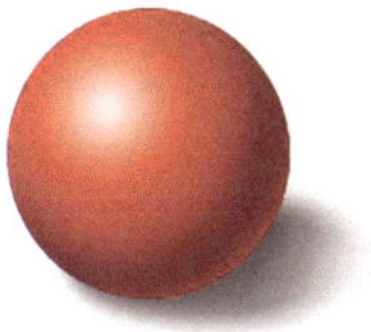

Special Guest

* The real GAMSAT may have advanced-level information presented (i.e. in a passage) but previous knowledge of said information is not required to answer the questions that would follow. Practice questions at the end of this chapter, as well as ACER and GS (HEAPS) practice GAMSATs can help you clarify this point.

2.1 Electronic Structure of an Atom

The modern view of the structure of atoms is based on a series of discoveries and complicated theories that were put forth at the turn of the twentieth century. The atom represents the smallest unit of a chemical element. It is composed of subatomic particles: protons, neutrons and electrons. At the centre of the atom is the nucleus composed of protons and neutrons surrounded by electrons forming an electron cloud.

The protons and neutrons have nearly identical masses of approximately 1 amu whereas electrons, by contrast, have an almost negligible mass. Protons and electrons both have electrical charges equal in magnitude but opposite in sign. Protons consist of a single positive (+1) charge, electrons consist of a single negative charge (−1) and neutrons have no charge (Physics Chapter 12).

Atoms have equal numbers of protons and electrons unless ionisation occurs in which ions are formed. Ions are defined as atoms with either a positive charge (*cation*) due to loss of one or more valence electrons or negative charge (*anion*) as a result of a gain in electron(s). An atom's valence electrons are electrons furthest from the nucleus and are responsible for an element's chemical properties and are instrumental in chemical bonding (*see* CHM 2.2 and 2.3 and Chapter 3).

Atoms of a given element all have an equal number of protons; however, they may vary in the number of neutrons. Atoms that differ only by neutron number are known as *isotopes*. Isotopes have the same atomic number but differ in atomic mass due to the differences in their neutron numbers. As they have the same atomic number, isotopes therefore exhibit the same chemical properties.

In the following paragraphs, we will only present the main ideas behind the findings that shaped our understanding of atomic structure. The first important idea is that electrons (as well as any subatomic particles) are in fact waves as well as particles; this concept is often referred to in textbooks as the "dual nature of matter" (cf. PHY 11.1).

Contrary to classical mechanics, in this modern view of matter, information on particles is not derived from the knowledge of their position and momentum at a given time but by the knowledge of the wave function (mathematical expression of the above-mentioned wave) and their energy. Mathematically, such information can be derived, in principle, by solving the master equation of quantum mechanics known as the Schrödinger equation. Moreover, the mathematical derivation of atomic orbitals and respective energies comes from solving the equation which includes the total energy profiles for the electrons as well as the wave function describing the wave-like nature of the electrons. Thus, the various solutions to the Schrödinger equation describes the atomic orbitals as complicated wave functions which may alternatively be graphically represented (*see* Figure III.A.2.1 and Figure III.A.2.2).

In the case of the hydrogen atom, this equation can be solved exactly. It yields the possible states of energy in which the

Low-level Importance

electron can be found within the hydrogen atom and the wave functions associated with these states. The square of the wave function associated with a given state of energy gives the probability to find the electron, which is in that same state of energy, at any given point in space at any given time. These wave functions as well as their geometrical representations are referred to as the *atomic orbitals*. We shall explain further below the significance of these geometrical representations.

Atoms of any element tend to exist toward a minimal energy level (= *ground state*) unless subjected to an external environmental change. Even for a hydrogen atom there is a large number of possible states in which its single electron can be found (when it is subjected to different external perturbations). A labelling of these states is necessary. This is done using the quantum numbers. Hence, any orbital may be completely described by four quantum numbers; n, *l*, m_l and m_s. The position and energy of an electron and each of the orbitals are therefore described by its quantum number or energy state. The four quantum numbers are thus described as follows:

(i) n: *the principal quantum number*. This number takes the integer values 1, 2, 3, 4, 5... The higher the value of n the higher the energy of the state labelled by this n. This number defines the atomic shells K (n = 1), L (n = 2), M (n = 3) etc... or the size of an orbital.

(ii) *l*: *the angular momentum quantum number*. It defines the shape of the atomic orbital in a way which we will discuss further below. For a given electronic state of energy defined by n, *l* takes all possible integer values between 0 and n – 1. For instance for a state with n = 0, there is only one possible shape of orbital, it is defined by *l* = 0. For a state defined by n = 3 there are 3 possible orbital shapes with *l* = 0, 1 and 2.

All orbitals with *l* = 0 are called "s"-shaped, all with *l* = 1 are "p"-shaped, those with *l* = 2 or 3 are "d" or "f"-shaped orbitals, respectively. The important shapes to remember are: **i)** s = spherical, and **ii)** p = 2 lobes or "dumbbell" (*see the following diagrams*). For values of *l* larger than 3, which occur with an n greater or equal to 4, the corresponding

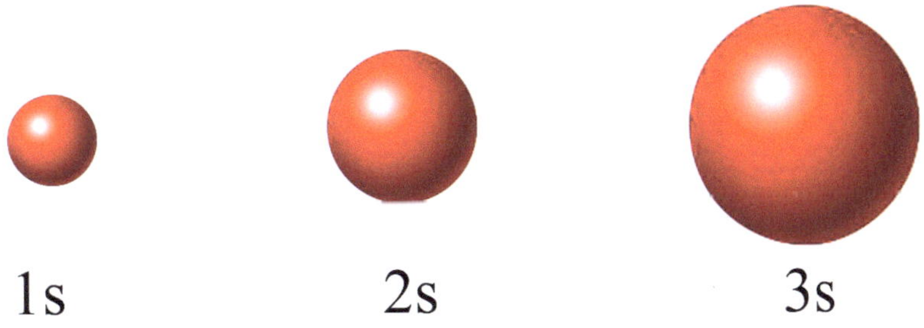

Figure III.A.2.1: Atomic orbitals where *l* = 0. Notice that the orbitals do not reveal the precise location (position) or momentum of the fast moving electron at any point in time (Heisenberg's Uncertainty Principle). Instead, we are left with a 90% chance of finding the electron somewhere within the shapes described as orbitals.

Low-level Importance

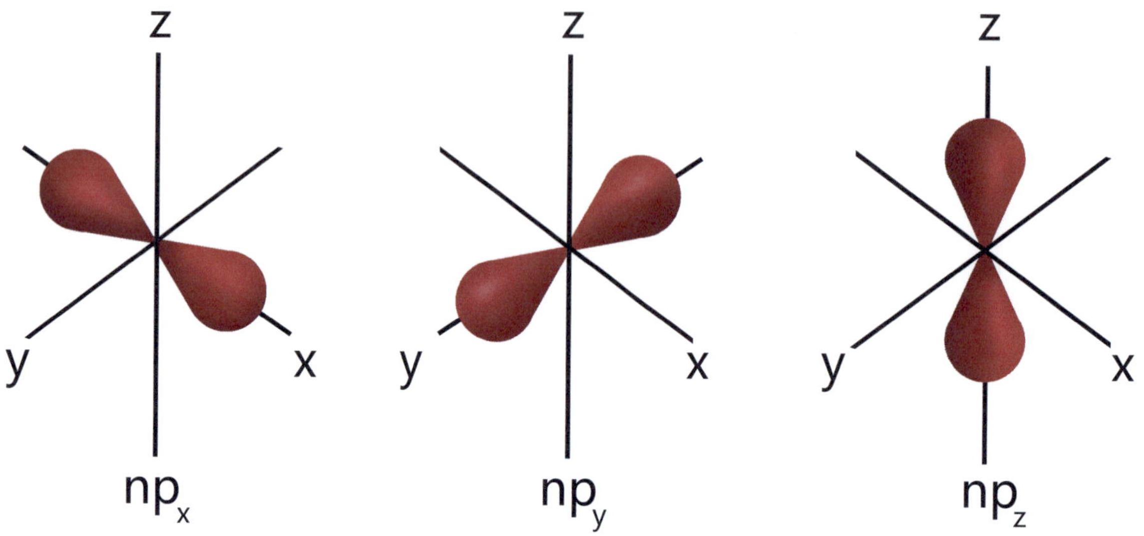

Figure III.A.2.2: Atomic orbitals where $l = 1$.

series of atomic orbitals follows the alphabetical order h, i, j, etc...

(iii) m_l: *the magnetic quantum number.* It defines the orientation of the orbital of a given shape. For a given value of l (given shape), m_l can take any of the $2l + 1$ integer values between $-l$ and $+l$. For instance for a state with n = 3 and $l = 1$ (3p orbital in notation explained in the previous paragraph), there are three possible values for m_l: –1, 0 and 1. These 3 orbitals are oriented along *x*, *y* or the *z*-axis of a coordinate system with its origin on the nucleus of the atom: they are denoted as $3p_x$, $3p_y$ and $3p_z$. Figure III.A.2.2 shows the representation of an orbital corresponding to an electron in a state ns, np_x, np_y, and np_z. These are the 3D volumes where there is 90% chance to find an electron which is in a state ns, np_x, np_y, or np_z, respectively. This type of diagram constitutes the most common geometrical representation of the atomic orbitals (besides looking at the diagrams, consider watching one of the chapter videos if you are having trouble visualising these facts).

(iv) m_s: *the spin quantum number.* This number takes the values +1/2 or –1/2 for the electron. Some textbooks present the intuitive, albeit wrong, explanation that the spin angular momentum arises from the spinning of the electron around itself, the opposite signs for the spin quantum number would correspond to the two opposite rotational directions. We do have to resort to such an intuitive presentation because the spin angular moment has, in fact, no classical equivalent and, as a result, the physics behind the correct approach is too complex to be dealt with in introductory courses.

Low-level Importance

2.2 Conventional Notation for Electronic Structure

As described in the previous section, the state of an electron in an atom is completely defined by a set of four quantum numbers (n, *l*, m_l, m_s). If two electrons in an atom share the same n, *l* and m_l numbers their m_s have to be of opposite signs: this is known as the Pauli's exclusion principle which states that no two electrons in an atom can have the same four quantum numbers. This principle along with a rule known as Hund's rule, which states that electrons fill orbitals singly first until all orbitals of the same energy are filled, constitutes the basis for the procedure that one needs to follow to assign the possible (n, *l*, m_l, m_s) quantum states to the electrons of a polyelectronic atom.

Orbitals are "filled" in sequence, according to an example shown below. When filling a set of orbitals with the same n and *l* (e.g., the three 2p orbitals: $2p_x$, $2p_y$ and $2p_z$ which differ by their m_l's) electrons are assigned to orbitals with different m_l's first with parallel spins (same sign for their m_s), until each orbital of the given group is filled with one electron, then, electrons are paired in the same orbital with antiparallel spins (opposite signs for m_s). This procedure is illustrated in an example which follows. The electronic configuration which results from orbitals filled in accordance with the previous set of rules corresponds to the atom being in its lowest overall state of energy. This state of lowest energy is referred to as the ground state of the atom.

Note: There are 2 periodic tables at the end of this chapter which you may want to consult from time to time.

The restrictions related to the previous set of rules lead to the fact that only a certain number of electrons is allowed for each quantum number:

- for a given n (given shell): the maximum number of electrons allowed is $2n^2$. The greater the value of n, the greater the energy level of the shell.
- for a given *l* (s, p, d, f...): this number is $4l + 2$.
- for a given m_l (given orbital orientation): a maximum of 2 electrons is allowed.

There is a **conventional notation** for the electronic structure of an atom:

(i) orbitals are listed in the order they are filled (see Figure III.A.2.3)

(ii) generally, in this conventional notation, no distinction is made between electrons in states defined by the same n and l but which do not share the same m_l.

For instance the ground state electronic configuration of oxygen is written as:

$$1s^2\ 2s^2\ 2p^4$$

When writing the electronic configuration of a polyelectronic atom, orbitals are filled (with electrons denoted as the superscripts of the configurations) in order of increasing energy: 1s 2s 2p 3s 3p 4s 3d ... according to the following figure:

Low-level Importance

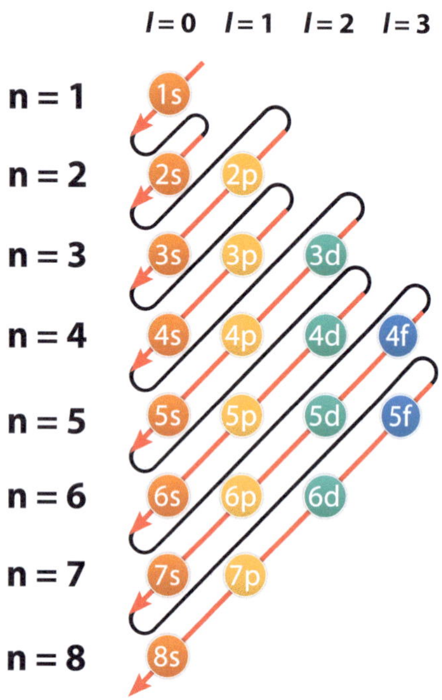

Figure III.A.2.3: The order for filling atomic orbitals: Follow the direction of successive arrows moving from top to bottom.

Thus, the electronic configuration or the pattern of orbital filling of an atom generally abides by the following rules or principles:

1. Always fill the lowest energy (or ground state) orbitals first (Aufbau principle);
2. No two electrons in a single atom can have the same four quantum numbers; if n, *l*, and m_l are the same, m_s must be different such that the electrons have opposite spins (Pauli exclusion principle);
3. Degenerate orbitals of the subshell are each occupied singly with electrons of parallel spin before double occupation of the orbitals occurs (Hund's rule).

An alternative way to write the aforementioned electronic configuration is based on the avoidance in writing out the inner core electrons. Moreover, this is an abbreviation of the previous longer configuration or otherwise known as a shorthand electronic configuration. Here, the core electrons are represented by a prior noble gas elemental symbol within brackets. As an example, calcium may be written in its expanded form or more commonly as a shorthand notation represented as $[Ar]4s^2$ shown with the prior noble gas symbol for argon [Ar] written within brackets.

Another illustrative notation is also often used. In this alternate notation orbitals are represented by boxes (hence the referring to this representation as "box diagrams"). Orbitals with the same *l* are grouped together and electrons are represented by vertical ascending or descending arrows (for the two opposite signs of m_s).

For instance for the series H, He, Li, Be, B, C we have the following electronic configurations:

H: $1s^1$ box diagram: [↑]

He: $1s^2$ box diagram: [↑↓] and not [↑↑]
(rejected by Pauli's exclusion principle)

Li: $1s^2$ $2s^1$
[↑↓] [↑]

Be: $1s^2$ $2s^2$
[↑↓] [↑↓]

B: $1s^2$ $2s^2$ $2p^1$
[↑↓] [↑↓] [↑][ ][ ]

C: $1s^2$ $2s^2$ $2p^2$
[↑↓] [↑↓] [↑][↑][ ]

(to satisfy Hund's rule of maximum spin)

To satisfy Hund's rule the next electron is put into a separate 2p "box". The 4th 2p

Low-level Importance

electron (for oxygen) is then put into the first box with an opposite spin.

O:	$1s^2$	$2s^2$	$2p^4$
	↑↓	↑↓	↑↓ ↑ ↑

Within a given subshell l, orbitals are filled in such a way to maximise the number of half-filled orbitals with parallel spins. An unpaired electron generates a magnetic field due to its spin. Consequently, when a material is composed of atoms with unpaired electrons, it is said to be *paramagnetic* as it will be attracted to an applied external magnetic field (i.e. Li, Na, Cs). Alternatively, when the material's atoms have paired electrons, it is weakly repelled by an external magnetic field and it is said to be *diamagnetic* (i.e. Cu, molecular carbon, H_2, H_2O). Non-chemists simply call diamagnetic materials "not magnetic". The strongest form of magnetism is a permanent feature of materials like Fe, Ni and their alloys and is said to be *ferromagnetic* (i.e. a fridge magnet).

For the main group elements, the valence electrons of an atom are those that are involved in chemical bonding and are in the outermost principal energy level or shell. For example, for Group IA and Group IIA elements, only electrons from the s subshell are valence electrons. For Group IIIA through Group VIIIA elements, electrons from s and p subshells are valence electrons. Under certain circumstances, elements from Group IIIA through Group VIIA may accept electrons into its d subshell, leading to more than 8 valence electrons.

Finally, as previously mentioned, we should point out that electrons can be promoted to higher, unoccupied (or partially occupied) orbitals when the atom is subjected to some external perturbation which inputs energy into the atom. The resulting electronic configuration is then called an excited state configuration (this concept was explored in PHY 12.5, 12.6).

2.3 Elements, Chemical Properties and The Periodic Table

Since most chemical properties of the atom are related to their outermost electrons (valence electrons), it is the orbital occupation of these electrons which is most relevant in the complete electronic configuration. The periodic table (there is one at the end of this chapter with a summary of trends) can be used to derive such information in the following way:

(i) the row or period number gives the "n" of the valence electrons of any given element of the period.

(ii) the first two columns or groups and helium (He) are referred to as the *s*-block. The valence electrons of elements in these groups are "s" electrons.

(iii) groups 3A to 8A (13th to 18th columns) are the *p*-block. Elements belonging to these groups have their ground state electronic configurations ending with "p" electrons.

Low-level Importance

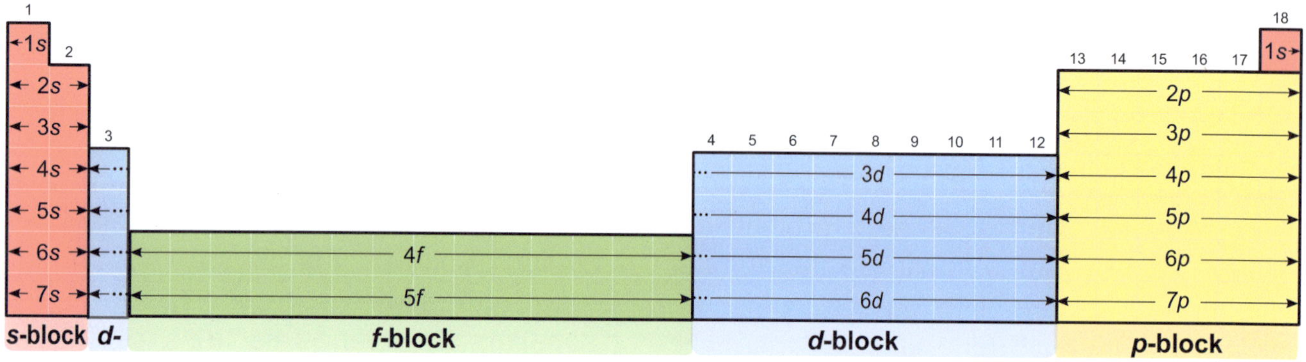

Figure III.A.2.4: Representation of s-, f-, d-, and p-blocks in the periodic table (cf. with the tables at the end of CHM 2.4.1). Each "block" refers to the sequence in which the electron shells of the elements are filled. Elements are assigned to blocks by what orbitals their valence electrons or vacancies lie in. The s-block comprises the first two groups (alkali metals and alkaline earth metals) as well as hydrogen and helium. The p-block comprises the last six groups, which includes nonmetals and metalloids. The d-block comprises groups 3 to 12 and contains all of the transition metals. The f-block comprises most of the lanthanides and actinides. (ref: α)

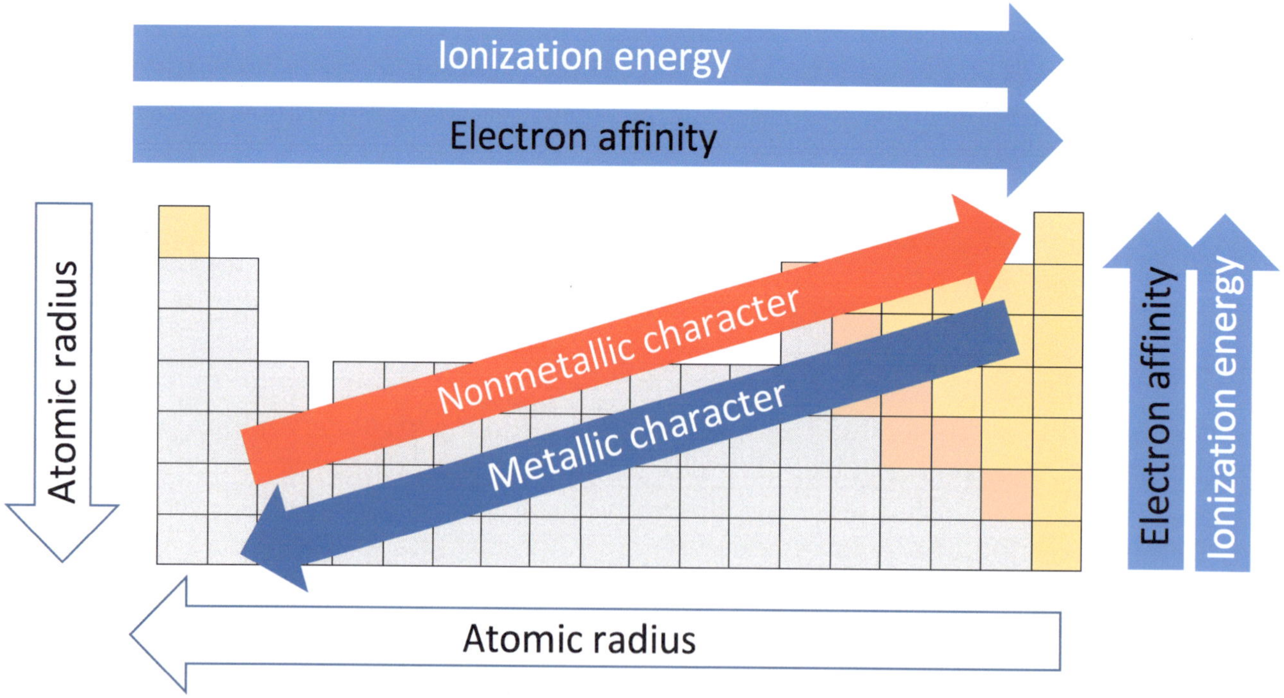

Figure III.A.2.5 Some of the trends in the periodic table with arrows illustrating increases. (ref: β)

Low-level Importance

(iv) Elements in groups 3B to 2B (columns 3 to 12) are called transition elements. Their electronic configurations end with $ns^2(n-1)d^x$ where n is the period number and x = 1 for column 3, 2 for column 4, 3 for column 5, etc… Note that these elements sometimes have unexpected or unusual valence shell electronic configurations.

This set of rules should make the writing of the ground-state, valence shell electronic configuration very easy. For instance: Sc being an element of the "d" group on the 4th period should have a ground-state, valence shell electronic configuration of the form: $4s^23d^x$. Since it belongs to group 3B (column 3) x = 1, the actual configuration is simply: $4s^23d^1$. However, half-filled (i.e. Cr) and filled (i.e. Cu, Ag, Au) d orbitals have remarkable stability. This stability behavior is essentially related to the closely spaced 3d and 4s energy levels with the stability associated with a half-filled (as in Cr) or completely filled (as in Cu) sublevel. Hence, this stability makes for unusual configurations (i.e. by the rules Cr = $4s^23d^4$, but in reality Cr = $4s^13d^5$ creating a half-filled d orbital). It can be noted that Cr therefore has an electronic configuration of $[Ar]4s^13d^5$, although four d electrons would be expected to be seen instead of five. This is because one electron from a s subshell jumps into the d orbital, giving the atom a half filled d subshell. As for Cu, it would have an electronic configuration of $[Ar]4s^23d^9$ by the rules. However, the Cu d shell is just one electron away from stability, and therefore, one electron from the s shell jumps into the d shell to convert it into $[Ar]4s^13d^{10}$.

Some metal ions form coloured solutions due to the transition energies of the d-electrons.

A number of physical and chemical properties of the elements are periodic, i.e. they vary in a regular fashion with atomic numbers. We will define some of these properties and explain their trends:

(A) Ionisation Energy

(i) The ionisation energy (IE) is defined as the energy required to remove an electron from a gaseous atom or ion. The first ionisation energy or potential (1st IE or IP) is the energy required to remove one of the outermost valence electrons from an atom in its gaseous state. The ionisation potential increases from left to right within a period and decreases from the top to the bottom of a group or column of the periodic chart. The 1st IP drops sharply when we move from the last element of a period (inert gas) to the first element of the next period. These are general trends. Elements located after an element with a half-filled shell, for instance, have a lower 1st IP than expected by these trends.

(ii) The second ionisation is the energy or potential (2nd IE or IP) required to remove a second valence electron from the ion to form a divalent ion. The previous trends can be used if one remembers the

Low-level Importance

relationship between 1st and 2nd ionisation processes of an atom of element X:

$$X + \text{energy} \rightarrow X^{+} + 1e^{-}$$
1st ionisation of X
$$X^{+} + \text{energy} \rightarrow X^{2+} + 1e^{-}$$
2nd ionisation of X

The second ionisation process of X can be viewed as the 1st ionisation of X^+. With this in mind it is very easy to predict trends of 2nd IP's. For instance, let us compare the 2nd IP's of the elements Na and Al. This is equivalent to comparing the 1st IP's of Na^+ and Al^+. These, in turn, have the same valence shell electronic configurations as Ne and Mg, respectively. Applying the previous general principles on Ne and Mg we arrive at the following conclusions:

- the 1st IP of Ne is greater than the 1st IP of Mg
- the 1st IP of Na^+ is therefore expected to be greater than the 1st IP of Al^+
- the latter statement is equivalent to the final conclusion that the 2nd IP of Na is greater than the 2nd IP of Al.

(B) Electron Affinity

(iii) Electron affinity (EA) is the energy change that accompanies the following process for an atom of element X:

$$X(gas) + 1e^{-} \rightarrow X^{-}(gas)$$

This property measures the ability of an atom to accept an electron. The stronger the attraction of a nucleus for electrons, the greater the electron affinity (EA) will be. The electron affinity becomes more negative for nonmetals than metals. Thus, halogen atoms (F, Cl, Br...) have a very negative EA because they have a great tendency to form negative ions. On the other hand, alkaline earth metals which tend to form positive rather than negative ions have very large positive EA's. The overall tendency is that EA's become more negative as we move from left to right across a period. They are more negative (less positive) for nonmetals than for metals and they do not change considerably within a group or column.

(C) Atomic Radii

(iv) The atomic radius generally decreases from left to right across a period since the effective nuclear charge increases as the number of protons within an atom increases. The effective nuclear charge is the net charge experienced by the valence electrons as a result of the nucleus (i.e. protons) and core electrons. Additionally, the atomic radius increases when we move down a group due to the shielding effect of the additional core electrons and the presence of another electron shell.

(D) Electronegativity

(v) Electronegativity is a parameter that measures the ability of an atom, when engaged in a molecular bond, to pull or repel the bond electrons. This parameter is determined from the 1st IE and the EA

Low-level Importance

of a given atom. Electronegativity follows the same general trends as the 1st IE. The greater the electronegativity of an atom, the greater its attraction for bonding electrons. In general, electronegativity is inversely related to atomic size. Moreover, the larger the atom, the less the ability for it to attract electrons to itself in chemical bonding.

In conclusion, as one moves to the right across a row in the periodic table, the atomic radii decreases, the ionisation energy (IE) increases and the electronegativity increases. As one moves down a column within the periodic table, the atomic radii increases, the ionisation energy (IE) decreases and electronegativity decreases.

2.3.1 Bond Strength

When there is a big difference in electronegativity between two atoms sharing a covalent bond then the bond is generally weaker as compared to two atoms with little electronegativity difference. This is because in the latter case, the bond is shared more equally and is thus more stable.

Bond strength is inversely proportional to bond length. Thus, all things being equal, a stronger bond would be shorter. Bonds and bond strength are further discussed in ORG 1.3-1.5.1.

2.4 Metals, Nonmetals and Metalloids

The elements of the periodic table belong in three basic categories: metals, nonmetals and metalloids (or *semimetals*).

Metals – Metals have high melting points and densities characterise metals. They are excellent conductors of heat and electricity due to their valence electrons being able to move freely. This fact also accounts for the major characteristic properties of metals: large atomic radius, low ionisation energy, low electron affinities and low electronegativity. Groups IA and IIA are the most reactive of all metal species.

Of course, metals tend to be shiny and solid (with the exception of mercury, Hg, a liquid at 'Standard Temperature and Pressure', STP). They are also *ductile* (they can be drawn into thin wires) and *malleable* (they can be easily hammered into very thin sheets).

Nonmetals – Nonmetals have high ionisation energies and electronegativities. As opposed to metals, they do not conduct heat or electricity. They tend to gain electrons easily contrarily to metals that readily lose electrons when forming bonds.

Low-level Importance

Metalloids – The metalloids share properties with both metals and nonmetals. Their densities, boiling points and melting points do not follow any specific trends and are very unpredictable. Ionisation energy and electronegativity values vary and can be found in between those of metals and nonmetals. Examples of metalloids are boron, silicon, germanium, arsenic, antimony and tellurium.

Table III A.2.1

*General characteristics of metals, nonmetals and metalloids		
Metals	**Nonmetals**	**Metalloids**
• Hard and Shiny	• Gases or dull, brittle solids	• Appearance will vary
• 3 or less valence electrons	• 5 or more valence electrons	• 3 to 7 valence electrons
• Form + ions by losing e^-	• Form – ions by gaining e^-	• Form + and/or – ions
• Good conductors of heat and electricity	• Poor conductors of heat and electricity	• Conduct better than nonmetals but not as well as metals

*These are general characteristics. There are exceptions beyond the scope of the exam.

2.4.1 The Chemistry of Groups

Low-level Importance

Alkali metals – The alkali metals are found in Group IA and are different than other metals in that they only have one loosely bound electron in their outermost shell. This gives them the largest ionic radius of all the elements in their respective periods. They are also highly reactive (especially with halogens) due to their low ionisation energies and low electronegativity and the relative ease with which they lose their valence electron.

Alkaline earth metals – The alkaline earth metals are found in Group IIA and also tend to lose electrons quite readily. They have two electrons in their outer shell and experience a stronger effective nuclear charge than alkali metals. This gives them a smaller atomic radius as well as low electronegativity values.

Halogens – The halogens are found in Group VIIA and are highly reactive nonmetals with seven valence electrons in their outer shell. This gives them extremely high electronegativity values and makes them reactive towards alkali metals and alkaline earth metals that seek to donate electrons to form a complete octet. Some halogens are gaseous at Standard Temperature and Pressure (F_2 and Cl_2) while others are liquid (Br_2) or solid (I_2).

Noble gases – The noble gases (= 'inert gases') are found in the last group and are characterised by being a mostly nonreactive species due to their complete valence shells. This energetically favorable configuration of electrons gives them high ionisation energies, low boiling points and no real electronegativities. They are all gaseous at room temperature.

Transition Elements – The transition elements are found in Groups IB to VIIIB and are characterised by high melting points and boiling points. Their key chemical characteristic is their ability to exist in a variety of different oxidation states. For the transition elements, the 4s shell gets filled prior to the 3d shell according to the Aufbau rule. However, electrons are lost from the 4s shell before the 3d shell. Thus, as the d electrons are held only loosely, this contributes to the high electrical conductivity and malleability of transition elements. This is because transition elements can lose electrons from both their s and d orbitals of their valence shell; the d electrons are held more loosely than the s electrons. They display low ionisation energies and high electrical conductivities.

PERIODIC TABLE OF THE ELEMENTS

1 H 1.008																	2 He 4.003
3 Li 6.941	4 Be 9.012											5 B 10.81	6 C 12.011	7 N 14.007	8 O 15.999	9 F 18.998	10 Ne 20.179
11 Na 22.990	12 Mg 24.305											13 Al 26.982	14 Si 28.086	15 P 30.974	16 S 32.06	17 Cl 35.453	18 Ar 39.948
19 K 39.098	20 Ca 40.08	21 Sc 44.956	22 Ti 47.90	23 V 50.942	24 Cr 51.996	25 Mn 54.938	26 Fe 55.847	27 Co 58.933	28 Ni 58.70	29 Cu 63.546	30 Zn 65.38	31 Ga 69.72	32 Ge 72.59	33 As 74.922	34 Se 78.96	35 Br 79.904	36 Kr 83.80
37 Rb 85.468	38 Sr 87.62	39 Y 88.906	40 Zr 91.22	41 Nb 92.906	42 Mo 95.94	43 Tc (98)	44 Ru 101.07	45 Rh 102.906	46 Pd 106.4	47 Ag 107.868	48 Cd 112.41	49 In 114.82	50 Sn 118.69	51 Sb 121.75	52 Te 127.60	53 I 126.905	54 Xe 131.30
55 Cs 132.905	56 Ba 137.33	57 *La 138.906	72 Hf 178.49	73 Ta 180.948	74 W 183.85	75 Re 186.207	76 Os 190.2	77 Ir 192.22	78 Pt 195.09	79 Au 196.967	80 Hg 200.59	81 Tl 204.37	82 Pb 207.2	83 Bi 208.980	84 Po (209)	85 At (210)	86 Rn (222)
87 Fr (223)	88 Ra 226.025	89 **Ac 227.028	104 Unq (261)	105 Unp (262)	106 Unh (263)												

*	58 Ce 140.12	59 Pr 140.908	60 Nd 144.24	61 Pm (145)	62 Sm 150.4	63 Eu 151.96	64 Gd 157.25	65 Tb 158.925	66 Dy 162.50	67 Ho 164.930	68 Er 167.26	69 Tm 168.934	70 Yb 173.04	71 Lu 174.967
**	90 Th 232.038	91 Pa 231.036	92 U 238.029	93 Np 237.048	94 Pu (244)	95 Am (243)	96 Cm (247)	97 Bk (247)	98 Cf (251)	99 Es (254)	100 Fm (257)	101 Md (258)	102 No (259)	103 Lr (260)

Low-level Importance

PERIODIC TABLE OF THE ELEMENTS

INCREASING IONIZATION ENERGY OR IONIZATION POTENTIAL
INCREASING NEGATIVITY OF ELECTRON AFFINITY
→
INCREASING ELECTRONEGATIVITY
DECREASING ATOMIC RADIUS

Periods move across →

Groups move down ↓

DECREASING IE/IP ↓
NO CONSIDERABLE CHANGES IN EA ↓
DECREASING ELECTRONEGATIVITY ↓
INCREASING ATOMIC RADIUS ↓

Key: atomic number / **Symbol** / atomic weight

	IA	IIA	IIIB	IVB	VB	VIB	VIIB	VIII	VIII	VIII	IB	IIB	IIIA	IVA	VA	VIA	VIIA	0
1	1 H 1.008																	2 He 4.003
2	3 Li 6.941	4 Be 9.012											5 B 10.81	6 C 12.011	7 N 14.007	8 O 15.999	9 F 18.998	10 Ne 20.179
3	11 Na 22.990	12 Mg 24.305											13 Al 26.982	14 Si 28.086	15 P 30.974	16 S 32.06	17 Cl 35.453	18 Ar 39.948
4	19 K 39.098	20 Ca 40.08	21 Sc 44.956	22 Ti 47.90	23 V 50.942	24 Cr 51.996	25 Mn 54.938	26 Fe 55.847	27 Co 58.933	28 Ni 58.70	29 Cu 63.546	30 Zn 65.38	31 Ga 69.72	32 Ge 72.59	33 As 74.922	34 Se 78.96	35 Br 79.904	36 Kr 83.80
5	37 Rb 85.468	38 Sr 87.62	39 Y 88.906	40 Zr 91.22	41 Nb 92.906	42 Mo 95.94	43 Tc (98)	44 Ru 101.07	45 Rh 102.906	46 Pd 106.4	47 Ag 107.868	48 Cd 112.41	49 In 114.82	50 Sn 118.69	51 Sb 121.75	52 Te 127.60	53 I 126.905	54 Xe 131.30
6	55 Cs 132.905	56 Ba 137.33	57 *La 138.906	72 Hf 178.49	73 Ta 180.948	74 W 183.85	75 Re 186.207	76 Os 190.2	77 Ir 192.22	78 Pt 195.09	79 Au 196.967	80 Hg 200.59	81 Tl 204.37	82 Pb 207.2	83 Bi 208.980	84 Po (209)	85 At (210)	86 Rn (222)
7	87 Fr (223)	88 Ra 226.025	89 **Ac 227.028	104 Unq (261)	105 Unp (262)	106 Unh (263)												

metals | non-metals

*	58 Ce 140.12	59 Pr 140.908	60 Nd 144.24	61 Pm (145)	62 Sm 150.4	63 Eu 151.96	64 Gd 157.25	65 Tb 158.925	66 Dy 162.50	67 Ho 164.930	68 Er 167.26	69 Tm 168.934	70 Yb 173.04	71 Lu 174.967
**	90 Th 232.038	91 Pa 231.036	92 U 238.029	93 Np 237.048	94 Pu (244)	95 Am (243)	96 Cm (247)	97 Bk (247)	98 Cf (251)	99 Es (254)	100 Fm (257)	101 Md (258)	102 No (259)	103 Lr (260)

Element categories in the periodic table

Metals						Metalloids	Nonmetals		
Alkali metals	Alkaline earth metals	Inner transition elements		Transition elements	Other metals		Other nonmetals	Halogens	Noble gases
		Lanthanides	Actinides						

Low-level Importance

Element	Symbol	Atomic Number
Actinium	Ac	89
Aluminium	Al	13
Americium	Am	95
Antimony	Sb	51
Argon	Ar	18
Arsenic	As	33
Astatine	At	85
Barium	Ba	56
Berkelium	Bk	97
Beryllium	Be	4
Bismuth	Bi	83
Boron	B	5
Bromine	Br	35
Cadmium	Cd	48
Calcium	Ca	20
Californium	Cf	98
Carbon	C	6
Cerium	Ce	58
Cesium	Cs	55
Chlorine	Cl	17
Chromium	Cr	24
Cobalt	Co	27
Copper	Cu	29
Curium	Cm	96
Dysprosium	Dy	66
Einsteinium	Es	99
Erbium	Er	68

Element	Symbol	Atomic Number
Europium	Eu	63
Fermium	Fm	100
Fluorine	F	9
Francium	Fr	87
Gadolinium	Gd	64
Gallium	Ga	31
Germanium	Ge	32
Gold	Au	79
Hafnium	Hf	72
Helium	He	2
Holmium	Ho	67
Hydrogen	H	1
Indium	In	49
Iodine	I	53
Iridium	Ir	77
Iron	Fe	26
Krypton	Kr	36
Lanthanum	La	57
Lawrencium	Lr	103
Lead	Pb	82
Lithium	Li	3
Lutetium	Lu	71
Magnesium	Mg	12
Manganese	Mn	25
Mendelevium	Md	101
Mercury	Hg	80
Molybdenum	Mo	42

Low-level Importance

Element	Symbol	Atomic Number
Neodymium	Nd	60
Neon	Ne	10
Neptunium	Np	93
Nickel	Ni	28
Niobium	Nb	41
Nitrogen	N	7
Nobelium	No	102
Osmium	Os	76
Oxygen	O	8
Palladium	Pd	46
Phosphorous	P	15
Platinum	Pt	78
Plutonium	Pu	94
Polonium	Po	84
Potassium	K	19
Praseodymium	Pr	59
Promethium	Pm	61
Protactinium	Pa	91
Radium	Ra	88
Radon	Rn	86
Rhenium	Re	75
Rhodium	Rh	45
Rubidium	Rb	37
Ruthenium	Ru	44
Samarium	Sm	62
Scandium	Sc	21

Element	Symbol	Atomic Number
Selenium	Se	34
Silicon	Si	14
Silver	Ag	47
Sodium	Na	11
Strontium	Sr	38
Sulfur	S	16
Tantalum	Ta	73
Technetium	Tc	43
Tellurium	Te	52
Terbium	Tb	65
Thallium	Tl	81
Thorium	Th	90
Thulium	Tm	69
Tin	Sn	50
Titanium	Ti	22
Tungsten	W	74
(Unnilhexium)	(Unh)	106
(Unnilpentium)	(Unp)	105
(Unnilquadium)	(Unq)	104
Uranium	U	92
Vanadium	V	23
Xenon	Xe	54
Ytterbium	Yb	70
Yttrium	Y	39
Zinc	Zn	30
Zirconium	Zr	40

Low-level Importance

CHAPTER 2: Electronic Structure and The Periodic Table

GOLD STANDARD GAMSAT-LEVEL PRACTICE QUESTIONS

CHM Chapter 2 (this chapter) and Chapter 3, due to the "Low-level Importance" of assumed knowledge, have no *Need for Speed* exercises, nor Foundational MCQs. We go straight to GAMSAT-level MCQs and you will continue to develop problem-solving skills that can apply to many other GAMSAT topics. Note that any page in the Masters Series with GAMSAT-level MCQs will have the label: High-level Importance.

Questions 1–3

The Danish scientist Niels Bohr astounded the chemical community when he published his ideas on electron distribution around the nuclei of atoms. What made it even more incredible was that it was the first theory to be based on Planck's revolutionary quantum theory. The theory states that matter cannot absorb energy continuously, but only in small discrete units which he called *quanta*.

Bohr postulated that the electrons are arranged around the atom in regions of space where they had energy corresponding to a whole number of quanta (*energy levels*). When an electron makes a transition from one energy level to the next, the wavelength of the radiation absorbed or emitted was determined by the energy difference between the two energy levels. The energy levels are numbered starting from the innermost energy level and moving outward.

When the emission spectrum of hydrogen, that is, the wavelengths of electromagnetic radiation emitted during energy level transitions in the molecules, was examined, a number of discrete lines were found, corroborating Planck's theory. These wavelengths corresponded to electron transitions from higher energy levels to lower ones. The Lyman series involves electron transitions to the n=1 energy level and had wavelengths in the ultraviolet region of the electromagnetic (e-m) spectrum. The Balmer series involved transitions to the n=2 energy level and the wavelengths corresponded to the visible range of the e-m spectrum.

The wavelength of radiation emitted in these transitions is given by the following formula:

$$1/L = R_H\,(1/n_1^2 - 1/n_2^2)$$

where L = wavelength of radiation emitted in centimetres; n_1 = lower energy level; n_2 = higher energy level; and R_H = Rydberg's constant. The wavelength of radiation emitted is inversely proportional to the energy difference between the two energy levels. The brightness of each line is related to how many of each type of transition occurred in the sample since transitions between two energy levels in different molecules of the same chemical species emits the same wavelength of radiation.

1) According to the information presented, the units of Rydberg's constant would be most consistent with:

A. cm^2
B. cm^{-2}
C. cm
D. cm^{-1}

2) Which of the following electronic transitions will result in the emission of electromagnetic radiation with the greatest energy?

A. n = 2 to n = 1
B. n = 3 to n = 1
C. n = 3 to n = 2
D. n = 4 to n = 2

3) What is the wavelength of the radiation emitted when an electron makes a transition from n = 2 to n = 1? (R_H = 110 000)

A. 82 500 cm
B. 182.82 cm
C. 6.57×10^{-5} cm
D. 1.21×10^{-5} cm

High-level Importance

Questions 4–10

The electronic configuration, or the pattern of orbital filling, of an atom generally abides by the following rules or principles:

1. Always fill the lowest energy (or ground state) orbitals first (Aufbau principle);
2. No two electrons in a single atom can have the same four quantum numbers; if n, *l*, and m_l are the same, m_s must be different such that the electrons have opposite spins (Pauli exclusion principle);
3. Degenerate orbitals of the subshell are each occupied singly with electrons of parallel spin before double occupation of the orbitals occurs (Hund's rule).

An illustrative notation is often used. Orbitals are represented by boxes (hence the referring to this representation as "box diagrams"). Orbitals are grouped together and electrons are represented by vertical ascending or descending arrows (for the two opposite signs of the magnetic spin m_s).

For instance, for the first six elements of the periodic table H, He, Li, Be, B, C, we have the following electronic configurations in their ground state:

H: $1s^1$ box diagram: [↑]

He: $1s^2$ box diagram: [↑↓] and not [↑↑] (rejected by Pauli's exclusion principle)

Li: $1s^2$ [↑↓] $2s^1$ [↑]

Be: $1s^2$ [↑↓] $2s^2$ [↑↓]

B: $1s^2$ [↑↓] $2s^2$ [↑↓] $2p^1$ [↑][ ][ ]

C: $1s^2$ [↑↓] $2s^2$ [↑↓] $2p^2$ [↑][↑][ ]

(to satisfy Hund's rule of maximum spin)

To satisfy Hund's rule: the next electron is put into a separate 2p "box". The 4th 2p electron (for oxygen, atomic number 8) is then put into the first box with an opposite spin.

O: $1s^2$ [↑↓] $2s^2$ [↑↓] $2p^4$ [↑↓][↑][↑]

4) Which electron configuration is most consistent with an atom in its ground state?

A. 1s [↑↓] 2s [↑↓] 2p [↑↓][ ][ ]

B. 1s [↑↑] 2s [↑↓] 2p [ ][ ][ ]

C. 1s [↑] 2s [↑↓] 2p [ ][ ][ ]

D. 1s [↑↓] 2s [↑↓] 2p [↑][ ][↑]

5) The word Aufbau means "built up" or "construction" in German. Which of the following is illustrated by the Aufbau principle?

A. Electrons with the same spin cannot build the same orbital.
B. Because electrons repel each other, electrons will occupy single orbitals within and energy level before doubling up.
C. Electrons fill lower energy levels first before occupying higher energy levels.
D. Neither **A**, nor **B**, nor **C** is correct.

6) Which ground state electron configuration represents a violation of the Aufbau principle?

A.

1s	2s	2p		
↑↓	↑↑	↑		

B.

1s	2s	2p		
↑↓	↑			

C.

1s	2s	2p		
↑	↑	↑	↓	↑

D.

1s	2s	2p		
↑↓	↑↓	↑↓		

7) Which electron configuration represents a violation of the Pauli exclusion principle?

A.

1s	2s	2p		
↑↓	↑↑	↑		

B.

1s	2s	2p		
↑↓	↑			

C.

1s	2s	2p		
↑↓	↑↓	↑↓		

D.

1s	2s	2p		
↑↓	↑↓	↑		↑

8) Which electron configuration represents a violation of the Pauli exclusion principle?

A.

1s	2s	2p		
↑	↑↓			

B.

1s	2s	2p		
↑↓	↑↓	↑		↑

C.

1s	2s	2p		
↑↓	↑↓	↑↓		

D.

1s	2s	2p		
↑↑	↑↓			

9) Which electron configuration represents a violation of Hund's rule for an atom in its ground state?

A.

1s	2s	2p		
↑↓	↑↓	↑↑	↑	↑

B.

1s	2s	2p		
↑↓	↑↓	↑	↑↓	

C.

1s	2s	2p		
↑↓	↑↓	↑	↑	

D.

1s	2s	2p		
↑↓	↑			

10) Nitrogen is atomic number 7 on the periodic table. Which one of the following is the correct electron configuration for a ground state, neutral nitrogen atom?

A.

1s	2s	2p		
↑↓	↑↓	↑	↑	↑

B.

1s	2s	2p		
↑↓	↑↑	↑	↑	↑

C.

1s	2s	2p		
↑↑	↑↓	↑	↑	↑

D.

1s	2s	2p		
↑↓	↑↓	↑↓	↑	

Questions 11–14

In the early 1900's, it was determined that if a beam of light is pointed at the negative end of a pair of charged plates, a current flow is measured. Thus, the beam of light must be liberating electrons from one metal plate, which are attracted to the other plate by electrostatic forces. This is the *photoelectric effect* as shown schematically in Figure 1.

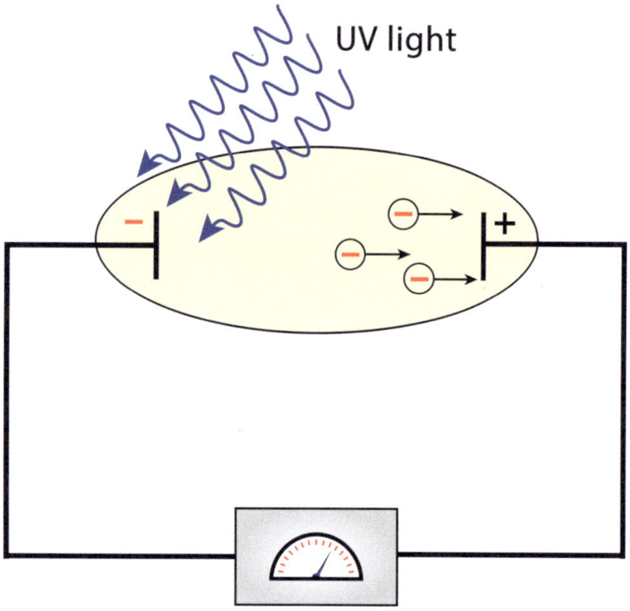

Figure 1: The photoelectric effect.

The photoelectric effect can be applied to ionise atoms in a gas, in a process often called *photoionisation*. Light is made to shine on an atom and the minimum frequency of light, corresponding to a minimum energy, is measured which will ionise an electron from an atom.

When the frequency of light is too low, the photons in that light do not have enough energy to ionise electrons from an atom. As the frequency of the light is increased, a threshold at which electrons begin to ionise is determined. Above this threshold, the energy hf, where h is Planck's constant, of the light of frequency f is greater than the energy required to ionise the atom, and the excess energy is retained by the ionised electron as kinetic energy.

By conservation of energy, the energy of the light is equal to the ionisation energy IE plus the kinetic energy KE of the ionised electron:

$$hf = IE + KE$$

Note that the velocity of light is a constant (c) and is related to frequency (f) and wavelength (λ) as follows:

$$c = \lambda f$$

Consider Table 1.

Element	Ionisation Energy (MJ/mol)					
H	1.31					
He	2.37					
Li	6.26	0.52				
Be	11.5	0.90				
B	19.3	1.36	0.80			
C	28.6	1.72	1.09			
Ne	84.0	4.68	2.08			
Na	104	6.84	3.67	0.50		
Mg	126	9.07	5.31	0.74		
Al	151	12.1	7.79	1.09	0.58	
Ar	309	31.5	24.1	2.82	1.52	
K	347	37.1	29.1	3.93	2.38	0.42
Ca	390	42.7	34.0	4.65	2.9	0.59

Table 1: Ionisation energies for various elements. The lowest number in any row is the first ionisation energy; if there is a higher number then it is the second ionisation energy; and if there is yet a higher number, then it is the third ionisation energy, and so on.

11) As part of the photoelectric effect experiments, it was determined that each photon of blue light released an electron but no matter how much red light was shone on the metal plate, no electrons were detected. What feature of blue light compared to red light is the most likely explanation for this?

A. Blue light has a longer wavelength.
B. Blue light has a greater velocity.
C. Blue light has a greater frequency.
D. Blue light has a greater ionisation energy.

12) If the wavelength of the beam of light incident to the negatively charged plate in Figure 1 is doubled, what happens to the energy of the photons?

A. It is halved.
B. It is doubled.
C. It remains the same.
D. It cannot be determined from the information provided.

13) X-rays of 1.06 MJ/mol are used to irradiate atoms of aluminium (Al). Which of the following would be consistent with the predicted kinetic energy of the emitted electrons?

A. 0.48 MJ/mol
B. 1.64 MJ/mol
C. 0.58 MJ/mol
D. 1.06 MJ/mol

14) Table 1 can be used to determine that hydrogen and helium have the highest first ionisation energies for their respective groups in the periodic table of the elements. The most likely reason for this is that for both of these atoms:

A. spherical orbitals are present.
B. the magnetic spin can be plus or minus 1/2.
C. the electron or electrons are in the innermost shell.
D. the d-shell electrons are relatively easy to ionise.

15) The energy of an electron (E_n) moving in the nth orbit of an element can be approximated by the following equation:

$$E_n = \frac{-13.6Z^2}{n^2}$$

where Z is the proton number of a chemical element.

If the value of n is held constant, the graph of E_n vs. Z^2 would be most consistent with which of the following?

A.

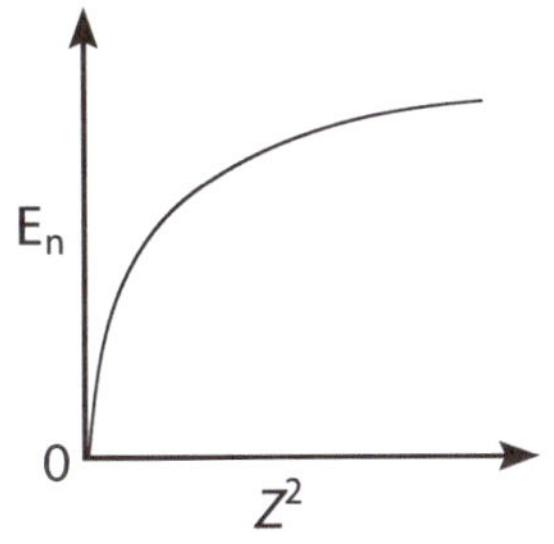

B.

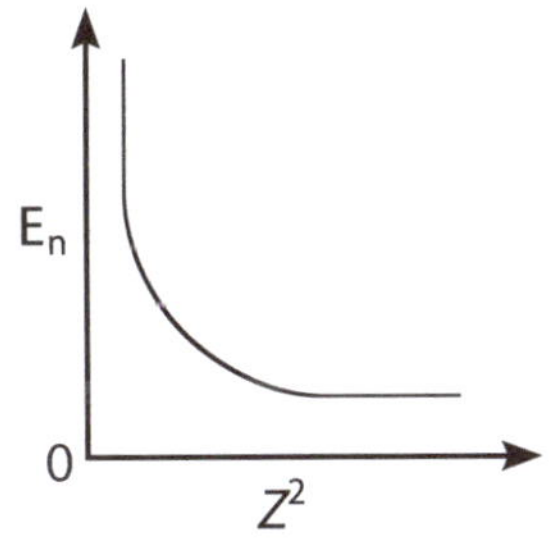

C.

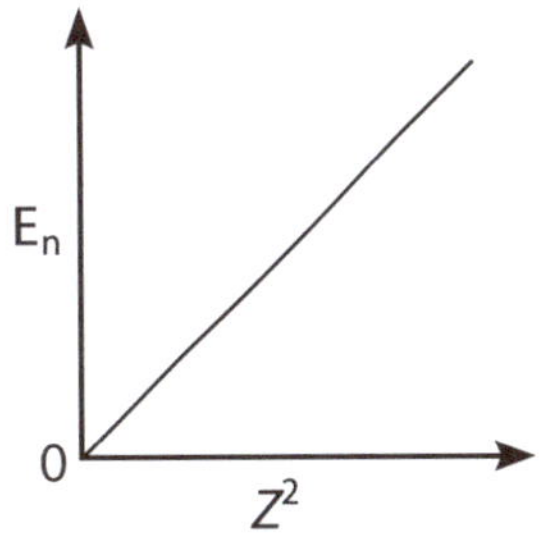

D.

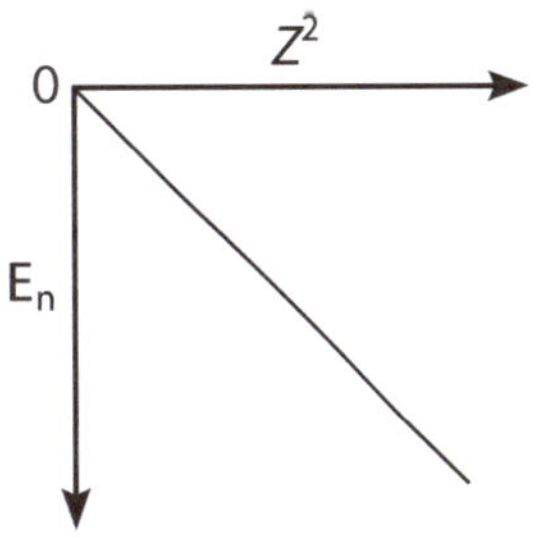

Questions 16–20

The quantum numbers describe the electronic configuration of atoms.

The state of each electron is determined by four quantum numbers:

- principal quantum number n determines the number of shells; possible values are identified by an integer or the letter in brackets: 1 (K), 2 (L), 3 (M), etc...
- angular momentum quantum number *l*, determines the subshell; possible values are identified by an integer or the letter in brackets: 0 (s), 1 (p), 2 (d), 3 (f), etc., up to a maximum value of n–1.
- magnetic momentum quantum number m_l, possible values are: ± *l*, ... , 0. For example, if *l* = 1, then the possible values are +1, 0, and –1.
- spin quantum number m_s, can be simplified to mean the direction of rotation of the electron, possible values are: ±1/2.

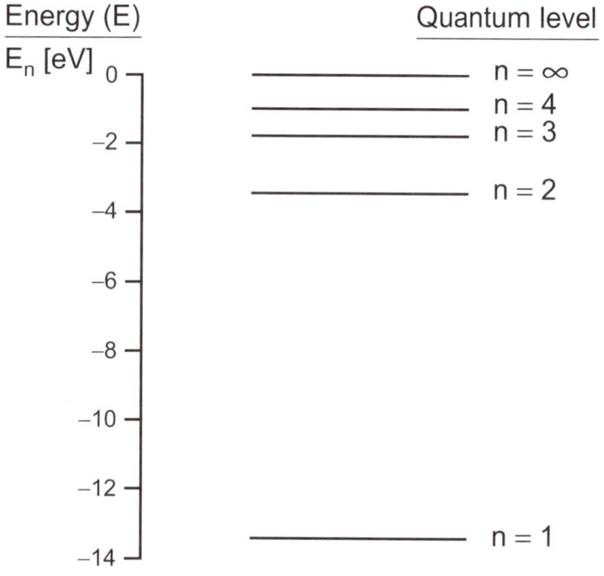

Figure 1: Energy levels. The energy E_n in each shell n is measured in electron volts (eV).

Each atomic shell has a maximum number of electrons that it can contain. For example, the first shell can contain two electrons, the second can contain eight electrons. The maximum number of electrons in each shell is given by the following formula:

$$N_{electrons} = 2n^2$$

$N_{electrons}$ designates the number of electrons in shell n.

16) Based on the information provided, what is the maximum number of electrons that can fit in a shell with an energy level of –1 eV?

A. 2
B. 8
C. 16
D. 32

17) What is the principle quantum number (n) of the first shell to have d-subshells?

A. K
B. L
C. M
D. N

18) How many possible values of the magnetic quantum number are there for d-subshells?

A. 1
B. 2
C. 3
D. 5

19) Based on the information provided, an electron transitioning between which of the following shells would be expected to have the greatest energy change?

A. d to s
B. N to K
C. M to N
D. L to N

20) Which one of the following represents an impossible set of quantum numbers for an electron in an atom? (arranged as n, l, m_l, and m_s, respectively)

A. 2, 1, –1, –1/2
B. 1, 0, 0, 1/2
C. 5, 4, –3, –1/2
D. 3, 3, 3, 1/2

High-level Importance

SPOILER ALERT

Gold Standard has cross-referenced the content in this chapter to examples from ACER's official GAMSAT practice materials. It is for you to decide when you want to explore these questions since you may want to preserve some of ACER's materials for timed mock-exam practice.

Examples – None that directly point to assumed knowledge from Chapter 2. Note that GAMSAT Organic Chemistry is a little different, in the sense that understanding the trends in electronegativity is sometimes (still, rarely) helpful. We will revisit this issue in ORG Chapter 1. Note that the Niels Bohr unit is from HEAPS-5; the unit with the box diagrams is from HEAPS-7; and the unit with the quantum numbers is from HEAPS-8.

Chapter Checklist

- ☐ Access your online account to view answers, worked solutions and discussion boards.
- ☐ Reassess your 'learning objectives' for this chapter: Go back to the first page of this chapter and re-evaluate the top 3 boxes and the Introduction.
- ☐ Complete a maximum of 1 page of notes using symbols/abbreviations to represent the entire chapter based on your learning objectives. These are your Gold Notes.
- ☐ Consider your multimedia options based on your optimal way of learning:
  - ☐ Download the free Gold Standard GAMSAT app for your Android device or iPhone.
  - ☐ Create your own, tangible study cards or try the free app: Anki.
  - ☐ Record your voice reading your Gold Notes onto your smartphone (audio files, e.g., *memo* or MP3s) and listen during exercise, transportation, etc.
  - ☐ Try out the Gold Standard GAMSAT online videos at gamsat-prep.com, or you can try other options on YouTube like Khan Academy or Crash Course Chemistry.
- ☐ Reassess your schedule for your full-length GAMSAT practice tests: ACER and/or HEAPS exams. Ensure that you have scheduled one full day to complete a practice test and 1-2 days for a thorough assessment of worked solutions while adding to your abbreviated Gold Notes.
- ☐ Reassess your progress in scheduling and/or evaluating stress reduction techniques such as regular exercise (sports), yoga, meditation and/or mindfulness exercises (*see* YouTube for suggestions).

References

α: Figure III.A.2.4
DePiep; Wikimedia Commons, 2021.

β: Figure III.A.2.5
Sandbh; Wikimedia Commons, 2021.

High-level Importance

BONDING

Chapter 3

Memorise	Understand (a little bit!)	Importance
* Nothing**	* Ionic, covalent bonds * VSEPR, resonance * Dipole, covalent polar bonds * Trends in the periodic table * Lewis structures, octet rule, formal charge * Molecular shapes (3 shapes will help in ORG: linear, 'flat triangle,' and tetrahedral)	**Low level: 2% of GAMSAT General Chemistry** questions released by ACER are related to content in this chapter (in our estimation). * Note that approximately 80% of the questions in GAMSAT General Chemistry are related to just 4 chapters: 4, 5, 6, and 9.

GAMSAT-Prep.com

Introduction

Attractive interactions between atoms and molecules involve a physical process called *chemical bonding*. In general, strong chemical bonding is associated with the sharing or transfer of electrons between atoms. Molecules, crystals and diatomic gases are held together by chemical bonds which makes up most of the matter around us.

This chapter lays down a lot of foundation for GAMSAT Organic Chemistry. However, with regards to what strategy to apply while studying this chapter from a GAMSAT General Chemistry perspective, please re-read the Introduction to Chapter 2. And, of course: Importance level does not apply to the GAMSAT-level practice questions at the end of the chapter which help you practice reasoning skills that apply to all of GAMSAT Sciences.

**The following would be normal to commit to memory for introductory-level chemistry: Hybrid orbitals, molecular shapes, Lewis structures (and Lewis acids/bases), the octet rule and formal charge. However, none of ACER's practice materials have any such assumed knowledge for GAMSAT General Chemistry, thus we cannot advise content for you to commit to memory for this chapter.

Multimedia Resources at GAMSAT-Prep.com

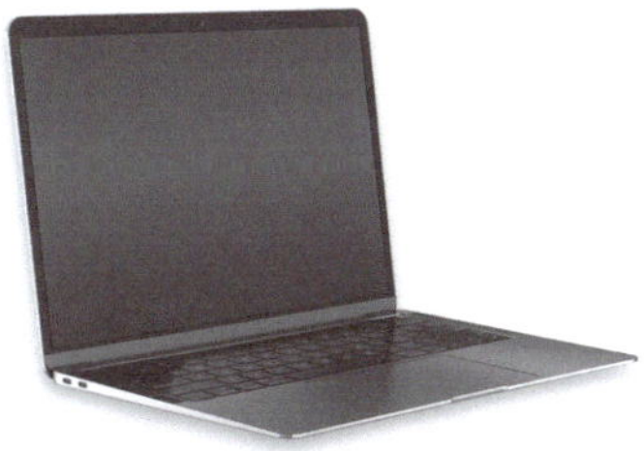

Open Discussion Boards
(gamsat-prep.com/forum)

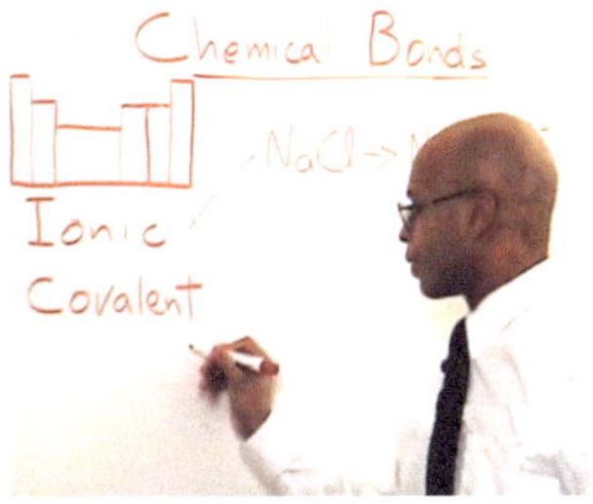

Science Preparation Videos

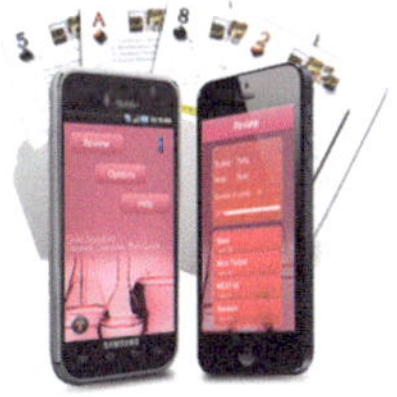

Flashcards

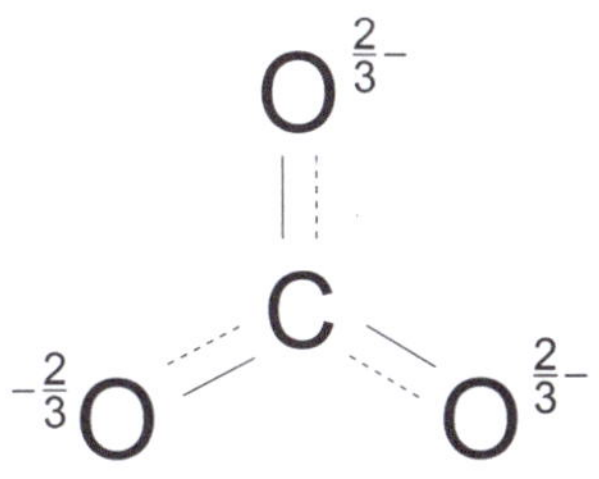

Special Guest

* The real GAMSAT may have advanced-level information presented (i.e. in a passage) but previous knowledge of said information is not required to answer the questions that would follow. Practice questions at the end of this chapter, as well as ACER and GS (HEAPS) practice GAMSATs can help you clarify this point.

3.1 Summary of Chemical Bonds

Chemical bonds are connections between atoms of the same element or between atoms of different elements. Primary (*strong*) chemical bonds are classified into three groups: ionic, covalent and metallic (we will explore secondary, *weak*, bonds in Chapter 4 such as London forces, H-bonds, etc.).

In summary, for primary bonds, if the electronegativity values of two atoms are:

- significantly different...
  - Ionic bonds are formed.
- similar...
  - Metallic bonds form between two metal atoms.
  - Covalent bonds form between two nonmetal atoms (or between metal and nonmetal atoms).
    - Non-polar covalent bonds form when the electronegativity values are very similar.
    - Polar covalent bonds form when the electronegativity values are somewhat further apart.

We will also see in this chapter that many bonds are formed according to the *octet rule*, which states that an atom tends to form bonds with other atoms until the bonding atoms obtain a stable electron configuration of eight valence electrons in their outermost shells, similar to that of Group VIIIA (noble gas) elements. There are certain exceptions to the octet rule such as, hydrogen forming bonds with two valence electrons; beryllium, which can bond to attain four valence electrons; boron, which can bond to attain six; and elements such as phosphorus and sulfur, which can incorporate d-orbital electrons to attain more than eight valence electrons.

3.1.1 The Ionic Bond

Low-level Importance

An *ion* is an atom, molecule or particle with a net electrical charge. Ionic bonds form when there is a complete transfer of one or more electrons between a metal and a nonmetal atom. When an element X with a low ionisation potential is combined with an element Y with a large negative electron affinity, one or more electrons are transferred from the atoms of X to the atoms of Y. This leads to the formation of cations (*positive charge*) X^{n+} and anions (*negative charge*) Y^{m-}. These ions of opposite charges are then attracted to each other through electrostatic forces (= "*opposites attract, like charges repel*") which then aggregate to form large stable spatial arrangements of ions: crystalline solids ("*crystals*"). The bonds that hold these ions together are called ionic bonds.

There exists a large difference in electronegativity between ionically bonded atoms. Electronegativity is defined as the ability of an atom to attract shared electrons in a covalent bond. Each atomic element is assigned a numerical electronegativity value with the greatest value of 4.0 assigned to the most electronegative element, fluorine. The higher the value of the electronegativity, the more strongly that element attracts the shared electrons. Ionic compounds are known to have high melting and boiling points and high electrical conductivity. In our general example, note that to maintain electrical neutrality the empirical formula of this ionic compound has to be of the general form: X_mY_n (the total positive charge: n × m is equal to the total negative charge: m × n in a unit formula). For instance, since aluminium tends to form the cation Al^{3+} and oxygen the anion O^{2-} the empirical formula for aluminium oxide is Al_2O_3 {*Some students call this* ***'drop and swap'*** *because the superscripts become subscripts while changing elements. See* CHM 5.3.4 *and the Chapter 5 Spoiler Alert.*}. Thus, the empirical or simplest formula is written for each of the formula units (Al_2O_3) which are part of a larger crystalline solid. The actual ionic solid lattice formed, however, consists of a large and equal number of ions packed together in a manner to allow maximal attraction of all the oppositely charged ions.

H	2.1												
Li	1.0	Be	1.5	B	2.0	C	2.5	N	3.0	O	3.5	F	4.0
Na	0.9	Mg	1.2	Al	1.5	Si	1.8	P	2.1	S	2.5	Cl	3.0
K	0.8	Ca	1.0	Ga	1.6	Ge	1.8	As	2.0	Se	2.4	Br	2.8
Rb	0.8	Sr	1.0	In	1.7	Sn	1.8	Sb	1.9	Te	2.1	I	2.5
Cs	0.7	Ba	0.9	Tl	1.8	Pb	1.9	Bi	1.9	Po	2.0	At	2.2

Table III.A.3.0: Pauling's values for the electronegativity of some important elements. Note that elements in the upper right hand corner of the periodic table have high electronegativities and those in the bottom left hand corner have low electronegativities (CHM 2.3, 2.4.1). Also note that Pauling's electronegativity is dimensionless since it measures electron-attracting ability on a relative scale. A difference in values greater than 2.0 suggests an ionic bond.

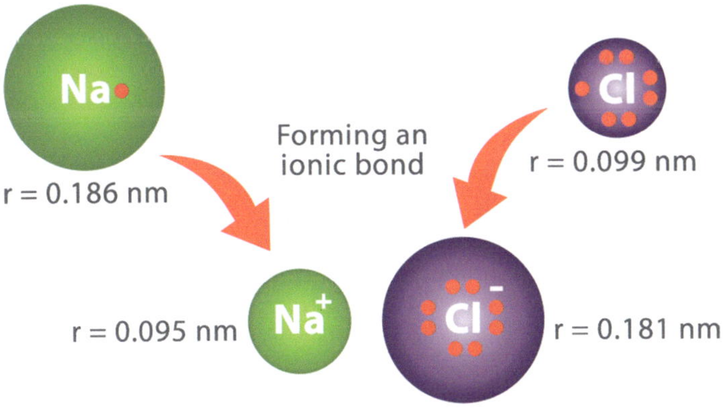

Figure III.A.3.0a: Forming an ionic bond. Note that when sodium loses an electron to form Na^+, its effective size decreases by about one half because it loses its outer shell (CHM 2.1-2.3). When chlorine gains an electron to produce the 8-electron (*octet*) structure within Cl^-, its size increases to almost double. As a result of the gain in charges, the ionic bond forms between Na^+ and Cl^- by electrostatic attraction (*opposites attract*; PHY 9.1). Again, due to the charges, ionic compounds conduct electricity when liquefied by heat (*molten*) or in solution, but typically not when solid. Ionic compounds generally have a high melting point, and tend to be soluble in water.

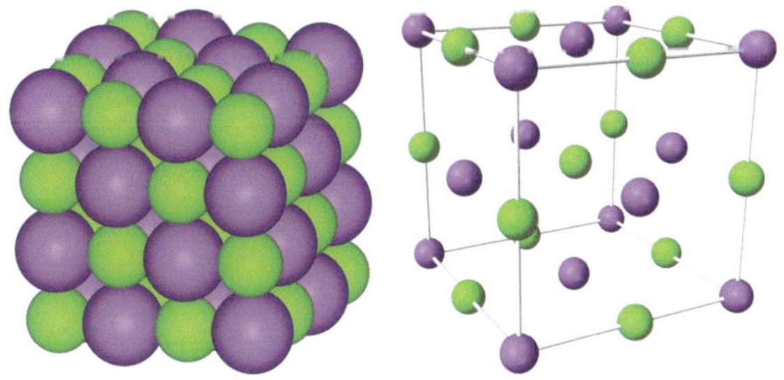

Figure III.A.3.0b: Two representations of the solid, crystal-lattice structure of table salt (sodium chloride, NaCl), a typical ionic compound. The Pauling's values for Na and Cl have a significant difference (*greater than 2.0*) leading to a complete transfer of an electron. On the left is the close-packing crystal; and on the right, an "exploded" version which is an easier way to see the arrangement of the most basic structure (*the unit cell*) that can repeat to make the entire crystal. The green spheres represent Na^+ which is strongly attracted to the purple spheres, Cl^-. A similar colour motif was used for the salt water in CHM 1.1 (a salt crystal dissolved in water thus separating the charged atoms).

Low-level Importance

3.2 The Covalent Bond

Atoms are held together in non-ionic molecules by covalent bonds. In this type of bonding, two valence electrons are shared between two atoms. Two atoms sharing one, two or three electron pairs form single, double or triple covalent bonds, respectively. As the number of shared electron pairs increases, the two atoms are pulled closer together, leading to a decrease in bond length and a simultaneous increase in bond strength. As opposed to ionic bonds, atoms in covalent bonds have similar electronegativity. Ionic and covalent bonding are thus considered as the two extremes in bonding types. Covalent bonding is further categorised into the following subclasses: non-polar, polar and coordinate types of covalent bonding.

Non-polar covalent bonding occurs when two bonding atoms have either equal or similar electronegativities or a calculated electronegativity difference of less than 0.4.

Polar covalent bonding occurs when there is a small difference in electronegativity between atoms in the range of approximately 0.4 up to 2.0. When the difference in electronegativity is greater than 2.0, ionic bonding occurs. In polar covalent bonding, the more electronegative atom will attract the bonding electrons to a larger extent. As a result, the more electronegative atom acquires a partial negative charge and the less electronegative atom acquires a partial positive charge.

Coordinate covalent bonding occurs when the shared electron pair comes from the lone pair of electrons of one of the atoms in the bonding component. Typically, coordinate bonds form between Lewis acids (electron acceptors) and Lewis bases (electron donors) as shown below.

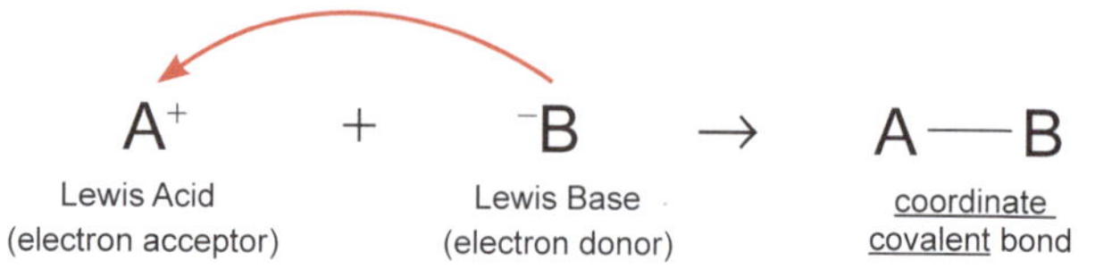

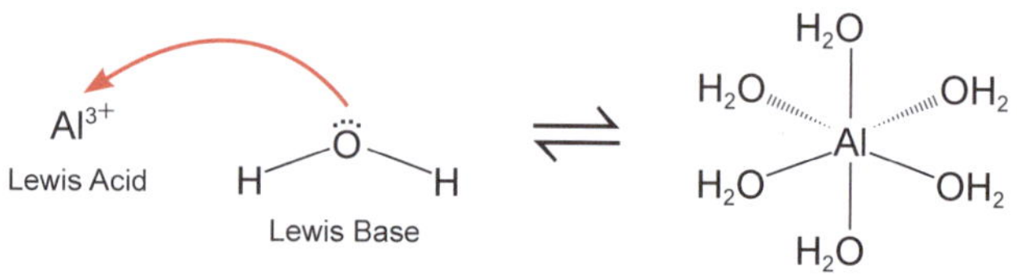

A Lewis structure is a representation of covalent bonding in which shared electrons are shown either as lines or as pairs of dots between two atoms. For instance, let us consider the H_2O molecule. The valence shell electronic configurations of the atoms that constitute this molecule are:

O: $2s^2 2p^4$
H: $1s^1$

Since hydrogen has only one electron to share with oxygen, there is only one possible covalent bond that can be formed between the oxygen atom and each of the hydrogen atoms. Four of the valence electrons of the oxygen atom do not participate in this covalent bonding; these are called non-bonding electrons or lone pairs. The Lewis structure of the water molecule is:

H:Ö:H or H-Ö-H

Lewis formulated the following general rule known as the octet rule concerning these representations: atoms tend to form covalent bonds until they are surrounded by 8 electrons (with few exceptions such as for hydrogen which can be surrounded by a maximum of only 2 electrons; *see* CHM 3.1 or the end of CHM 3.2 for details). To satisfy this rule (and if there is a sufficient number of valence electrons), two atoms may share more than one pair of electrons thus forming more than one covalent bond at a time. In such instances the bond between these atoms is referred to as a double or a triple bond depending on whether there are two or three pairs of shared electrons, respectively.

Some molecules cannot fully be described by a single Lewis structure. For instance, for the carbonate ion: CO_3^{2-}, the octet rule is satisfied for the central carbon atom if one of the C...O bonds is double (*see* the following diagrams). While this leads us to thinking that the three C...O bonds are not equivalent, every piece of experimental evidence concerning this molecule shows that the three bonds are in fact the same (same length, same polarity, etc...). This suggests that in such instances a molecule cannot be described fully by a single Lewis structure. However, a molecule may in fact be represented by two or more valid Lewis structures. Indeed, since there is no particular reason to choose one oxygen atom over another, we can write three equivalent Lewis structures for the carbonate ion. These three structures are called **resonance structures** represented with a double-headed arrow between each resonance structure. The carbonate ion (CO_3^{2-}) actually exists as a hybrid of the three equivalent structures. It is the full set of resonance structures that describes such a molecule. In this picture, the C...O bonds are neither double nor single, they are intermediate and have both a single and a double bonded character (*see* the following diagrams).

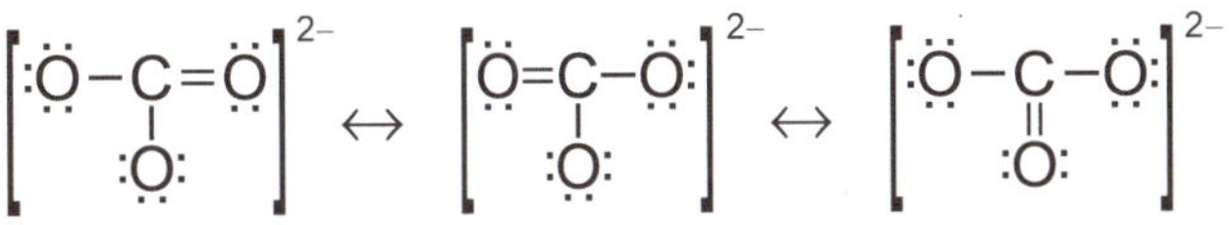

The actual structure of the carbonate ion is therefore one which is intermediate between the three resonance structures and is known as a *resonance hybrid*:

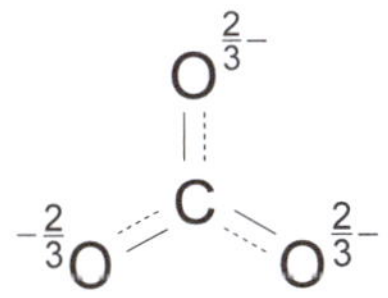

In many molecular structures, all of the respective resonance structures contribute equally to the hybridised representation. However, for some, resonance structures may not all contribute equally. Moreover, the more stable the resonance structure, the more contribution of that structure to the true hybrid structure based on formal charges.

Thus, based on their stabilities, non-equivalent resonance structures may contribute differently to the true overall hybridised structure representation of a molecule.

It is often interesting to compare the number of valence electrons that an atom

Low-level Importance

possesses when it is isolated and when it is engaged in a covalent bond within a given molecule. This is often quantitatively described by the concept of formal charge.

Generally, a formal charge is a calculated conjured charge assigned to each individual atom within a Lewis structure allowing one to distinguish amongst various possible Lewis structures. The formal charge on any individual atom is calculated based on the difference between the atom's actual number of valence electrons and the number of electrons the atom possesses as part of a Lewis structure.

Moreover, the number of electrons attributed to an atom within a Lewis structure (covalently bonded) is not necessarily the same as the number of valence electrons that would be isolated within that free atom, and the difference is thus referred to as the "formal charge" of that atom. This concept is defined as follows:

Formal charge (of atom X) = Total number of valence electrons in a free atom (V) – [(total number of non-bonding electrons (N) + ½ total number of bonding electrons (B) in a Lewis structure)].

Where, V is the number of valence electrons of the atom in isolation (*atom in the ground state*); N is the number of non-bonding valence electrons on this atom in the molecule; and B is the total number of bonding electrons shared in covalent bonds with other atoms in the molecule (*see* structure of CO_3^{2-} in the previous illustrations).

Let us apply this definition to the two previous examples: H_2O and CO_3^{2-}. This process is fairly straightforward in the case of the water molecule:

total # of valence e^-'s in free O:	6
– total # of non-bonding e^-'s on O in H_2O:	4
– 1/2 (total # of bonding e^-'s) on O in H_2O:	2
Formal charge of O in H_2O = 0	

In the case of the CO_3^{2-} ion, it is not as obvious. If we consider one of the three equivalent resonance forms, that of the oxygen with a double bond to carbon we have:

total # of valence e^-'s in free O:	6
– total # of non-bonding e^-'s on O in the ion:	4
– 1/2 (total # of bonding e^-) on O in the ion:	2
Formal charge of O of C = O in the ion = 0	

Similarly, the calculation of the formal charge for one of the two singly bonded oxygen's of C–O in the same ion leads to the following: 6 – 6 – 1/2(2) = –1. Considering that CO_3^{2-} is represented by three resonance forms, the actual formal charge of the oxygen atom is 1/3 (–1 –1 + 0) = –2/3. This value formally reflects the idea that the oxygen atoms are equivalent and that any one of them has a –1 charge in 2 out of three of the resonance forms of this ion. Here are some simple rules to remember about formal charges:

(i) For neutral molecules, the formal charges of all the atoms should add up to zero.

(ii) For an ion, the sum of the formal charges must equal the ion's charge.

Low-level Importance

The following rules should help you select a plausible Lewis structure:

(i) If you can write more than one Lewis structure for a given neutral molecule, the most plausible one is the one in which the formal charges of the individual atoms are zero.

(ii) Lewis structures with the smallest formal charges on each individual atom are more plausible than the ones that involve large formal charges.

(iii) Out of a range of possible Lewis structures for a given molecule, the most plausible ones are the ones in which negative formal charges are found on the most electronegative atoms and positive charges on the most electropositive ones.

In addition to these rules, remember that some elements have a tendency to form molecules that do not satisfy the octet rule:

(i) When sulfur is the central atom in a molecule or a polyatomic ion, it almost invariably does not fulfill the octet rule.

(ii) The number of electrons around S in these compounds is usually 12 (e.g. SF_6, SO_4^{2-}). This situation (expanded octets) also occurs in other elements in and beyond the third period.

(iii) Molecules that have an element from the 3A group (B, Al, etc...) as their central atom do not generally obey the octet rule. In these molecules there are less than 8 electrons around the central atom (e.g. AlI_3 and BF_3).

(iv) Some molecules with an odd number of electrons can clearly not obey the octet rule (e.g. NO and NO_2).

3.3 Partial Ionic Character: Polar Covalent Bonds

Except for homonuclear molecules (molecules made of atoms of the same element, e.g. H_2, O_3, etc...), bonding electrons are not equally shared by the bonded atoms. Thus a diatomic (= *two atoms*) compound like Cl_2 shares its bonding electrons equally; whereas, a binary (= *two* different *elements*) compound like CaO (calcium oxide) or NaCl (sodium chloride) does not. Indeed, for the great majority of molecules, one of the two atoms between which the covalent bond occurs is necessarily more electronegative than the other. This atom will attract the bonding electrons to a larger extent (*see* CHM 3.2). Although this phenomenon does not necessarily lead to the formation of two separate ionic species, it does result in a molecule in which there are partial charges on these particular atoms: the corresponding covalent bond is said to possess partial ionic character. This **polar bond** will also have a dipole moment given by:

$$D = q \cdot d$$

Low-level Importance

where q is the absolute value of the partial charge on the most electronegative or the most electropositive bonded atom and d is the distance between these two atoms. To obtain the total dipole moment of a molecule one must add the individual dipole moment vectors present on each one of its bonds. Since this is a vector addition (*see* ORG 1.5), the overall result may be zero even if the individual dipole moment vectors are very large.

Non-polar bonds are generally stronger than polar covalent and ionic bonds, with ionic bonds being the weakest. However, in compounds with ionic bonding, there is generally a large number of bonds between molecules and this makes the compound as a whole very strong. For instance, although the ionic bonds in one compound are weaker than the non-polar covalent bonds in another compound, the ionic compound's melting point will be higher than the melting point of the covalent compound. Polar covalent bonds have a partially ionic character, and thus the bond strength is usually intermediate between that of ionic and that of non-polar covalent bonds. The strength of bonds generally decreases with increasing ionic character.

3.4 Lewis Acids and Lewis Bases

The Lewis model of acids and bases focuses on the transfer of an electron pair. Generally, a Lewis acid is defined as any substance that may accept an electron pair to form a covalent bond, while a Lewis base is defined as any substance that donates an electron pair to form a respective covalent bond. Hence, as per the Lewis definition of an acid or base, a substance need not contain a hydrogen as defined by either Arrhenius or Bronsted-Lowry to be an acid, nor is a hydroxyl group (OH^-) needed to be a base (*see* CHM 6.1). A Lewis acid therefore generally has an empty electronic orbital that can accept an electron pair whereas a Lewis base will contain a full electronic orbital or lone pair of electrons ready to be donated.

In CHM 3.2, we pointed out some exceptions to the Lewis' octet rule. Among these were molecules that had a deficiency of electrons around the central atom as described previously (e.g. BF_3). When such a molecule is put into contact with a molecule with lone pairs (e.g. NH_3) a reaction occurs. Such a reaction can be interpreted as a donation of a pair of electrons from the second type of molecule (Lewis base) to the first type of molecule

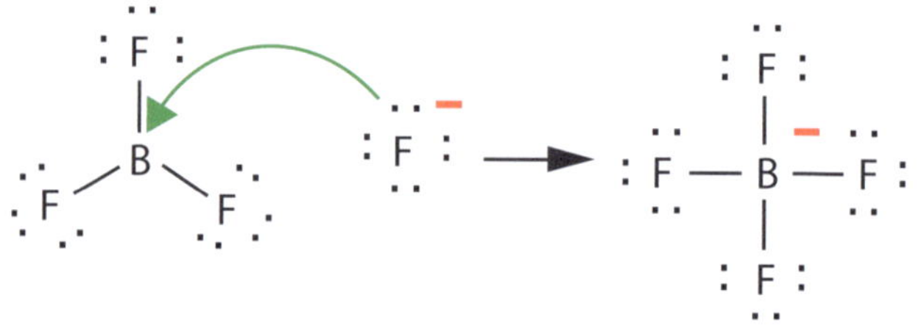

The Lewis acid BF_3: Notice that the green arrow follows the flow of electrons.

Low-level Importance

(Lewis acid), or alternately by an acceptance of a pair of electrons by the first type of molecule. Thus, as previously shown, molecules such as BF_3 are referred to as Lewis acids while molecules such as NH_3 are known as Lewis bases. Thus some examples of Lewis acids are: BF_3, H^+, Cu^{2+}, and Cr^{3+} and Lewis bases are: NH_3, OH^-, and H_2O. {lEwis Acids: Electron pair Acceptors}.

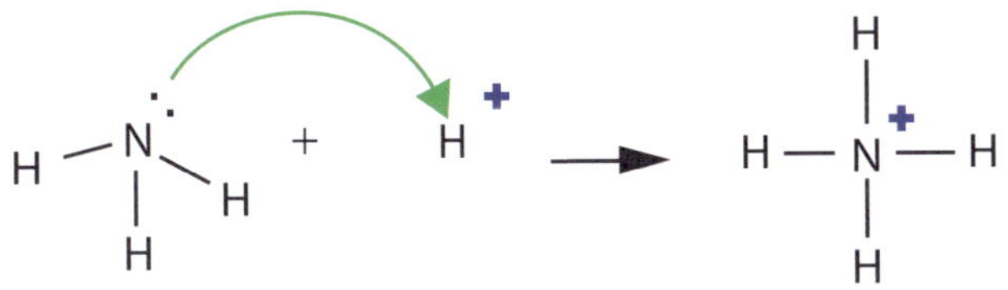

The Lewis base NH_3: Notice that the green arrow follows the flow of electrons.

3.5 Valence Shell Electron Pair Repulsions (VSEPR Models)

One of the shortcomings of Lewis structures is that they cannot be used to predict molecular geometries. In this context a model known as the valence shell electron pair repulsion or VSEPR model is very useful. In this model, the geometrical arrangement of atoms or groups of atoms bound to a central atom A is determined by the number of pairs of valence electrons around A. VSEPR procedure is based on the principle that these electronic pairs around the central atom are arranged in such a way that the repulsions between them are minimised. The general VSEPR procedure starts with the determination of the number of electronic pairs around A:

  # of valence electrons in a free atom of A
\+ # of sigma (or single) bonds involving A
− # of pi (or double) bonds involving A

= (total # of electrons around A)

The division of this total number by 2 yields the total number of electron pairs around A. Note the following important points:

(i) A single bond counts for 1 sigma bond, a double bond for 1 sigma bond and 1 pi bond and a triple bond for 1 sigma and two pi bonds.

(ii) The general calculation that we have presented is performed for the purposes of VSEPR modeling; its result can be quite different from the one obtained in the corresponding Lewis structure.

(iii) For all practical purposes, one always assigns a double bond (i.e. 1 sigma bond and one pi bond) to a terminal oxygen (an oxygen which is not a central atom and is not attached to any other atom besides the central atom).

(iv) A terminal halogen is always assigned a single bond.

Once the number of pairs around the central atom is determined, the next step is to use Table III.A.3.1 to predict the geometrical arrangement of these pairs around the central atom.

Low-level Importance

Table III.A.3.1: Geometry of simple molecules in which the central atom A has one or more lone pairs of electrons (= e⁻).

Total number of e⁻ pairs	Number of lone pairs	Number of bonding pairs	Electron Geometry, Arrangement of e⁻ pairs	Molecular Geometry (Hybridisation State)	Examples
3	1	2	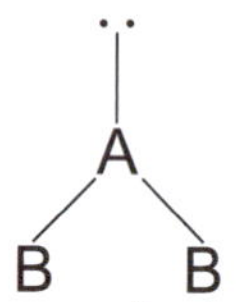 Trigonal planar	Bent (sp^2)	SO_2
4	1	3	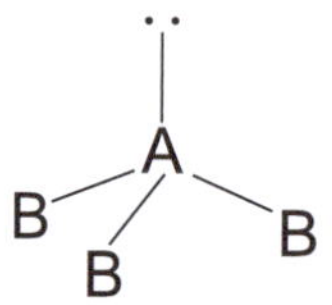 Tetrahedral	Trigonal pyramidal (sp^3)	NH_3
4	2	2	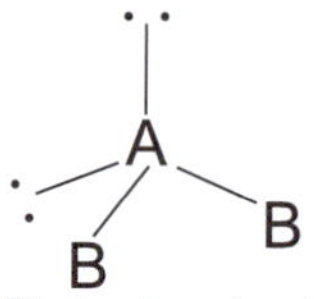 Tetrahedral	Bent (sp^3)	H_2O
5	1	4	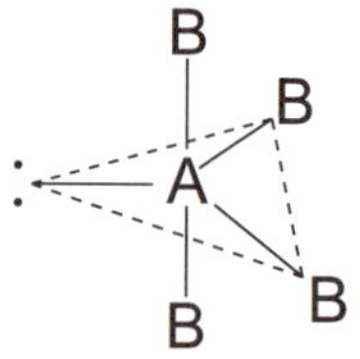 Trigonal bipyramidal	Seesaw (sp^3d)	SF_4
5	2	3	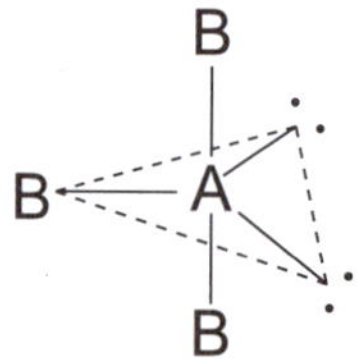 Trigonal bipyramidal	T-shaped (sp^3d)	ClF_3

Note: dotted lines only represent the overall molecular shape and not molecular bonds. In brackets under "Molecular Geometry" is the hybridisation, to be discussed in ORG 1.2.

Low-level Importance

The next step is to consider the previous arrangement of the electronic pairs and place the atoms or groups of atoms that are attached to the central atom in accordance with such an arrangement. The pairs of electrons which are not involved in the bonding between these atoms and the central atom are known as lone pairs. If we subtract the number of lone pairs from the total number of pairs of electrons, we readily obtain the number of bonding electron pairs. It is the number of bonding electron pairs which ultimately determines the molecular geometry in the VSEPR model according to Table III.A.3.1.

On the other hand, as for the *electronic* geometrical arrangement of a molecule, one is also to consider the free lone pair(s) of electrons. Consequently, a simple molecule such as SO_2 (*see* Table III.A.3.1) will have a trigonal planar electronic geometry with a bent molecular geometry with the respective differences in geometrical arrangement based solely on the lone pair of the central sulfur atom. Thus, the electron and molecular geometry of a molecule may be different. (Note: *electron geometry is based on the geometrical arrangement of electron pairs around a central atom, whereas, molecular geometry is based on the geometrical arrangement of the atoms surrounding a central atom*). Let us consider three classic examples: CH_4, H_2O and CO_2.

1 – CH_4:

# of valence electrons on C:	4
+ # of sigma bonds:	+ 4
– # of pi bonds:	– 0
	= 8/2 = 4 pairs

According to Figure III.A.3.1, CH_4 corresponds to a tetrahedral arrangement. Each of these four pairs of electrons corresponds to a H atom bonded each to the central atom of carbon. Therefore, all 4 pairs of electrons are bonding pairs with a tetrahedral molecular and electronic geometry, respectively (due to a lack in lone pairs).

2 – H_2O:

# of valence electrons on O:	6
+ # of sigma bonds on the central O:	+ 2
– # of pi bonds on the central O:	– 0
	= 8/2 = 4 pairs

For the H_2O geometry, it also corresponds to a tetrahedral arrangement (i.e. 4 pairs). However, due to lone pairs surrounding each of the oxygen atoms, the molecular geometry is of a bent geometrical shape with a tetrahedral electronic geometrical configuration.

3 – CO_2:

# of valence electrons on C:	4
+ # of sigma bonds for terminal O's:	+ 2
– # of pi bonds for terminal O's:	– 2
	= 4/2 = 2 pairs

This total number of pairs corresponds to a linear arrangement. Since both of these electron pairs are used to connect the central C atom to the terminal O's there are no lone pairs left on C. Therefore, the number of bonding pairs is also 2 and both the molecular and electronic geometries are also linear.

Low-level Importance

Here are some additional rules when applying the VSEPR model:

(i) When dealing with a cation (positive ion) subtract the charge of the ion from the total number of electrons.

(ii) When dealing with an anion (negative ion) add the charge of the ion to the total number of electrons.

(iii) A lone pair repels another lone pair or a bonding pair very strongly. This causes some deformation in bond angles. For instance, the H–O–H angle is smaller than the normal tetrahedral angle of 109.5° (*see* below).

(iv) The previous rule also holds for a double bond. Note that in one of our previous examples (CO_2), the angle is still 180° since there are two double bonds and no lone pairs. Indeed, in this geometry, the strong repulsions between the two double bonds are symmetrical.

(v) The VSEPR model can be applied to polyatomic molecules. The procedure is the

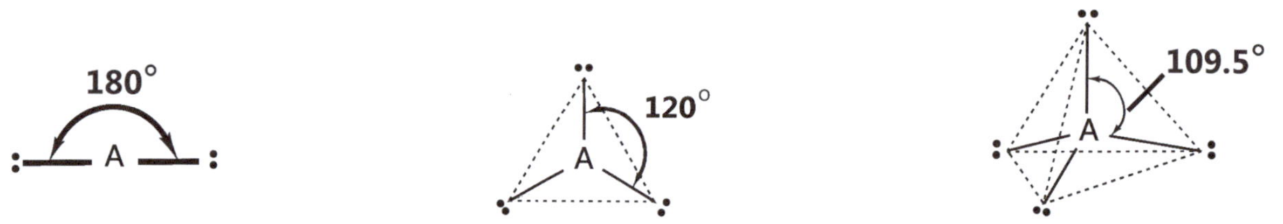

linear arrangement of 2 electron pairs around central atom A

trigonal planar arrangement of 3 electron pairs around central atom A

tetrahedral arrangement of 4 electron pairs around central atom A

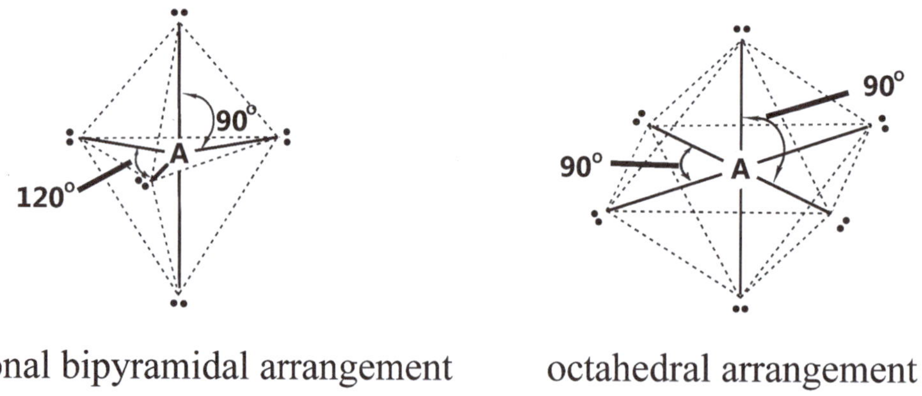

trigonal bipyramidal arrangement of 5 electron pairs around central atom A

octahedral arrangement of 6 electron pairs around central atom A

Figure III.A.3.1: Molecular arrangement of electron pairs around a central atom A. Dotted lines only represent the overall molecular shape and not molecular bonds.

Low-level Importance

same as above except that one can only determine the arrangements of groups of atoms around one given central atom at a time. For instance, you could apply the VSEPR model to determine the geometrical arrangements of atoms around C or around O in methanol (CH_3OH). In the first case the molecule is treated as CH_3–X (where –X is –OH) and in the second it is treated as HO–Y (where –Y is $-CH_3$). The geometrical arrangement is tetrahedral in the first case which gives HCX or HCH angles close to 109°. The second case corresponds to a bent arrangement (with two lone pairs on the oxygen) and gives an HOY angle close to 109° as well. This also corresponds to a tetrahedral arrangement; however, only two of these pairs are bonding pairs (connecting the H atoms to the central oxygen atom); therefore, the actual geometry according to Table III.A.3.1 is bent or V-shape geometry.

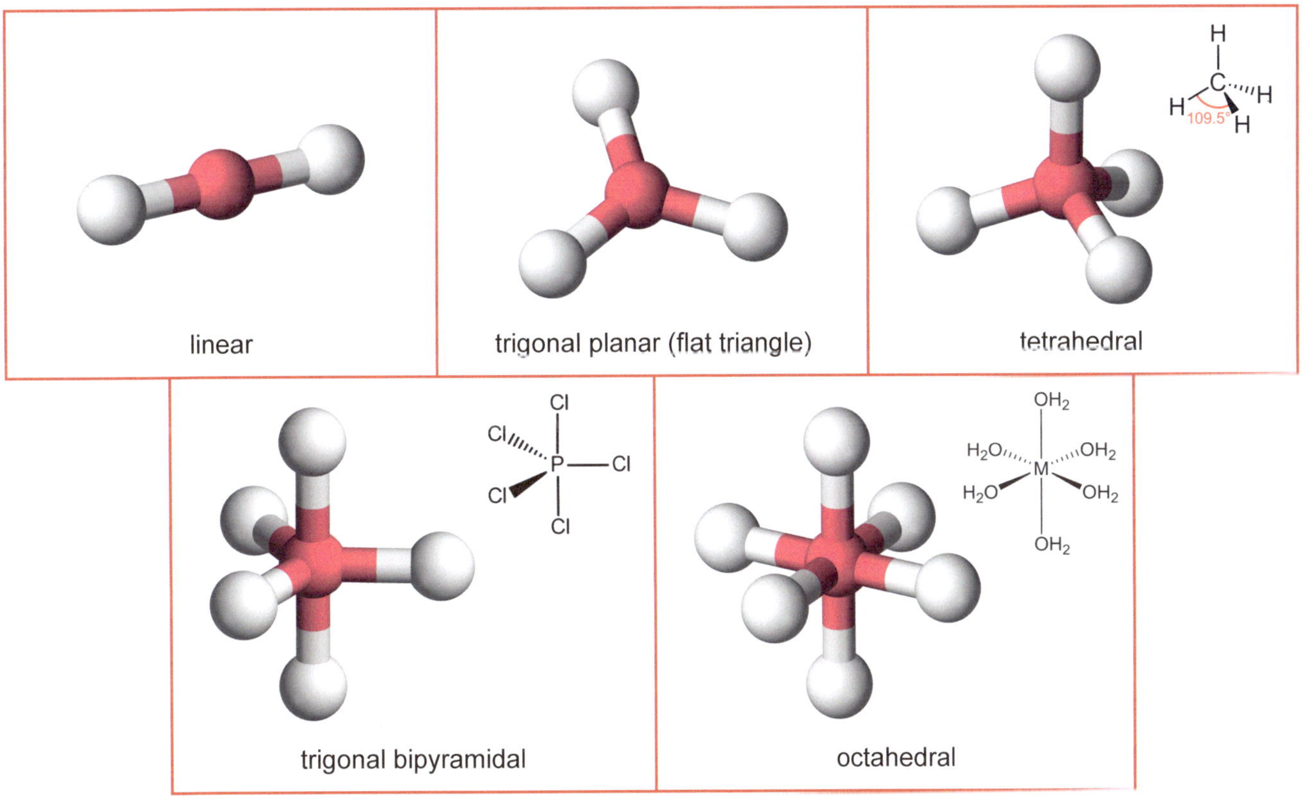

Figure III.A.3.2: 3D-illustration of molecular arrangement/geometry. Please note that the first 3 structures will be revisited continuously in GAMSAT Organic Chemistry. Regarding the insets for the last 3 structures: A dark triangle symbolises a bond that projects towards you, whereas a broken bond symbolises a projection away from the viewer. In the inset for octahedral, M represents a metal; for example, aluminium Al which we saw in the same structure in CHM 3.2. Note that 'trigonal' refers to the triangular aspect of the shape; 'planar' means flat; 'bipyramidal' refers to there being 2 pyramids; and, 'octahedral' is a square bipyramid with only 6 bonds to the central atom, but it creates a 3D shape with 8 triangular faces. The 3D aspect of molecules will be explored more deeply in GAMSAT Organic Chemistry Chapter 2: Stereochemistry.

High-level Importance

CHAPTER 3: Bonding

GOLD STANDARD GAMSAT-LEVEL PRACTICE QUESTIONS

CHM Chapter 2 and Chapter 3 (this chapter), due to the "Low-level Importance" of assumed knowledge, have no *Need for Speed* exercises, nor Foundational MCQs. We go straight to GAMSAT-level MCQs and you will continue to develop problem-solving skills that can apply to many other GAMSAT topics.

Questions 1–9

Many chemical bonds are neither purely ionic nor purely covalent, rather they are polar covalent. This type of bond results from the shift of the electrons which make up the bond toward the atom with the more negative electron affinity. The magnitude of the charge displacement in a polar covalent bond is measured by a quantity called the dipole moment, μ. The dipole moment of a molecule increases as the quantity of charge which is separated increases, or as the distance between the positive and negative centres increases:

$$\mu = \text{charge} \times \text{separation distance}$$

Dipole moments are usually measured in debyes (D), where 1 debye $= 3.34 \times 10^{-30}$ coulombs • metre.

In a molecule with several chemical bonds, the overall dipole moment is the sum of all the individual bond dipole moments. Equal bond dipole moments pointing in opposite directions cancel. As a result, the overall dipole moment sometimes indicates nothing about the bond polarities.

The molecular geometry of some simple molecules can be determined based on the presence or absence of an overall dipole moment in the molecule. Table 1 gives the electronegativity difference, dipole moment, and bond energy of the hydrogen halides. Table 2 lists the dipole moments of other compounds.

Note that: Electronegativity difference is dimensionless since it measures electron-attracting ability on a relative scale.

Compound	Electronegativity Difference	Dipole Moment (debye)	Bond Energy (kJ/mol)
HF	1.8	1.91	565
HCl	1.0	1.03	431
HBr	0.8	0.75	364
HI	0.5	0.38	297

Table 1

Compound	Dipole Moment
CCl_4	0
$HgBr_2$	0
SO_2	1.47
HNO_3	2.17
BaO	7.95
KCl	10.27

Table 2

The polarity of bonds is determined by electronegativity differences ($\Delta\chi$). As a guideline, bonds can be defined as:

- **ionic** if $\Delta\chi > 2.0$
- **polar covalent** if $2.0 > \Delta\chi > 0.4$
- **nonpolar covalent** if $0.4 > \Delta\chi$.

1) If the charge is halved and the distance between 2 atoms that are bonded is tripled, the chance that the bond has changed to become ionic has:

A. increased.
B. decreased.
C. definitely stayed the same.
D. either increased or decreased is equally likely.

2) The relationship between the difference in the electronegativity between atoms and their bond energy can be regarded as which of the following?

A. Direct
B. Indirect
C. One decreases the other
D. Cannot be determined based on the information provided.

3) Given a charge of 1.5×10^{-20} coulombs, what is the approximate distance, in metres, between the hydrogen and bromine atoms in the molecule HBr?

A. 1.7×10^{-9} m
B. 1.7×10^{-10} m
C. 1.7×10^{-11} m
D. 1.7×10^{-12} m

4) Bromine (Br) is much more electronegative than mercury (Hg). Which of the following best explains the observed molecular dipole moment (*see* Table 2) of the molecule $HgBr_2$?

A. Hg and Br have the same effective nuclear charge.
B. Hg and Br have similar atomic radii.
C. Br has a greater electron affinity than Hg.
D. The geometry of the molecule causes the bond moments to cancel.

5) All of the hydrogen halides in Table 1 are strong acids except HF. Which of the following statements best explains why HF is not a strong acid like the other hydrogen halides?

A. HF has the largest electronegativity difference.
B. HF has the largest dipole moment.
C. HF has the greatest bond energy.
D. HF can form intermolecular hydrogen bonds.

6) Based on the information provided, which of the following best characterises the bond between hydrogen and bromine in HBr?

A. Nonpolar covalent
B. Polar covalent
C. Ionic
D. Nonpolar covalent with ionic character

7) Given the information in the passage, what type of bond would most likely form between iodine (I) and chlorine (Cl)?

A. Polar covalent
B. Covalent
C. Ionic
D. Neither **A**, nor **B**, nor **C** would be likely.

8) Water (H_2O) has a net dipole moment of 1.84 D. Since oxygen is the central atom and there are 2 hydrogens attached to it, one might predict that the bond moments would be in opposite directions and there would be no resultant dipole moment. Which of the following most reasonably accounts for the observed net dipole moment of H_2O?

A. The angle between the bonds is less than 180°.
B. There is an electronegativity difference between hydrogen and oxygen.
C. H_2O can form intramolecular hydrogen bonds.
D. The atomic radius of oxygen is larger than the atomic radius of hydrogen.

9) Based on the information provided, a bond between chlorine and bromine is likely to be which of the following?

A. Ionic
B. Polar covalent
C. Nonpolar covalent
D. Hydrogen

High-level Importance

Questions 10–13

The valence-shell electron-pair repulsion (VSEPR) model is used to predict the shapes of molecules and ions (*see* Table 1). Electron pairs, whether as bonding pairs or as lone pairs, repel each other, and the shape that allows the maximum distances between electron pairs is the shape that a molecule or ion assumes.

Note that:

- a lone pair of electrons refers to a pair of valence electrons that are not shared with another atom in a covalent bond; the pair can be symbolised by 2 dots. The presence of lone pair electrons can affect molecular geometry. Their absence means that the electron geometry is the same as the molecular geometry.
- a hybrid orbital is an orbital formed by the combination of two or more atomic orbitals. For example, a combination of 1 s and 3 p orbitals may form sp^3 hybrid orbitals.

Table 1: Geometry of simple molecules in which the central atom A has one or more lone pairs of electrons (= e^-).

Total number of e^- pairs	Number of lone pairs	Number of bonding pairs	Electron Geometry, Arrangement of e^- pairs	Molecular Geometry (Hybridisation State)	Examples
3	1	2	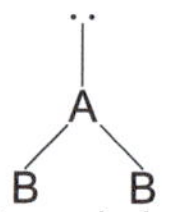 Trigonal planar	Bent (sp^2)	SO_2
4	1	3	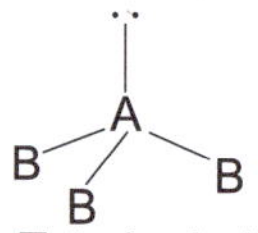 Tetrahedral	Trigonal pyramidal (sp^3)	NH_3
4	2	2	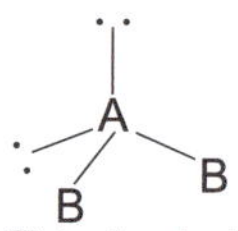 Tetrahedral	Bent (sp^3)	H_2O
5	1	4	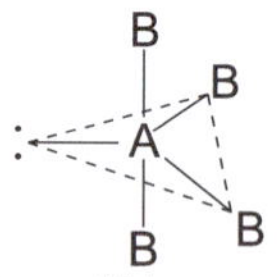 Trigonal bipyramidal	Seesaw (sp^3d)	SF_4
5	2	3	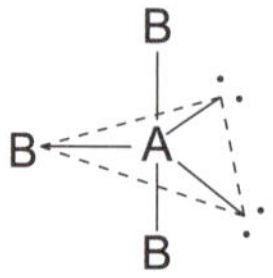 Trigonal bipyramidal	T-shaped (sp^3d)	ClF_3

10) What are the total number of bonding and non-bonding (lone) electrons in ClF_3?

A. 2
B. 3
C. 5
D. 10

11) Consider the annotated structure of phosphine (PH_3) with lone pair electrons, bond angle and bond length.

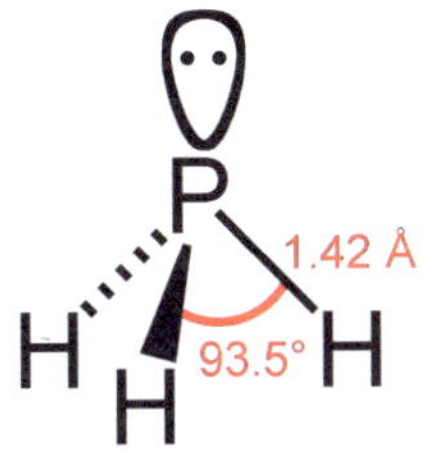

Using the VSEPR model, what is the molecular hybridisation state of the central atom in PH_3?

A. sp^2
B. sp^3
C. sp^3d
D. Both **B** and **C** are possible.

12) Using the VSEPR model, what is the molecular geometry of oxygen difluoride (OF_2)?

Note that: Oxygen has 2 lone pairs of electrons.

A. Trigonal planar
B. Tetrahedral
C. Bent
D. Trigonal bipyramidal

13) Consider the annotated structure for phosphorus pentachloride (PCl_5) with bond angles and bond lengths.

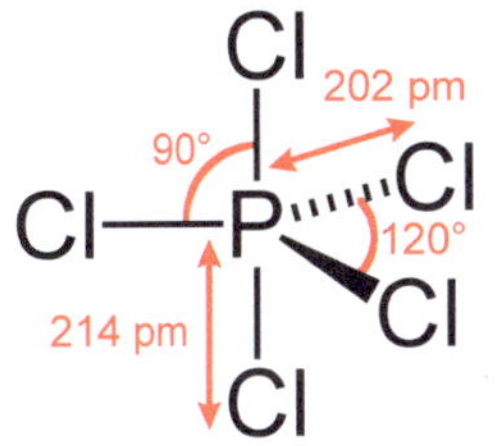

Using the VSEPR model, the shape of phosphorus pentachloride is likely to be:

A. tetrahedral.
B. T-shaped
C. trigonal bipyramidal.
D. seesaw.

High-level Importance

Questions 14–15

Both diamond and silicon (*see* Figure 1) form a diamond crystal lattice. The crystal lattice can be thought of as an array of 'small boxes', or *unit cells*, infinitely repeating in all three spatial directions: *x*, *y* and *z*.

Continuing with the box analogy, consider that an atom in, for example, a top corner is shared by 3 other boxes at the same level plus another 4 boxes above. Fractions of atoms can be added to be equivalent to a full atom or atoms. There are 4 atoms completely within the lattice (grey spheres in Figure 1), while all other atoms are shared between boxes to one degree or another. The length of one side of a crystal lattice for silicon is 0.543 nm.

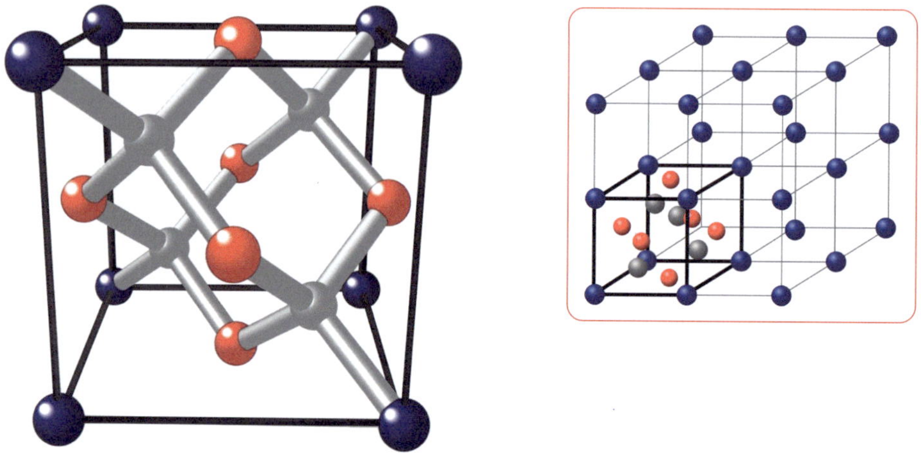

Figure 1: The unit cell (*on the left*) and the unit cell within an incomplete diamond crystal lattice (*inset on the right*). The unit cell is like a small cube or box that constitutes a repeating structure. Atoms are represented as spheres. Each of the 6 faces of the unit cell has 1 centrally-located (*red*) atom which is equally shared with 1 adjacent unit cell.

14) To calculate the number of atoms per unit cell, the degree to which atoms at the surface or corners are shared, as well as the number of whole atoms within the cell, must be taken into account. Considering the information in the passage and Figure 1, how many silicon atoms are there per unit cell?

- **A.** 4
- **B.** 8
- **C.** 16
- **D.** 18

15) Given the information provided, which of the following is most consistent with an estimate of the number of silicon atoms per cm^3?

- **A.** $8\left(\frac{1}{(5.43 \times 10^{-8})^3}\right)$
- **B.** $16\left(\frac{1}{(5.43 \times 10^{-8})^3}\right)$
- **C.** $8\left(\frac{1}{(5.43 \times 10^{-10})^3}\right)$
- **D.** $16\left(\frac{1}{(5.43 \times 10^{-10})^3}\right)$

SPOILER ALERT

Gold Standard has cross-referenced the content in this chapter to examples from ACER's official GAMSAT practice materials. It is for you to decide when you want to explore these questions since you may want to preserve some of ACER's materials for timed mock-exam practice.

This is complicated! Chapter 3 lays the groundwork for hydrogen bonds (for which we added a question in the dipole-moment unit), which will be explored in Chapter 4, and you will see that there are recent ACER practice questions exploring hydrogen bonds listed in the Spoiler Alert for Chapter 4. Also, and perhaps most importantly, Chapter 3 lays the groundwork for GAMSAT Organic Chemistry: Resonance, Lewis structures, molecular shapes [especially: linear, trigonal planar (= flat triangle), and the very famous tetrahedron], and the octet rule – all of which will be revisited in the Masters Series Organic Chemistry book. The 15 full-length GAMSAT practice tests by Gold Standard, HEAPS-1 through HEAPS-15, contain specific cross-references to this chapter within the worked solutions. Note that the diamond crystal lattice is from HEAPS-6, and the unit with electronegativity (debyes) is from HEAPS-9.

Chapter Checklist

- ☐ Access your online account to view answers, worked solutions and discussion boards.
- ☐ Reassess your 'learning objectives' for this chapter: Go back to the first page of this chapter and re-evaluate the top 3 boxes and the Introduction.
- ☐ Complete a maximum of 1 page of notes using symbols/abbreviations to represent the entire chapter based on your learning objectives. These are your Gold Notes.
- ☐ Consider your multimedia options based on your optimal way of learning:
  - ☐ Download the free Gold Standard GAMSAT app for your Android device or iPhone.
  - ☐ Create your own, tangible study cards or try the free app: Anki.
  - ☐ Record your voice reading your Gold Notes onto your smartphone (audio files, e.g., *memo* or MP3s) and listen during exercise, transportation, etc.
  - ☐ Try out the Gold Standard GAMSAT online videos at gamsat-prep.com, or you can try other options on YouTube like Khan Academy or Crash Course Chemistry.
- ☐ Reassess your schedule for your full-length GAMSAT practice tests: ACER and/or HEAPS exams. Ensure that you have scheduled one full day to complete a practice test and 1-2 days for a thorough assessment of worked solutions while adding to your abbreviated Gold Notes.
- ☐ Reassess your progress in scheduling and/or evaluating stress reduction techniques such as regular exercise (sports), yoga, meditation and/or mindfulness exercises (*see* YouTube for suggestions).

PHASES AND PHASE EQUILIBRIA
Chapter 4

Memorise

* Define: Temperature (°C, K, conversion), gas pressure and weight
* Define: Hydrogen bonds, dipole forces

Understand

* Kinetic molecular theory of gases
* Maxwell distribution plot, hydrogen bonds, dipole forces
* Deviation from ideal gas behavior
* Equations: ideal gas/Charles'/Boyle's
* Partial Press., mole fraction, Dalton's
* Intermolecular forces, phase change/diagrams

Importance

High level: 15% of GAMSAT General Chemistry

questions released by ACER are related to content in this chapter (in our estimation).

* Note that approximately 80% of the questions in GAMSAT General Chemistry are related to just 4 chapters: 4, 5, 6, and 9.

GAMSAT-Prep.com

Introduction

A phase, or state of matter, is a uniform, distinct and usually separable region of material. For example, for a glass of water: the ice cubes are one phase (solid), the water is a second phase (liquid), and the humid air over the water is the third phase (gas = vapor). This chapter will focus on the 3 phases of matter that dominate everyday life.

You have likely witnessed liquid water evaporate from a container or puddle (liquid $\rightarrow$ vapor) that went *to completion,* signified by the one-way arrow. You have also likely witnessed a closed bottle of water which contains liquid and vapor in *dynamic equilibrium* (plural: *equilibria*; liquid $\rightleftharpoons$ vapor), signified by the two-way arrow, thus the forward reaction is reversible. In the bottle, there is surely no net creation of vapor and the water level does not suddenly increase on its own! However, there is a constant interplay between evaporating liquid and condensing vapor applying pressure on the liquid's surface (*vapor pressure*). Pressure, volume, temperature and the number of particles (*moles*) are often key parameters when examining the phases of matter.

This is the first of the four High-importance Level chapters in this textbook. For some, this will be revision, for others, exploring solids, liquids and gases will be very challenging. However, please understand that most of what you read will be provided to you, if necessary, in the passage during the exam. You are just trying to get a sense of some of the relationships and then practice, practice, practice.

Multimedia Resources at GAMSAT-Prep.com

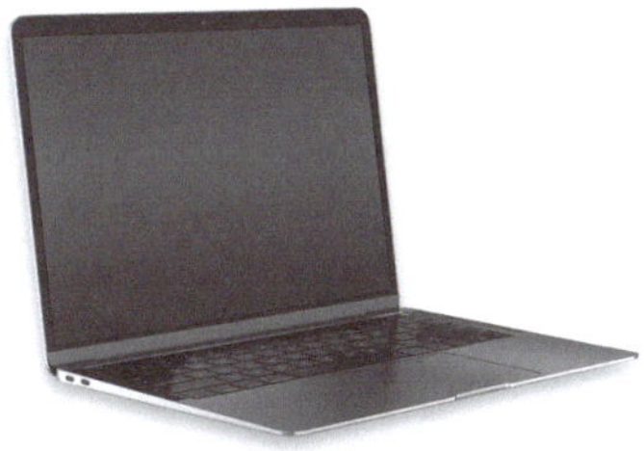

Open Discussion Boards
(*gamsat-prep.com/forum*)

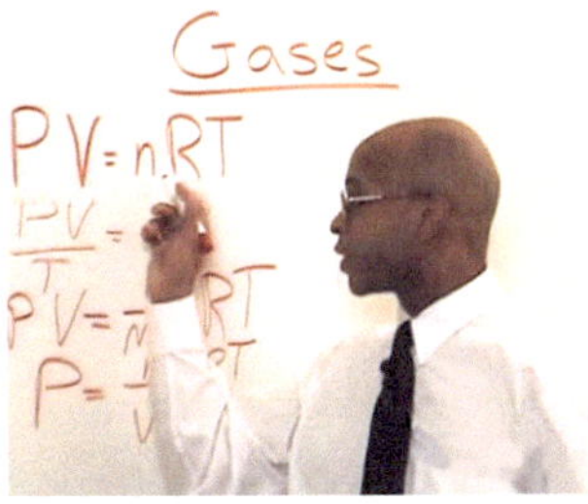

Science Preparation Videos

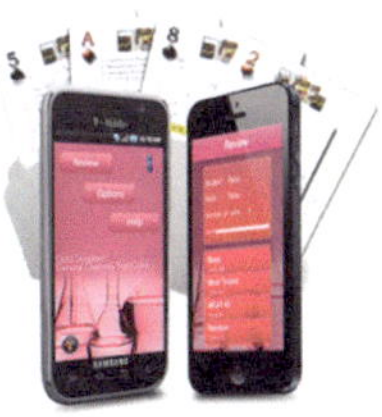

Flashcards

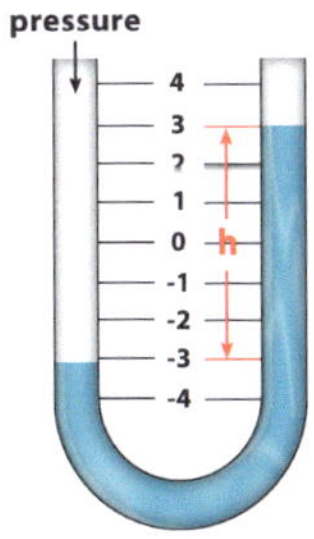

Special Guest

* The real GAMSAT may have advanced-level information presented (i.e. in a passage) but previous knowledge of said information is not required to answer the questions that would follow. Practice questions at the end of this chapter, as well as ACER and GS (HEAPS) practice GAMSATs can help you clarify this point.

4.0 GAMSAT has a *Need for Speed*!

High-level Importance

Section	GAMSAT General Chemistry *Need for Speed* Exercises
4.1.2	Consider the graph below. Which temperature must be higher: T_1 or T_2? 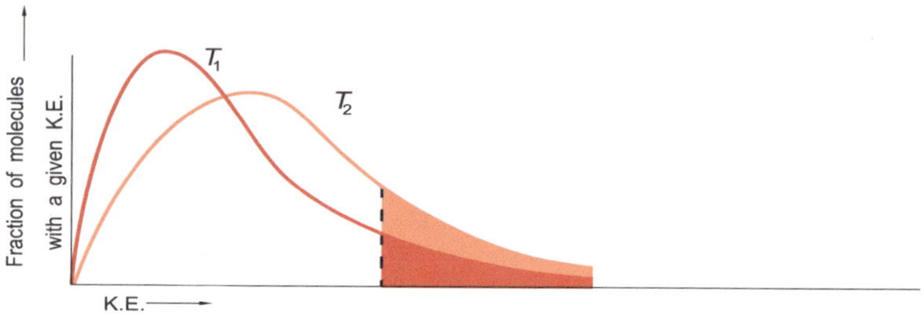
4.1.3	For the exercises below, compare 2 gases (gas 1 and gas 2), and identify them by using the subscripts 1 and 2, respectively. Given that the rate at which a gas diffuses is inversely proportional to the square root of its molar mass (M), complete the equation below. $\frac{\text{Rate}_1}{\text{Rate}_2} =$
4.1.4	$V = \text{Constant} \times T$ *means that* $V_1/V_2 =$ *or* $V_1/T_1 =$
4.1.5	$V = \text{Constant} \times 1/P$ *means that* $P_1V_1 =$
4.1.6	$V/n = \text{Constant}$ *means that* $V_1/n_1 =$
4.1.7	$\frac{PV}{T} = \text{Constant}$ *means that* $\frac{P_1V_1}{T_1} =$
4.1.8	State the ideal gas law (*optional*):
	How is the density of a gas related to its mass and volume?

4.2

Name 3 atoms with which hydrogen could engage in the "famous" intermolecular attraction: *hydrogen bonding*.

Electrons are not shared equally within the molecules below. Atoms that are partially positive (δ^+) or partially negative (δ^-) are identified. Use dash lines (-----) or short parallel lines (| | | | |) between atoms of molecules to demonstrate intermolecular (*between different molecules*) bonding:

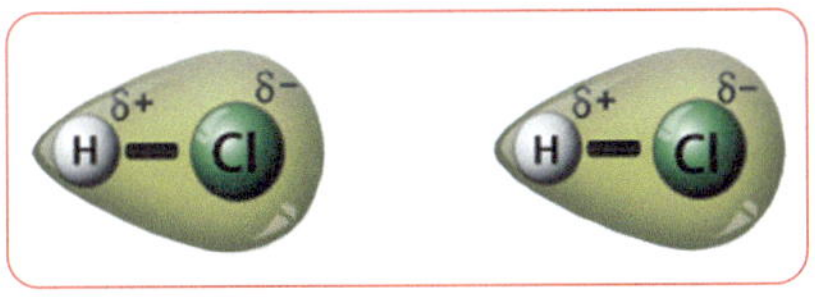

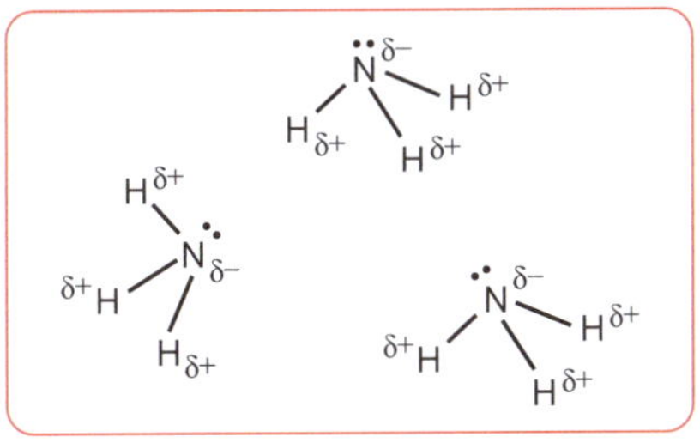

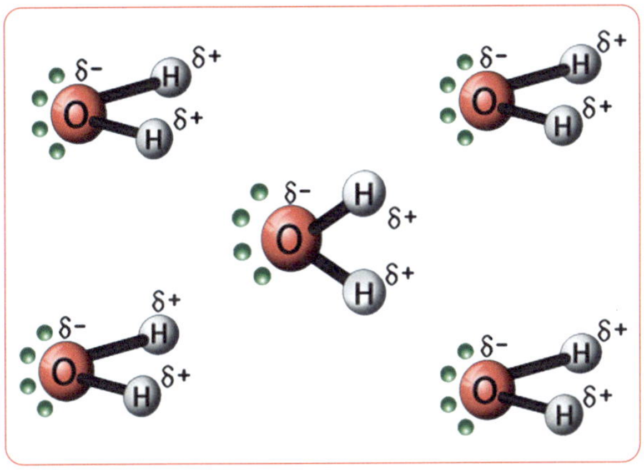

Of the following, circle the one that would be expected to have the highest boiling point:

ammonia   water   hydrogen fluoride   methanol

One molecule of H_2O can potentially form hydrogen bonds with up to how many surrounding H_2O molecules?

4.4.2

A liquid can be converted to a gas by the process of vaporisation. Define "boiling point."

4.1 The Gas Phase

High-level Importance

Elements and compounds largely exist in one of three states: the gaseous state (CHM 4.1), the liquid state (CHM 4.2), or the solid state (CHM 4.3).

A substance in the gaseous state (*gas phase*) has neither fixed volume nor fixed shape: it spreads itself uniformly throughout any container in which it is placed.

4.1.1 Standard Temperature and Pressure, Standard Molar Volume

Any given gas can be described in terms of four fundamental properties: mass, volume, temperature and pressure. To simplify comparisons, the volume of a gas is normally reported at 0 °C (273.15 K) and 1.00 atm (101.33 kPa = 760 mmHg = 760 torr); these conditions are known as the standard temperature and pressure (STP).

The SI unit of pressure is the pascal (Pa). The old-fashioned Imperial unit is the pound per square inch since pressure is defined as *force per unit area* (PHY 6.1.2). If we enclose a gas within a container, we detect the pressure in the gas from the force of the molecules colliding with a unit area of the walls of the container.

The volume occupied by one mole of any gas at STP is referred to as the standard molar volume and is equal to 22.4 L.

4.1.2 Kinetic Molecular Theory of Gases (A Model for Gases)

The kinetic molecular theory of gases describes the particulate behavior of matter in the gaseous state. A gas that fits this theory exactly is called an ideal gas. The essential points of the theory are as follows:

1. Gases are composed of extremely small particles (*either molecules or atoms depending on the gas*) separated by distances that are relatively large in comparison with the diameters of the particles.
2. Particles of gas are in constant motion, except when they collide with one another.
3. Particles of an ideal gas exert no attractive or repulsive force on one another.
4. The collisions experienced by gas particles do not, on the average, slow them down; rather, they cause a change in the direction in which the particles are moving. If one particle loses energy as a result of a collision, the energy is gained by the particle with which it collides. Collisions of the particles of an ideal gas with the walls of the container result in no loss of energy.

5. The average kinetic energy of the particles ($KE = 1/2\ mv^2$) increases in direct proportion to the temperature of the gas ($KE = 3/2\ kT$) when the temperature is measured on an absolute scale (i.e. the Kelvin scale) and k is a constant (the Boltzmann constant). The typical speed of a gas particle is directly proportional to the square root of the absolute temperature. Summary: Increased temperature = more energy = more speed.

The plot of the distribution of collision energies of gases is similar to that of liquids. However, molecules in liquids require a minimum escape kinetic energy in order to enter the vapor phase (*see* figure below).

The properties of gases can be explained in terms of the kinetic molecular theory of ideal gases.

Experimentally, we can measure four properties of a gas:

1. The weight of the gas, from which we can calculate the number (*N*) of molecules or atoms of the gas present;

2. The pressure (*P*), exerted by the gas on the walls of the container in which this gas is placed (N.B.: a vacuum is completely devoid of particles and thus has *no* pressure);

3. The volume (*V*), occupied by the gas;

4. The temperature (*T*) of the gas.

In fact, if we know any three of these properties, we can calculate the fourth. So the minimum number of these properties required to fully describe the state of an ideal gas is three.

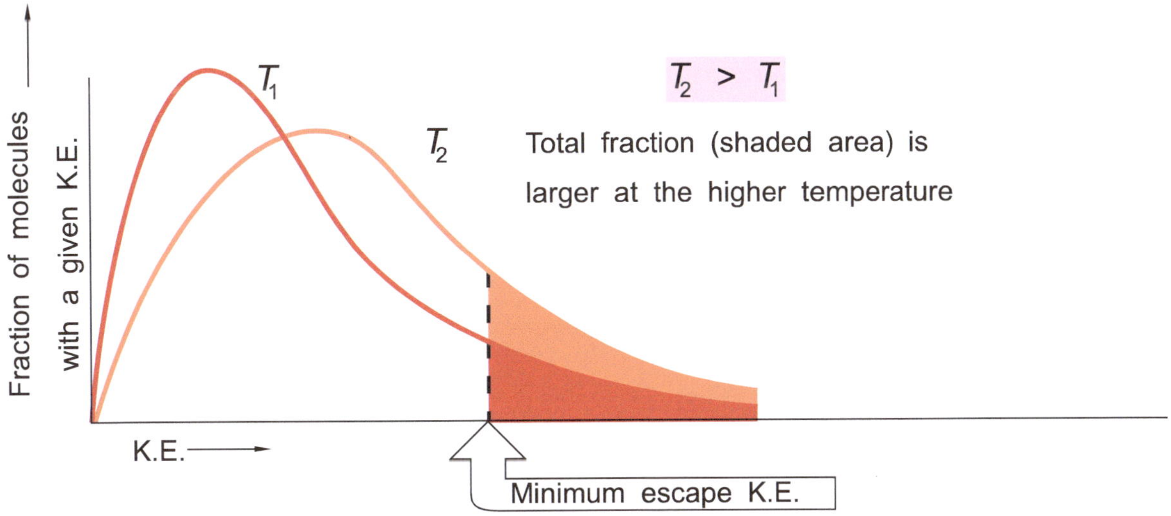

Figure III.A.4.1: The Maxwell Distribution Plot. At a higher temperature T_2, more particles have a higher kinetic energy and so the curve shifts to the right; note also that the curve's peak is flattened, which means that gas particles within the sample are travelling at a wider range of velocities. Additionally, the larger shaded area at a temperature T_2 means that a greater proportion of molecules will possess the minimum escaping kinetic energy (KE) required to evaporate (note: the Maxwell distribution plot makes an appearance in GAMSAT-level practice questions in Physics Chapter 2).

4.1.3 Graham's Law (Diffusion and Effusion of Gases)

Graham's law describes the mean (average) free path of any typical gas particle taken per unit volume. The process taken by such gas particles is known as *diffusion* and its related process *effusion* which are defined as follows:

Diffusion is the flow of gas particles spreading out evenly through random motion. Gas particles diffuse from regions of high concentration to regions of low concentration. The rate at which a gas diffuses is inversely proportional to the square root of its molar mass. The ratio of the diffusion rates of two different gases is inversely proportional to the square root of their respective molar masses. $Rate_1/Rate_2$ and M_1/M_2 represents diffusion rates of gases 1 and 2 and the molar mass of gases 1 and 2. Lighter particles diffuse quicker than heavier particles.

Effusion is the movement of a gas through a small hole or pore into another gaseous region or into a vacuum. If the hole is large enough, the process may be considered diffusion instead of effusion. The rates at which two gases effuse are inversely proportional to the square root of their molar masses, the same as that for diffusion:

$$\frac{Rate_1}{Rate_2} = \sqrt{\frac{M_2}{M_1}}$$

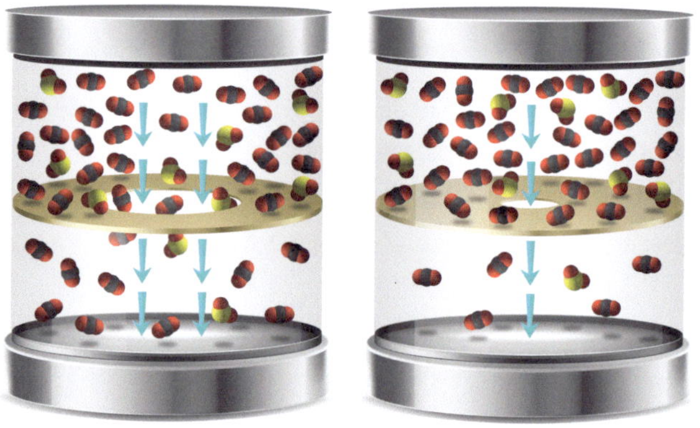

Figure III.A.4.1.1: Diffusion and effusion. The gases carbon dioxide (CO_2) and the heavier, and thus slower, sulfur dioxide (SO_2) shown diffusing on the left, and effusing on the right (carbon: a graphite grey/black colour; oxygen: red; sulfur: yellow). The arrows indicate the net movement of molecules.

4.1.4 Charles' Law

The volume (*V*) of a gas is directly proportional to the absolute temperature (*expressed in kelvin*) when *P* and *N* are kept constant.

$$V = \text{Constant} \times T \quad \text{or} \quad V_1/V_2 = T_1/T_2$$
$$\text{or} \quad V_1/T_1 = V_2/T_2$$

NOTE: For Charles' Law and all subsequent laws, the subscripts 1 and 2 refer to both initial and final values, respectively, of all variables for the gas in question. Also note that if V = cT, where c is constant, then divide both sides by T to get V/T = c, meaning $V_1/T_1 = V_2/T_2$; cross multiply (GM 1.6.2) to get:

$$V_1/V_2 = T_1/T_2$$

4.1.5 Boyle's Law

The volume (V) of a fixed weight of gas held at constant temperature (T) varies inversely with the pressure (P).

$$V = \text{Constant} \times 1/P \quad \text{or} \quad P_1V_1 = P_2V_2$$

4.1.6 Avogadro's Law

The volume (V) of a gas at constant temperature and pressure is directly proportional to the number of particles or moles (n) of the gas present.

$$V/n = \text{Constant} \quad \text{or} \quad V_1/n_1 = V_2/n_2$$

4.1.7 Combined Gas Law

For a given constant mass of any gas, the product of its pressure and volume divided by its kelvin temperature is equal to a constant. Therefore, by using the combined gas law, one may calculate any of the three variables of a gas exposed to two separate conditions as follows:

This relationship depicts how a change in pressure, volume, and/or temperature of any gas (at constant mass) will be affected as a function of the other quantities (P_2, V_2 or T_2).

$$\frac{PV}{T} = \text{Constant} \quad \text{or} \quad \frac{P_1V_1}{T_1} = \frac{P_2V_2}{T_2} \quad \text{(at constant mass)}$$

4.1.8 Ideal Gas Law

The combination of Boyle's law, Charles' law and Avogadro's law yields the *ideal gas law*, the equation of state for a hypothetical ideal gas:

$$PV = nRT$$

where R is the universal gas constant and n is the number of moles of gas particles.

$$R = 0.0821 \text{ atm•L/K•mol}$$
$$= 8.31 \text{ kPa•dm}^3\text{/K•mol}$$

A typical ideal gas problem is as follows: an ideal gas at 27 °C and 380 torr occupies a volume of 492 cm^3. What is the number of moles of gas? {*Consider trying to solve the problem before looking at the solution.*}

High-level Importance

High-level Importance

Ideal Gas Law problems often amount to mere exercises of unit conversions. The easiest way to do them is to convert the units of the values given to the units of the R gas constant.

$$P = 380 \text{ torr} = \frac{380 \text{ torr}}{(760 \text{ torr/atm})} = 0.500 \text{ atm}$$

$$T = 27\,°\text{C} = 273 + 27\,°\text{C} = 300 \text{ K}$$

$$V = 492 \text{ cm}^3 = 492 \text{ cm}^3 \times (1 \text{ litre}/1000 \text{ cm}^3)$$

$$= 0.492 \text{ litre}$$

$$PV = n\text{RT}$$

$$n = \text{PV/RT}$$

$$n = \frac{(0.500 \text{ atm} \times 0.492 \text{ L})}{(0.0821 \text{ L-atm/K-mole} \times 300 \text{ K})}$$

$$n = 0.0100 \text{ mole}$$

Also note that the ideal gas law could be used in the following alternate ways (Mwt = molecular weight):

(i) since n = (mass m of gas sample)/(Mwt M of the gas) [*see* CHM 1.3]

$$PV = (m/M)\text{R}T$$

(ii) since m/V equals the density (d) of a gas:

$$P = \frac{d\text{RT}}{M}$$

The calculations and variable manipulations in this section (CHM 4.1.8) are based on dimensional analysis (GM 2.2) which is of fundamental importance for all GAMSAT sciences.

4.1.9 Partial Pressure and Dalton's Law

In a mixture of unreactive gases, each gas distributes evenly throughout the container. All particles exert the same pressure on the walls of the container with equal force. If we consider a mixture of gases occupying a total volume (V) at a temperature (T) the term partial pressure is used to refer to the pressure exerted by one component of the gas mixture if it were occupying the entire volume (V) at the same temperature (T). Dalton's law states that the total pressure observed for a mixture of gases is equal to the sum of the pressures that each individual component would exert were it alone in the container.

$$P_T = P_1 + P_2 + \ldots + P_i$$

where P_T is the total pressure and P_i is the partial pressure of any component (i).

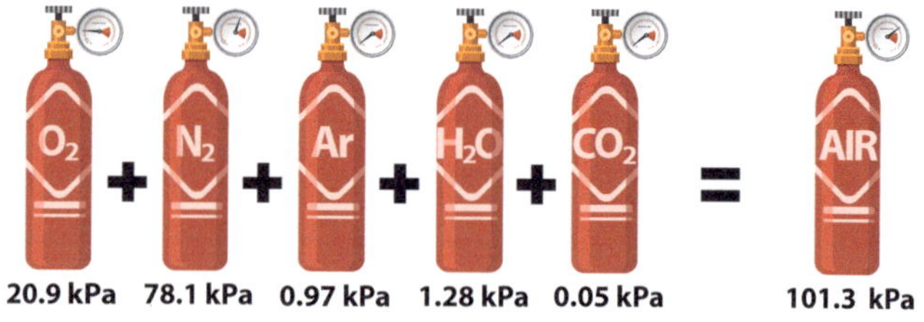

The mole fraction (X_i) of any one gas present in a mixture is defined as follows:

$$X_i = n_i / n_{(total)}$$

where n_i = moles of that gas present in the mixture and $n_{(total)}$ = sum of the moles of all gases present in the mixture (*see* CHM 5.3.1).

Of course, the sum of all mole fractions in a mixture must equal one:

$$\Sigma X_i = 1$$

The partial pressure (P_i) of a component of a gas mixture is equal to:

$$P_i = X_i P_T$$

The ideal gas law applies to any component of the mixture:

$$P_i V = n_i RT$$

4.1.10 Deviation of Real Gas Behavior from the Ideal Gas Law

The particles of an ideal gas have zero volume and no intermolecular forces. It obeys the ideal gas law. Its particles behave as though they were moving points exerting no attraction on one another and occupying no space. Real gases deviate from ideal gas behavior particularly when the gas particles are forced into close proximity under high pressure and low temperature, as follows:

1. They do not obey $PV = nRT$. We can calculate n, P, V and T for a real gas on the assumption that it behaves like an ideal gas but the calculated values will not agree with the observed values.

2. Their particles are subject to intermolecular forces (i.e. forces of attraction between different molecules like Van der Waal forces; CHM 4.2) which are themselves independent of temperature. But the deviations they cause are more pronounced at low temperatures because they are less effectively opposed by the slower motion of particles at lower temperatures. Similarly, an increase in pressure at constant temperature will crowd the particles closer together and reduce the average distance between them. This will increase the attractive force between the particles and the stronger these forces, the more the behavior of the real gas will deviate from that of an ideal gas. Thus, a real gas will act less like an ideal gas at higher pressures than at lower pressures. {Mnemonic: an ideal Plow and Thigh = an ideal gas exists when **P**ressure is **low** and **T**emperature is **high**}

3. The particles (i.e. molecules or atoms) occupy space. When a real gas is subjected to high pressures at ordinary temperatures, the fraction of the total volume occupied by the particles increases. At moderately high pressure, gas particles are pushed closer together and intermolecular attraction causes the gas to have a smaller volume than would be predicted by the ideal gas law. At extremely high pressure, gas particles are pushed even closer in such a way that the distance between them are becoming insignificant compared to the size of the particles, therefore causing the gas to take up a smaller volume than would be predicted by the ideal gas law. Under these conditions, the real gas deviates appreciably from ideal gas behavior.

High-level Importance

4. Their <u>size and mass</u> also affect the speed at which they move. At constant temperature, the kinetic energy (KE = 1/2 mv^2) of all particles – light or heavy – is nearly the same. This means that the heavier particles must be moving more slowly than the lighter ones and that the attractive forces between the heavier particles must be exercising a greater influence on their behavior. The greater speed of light particles, however, tends to counteract the attractive forces between them, thus producing a slight deviation from ideal gas behavior. Thus, a heavier particle (molecule or atom) will deviate more widely from ideal gas behavior than a lighter particle. At low temperature, the average velocity of gas particles decreases and the intermolecular attraction becomes increasingly significant, causing the gas to have a smaller volume than would be predicted by the ideal gas law. {The preceding is given by Graham's law, where the rate of movement of a gas (*diffusion* or streaming through a fine hole – *effusion*) is inversely proportional to the square root of the molecular weight of the gas (*see* CHM 4.1.3)}

4.2 Liquid Phase (Intermolecular Forces)

A liquid is composed of tiny vibrating particles of matter, such as atoms or molecules, held together by *inter*molecular (*between* molecules) forces (*bonds*). Liquids have the ability to mix with one another - and with other phases - to form *solutions*. The degree to which two liquids can mix is called their *miscibility*. Substances are said to be *immiscible* if there are certain proportions in which the mixture does *not* form a solution (i.e. *remain separated like oil and water*).

Other important characteristics of liquids: **(i)** definite volume, but no definite shape; **(ii)** viscosity and surface tension (CHM 4.2.1, 4.2.2); **(iii)** cohesion and adhesion (CHM 4.2.2); **(iv)** as compared to gases, liquids are relatively incompressible (CHM 4.3).

We previously discussed primary (*strong*) bonds (CHM 3.1) and molecules with charge separation (*dipoles*; CHM 3.3). We will now explore secondary (*weak*) bonds which are just strong enough to hold molecules together to form a liquid. These intermolecular forces are effective over short distances only.

Van der Waal forces include *dipole-dipole*, *dipole-induced dipole* and *London forces*. Dipole-dipole forces are attractive forces between the positive end of one polar molecule and the negative end of another polar molecule. By far, the strongest of the *electrostatic* (CHM 3.1.1, 4.3), dipole-dipole interactions is the *hydrogen* bond.

To summarise, the most important intermolecular forces are: **1.** Dipole-dipole forces; **2.** London forces; and, **3.** Hydrogen bonds.

1. Dipole-dipole forces depend on the orientation as well as on the distance between the molecules; they are inversely proportional to the third power of the distance. In addition to the forces between permanent dipoles, a dipolar molecule induces in a neighboring molecule an electron distribution that results in another attractive force, the dipole-induced dipole force, which is inversely proportional to the sixth power of the distance and which is relatively independent of orientation.

2. London forces (or *dispersive* forces) are attractive forces acting between nonpolar molecules. They are due to the unsymmetrical instantaneous electron distribution which induces a dipole in neighboring molecules with a resultant attractive force. This instantaneous unsymmetrical distribution of electrons causes rapid polarisation of the electrons and formation of short-lived dipoles. These dipoles then interact with neighboring molecules, inducing the formation of more dipoles. Dispersion forces are thus responsible for the liquefaction of noble gases to form liquids at low temperatures (and high pressures).

3. Hydrogen bonds occur whenever hydrogen (H) is covalently bonded to an atom

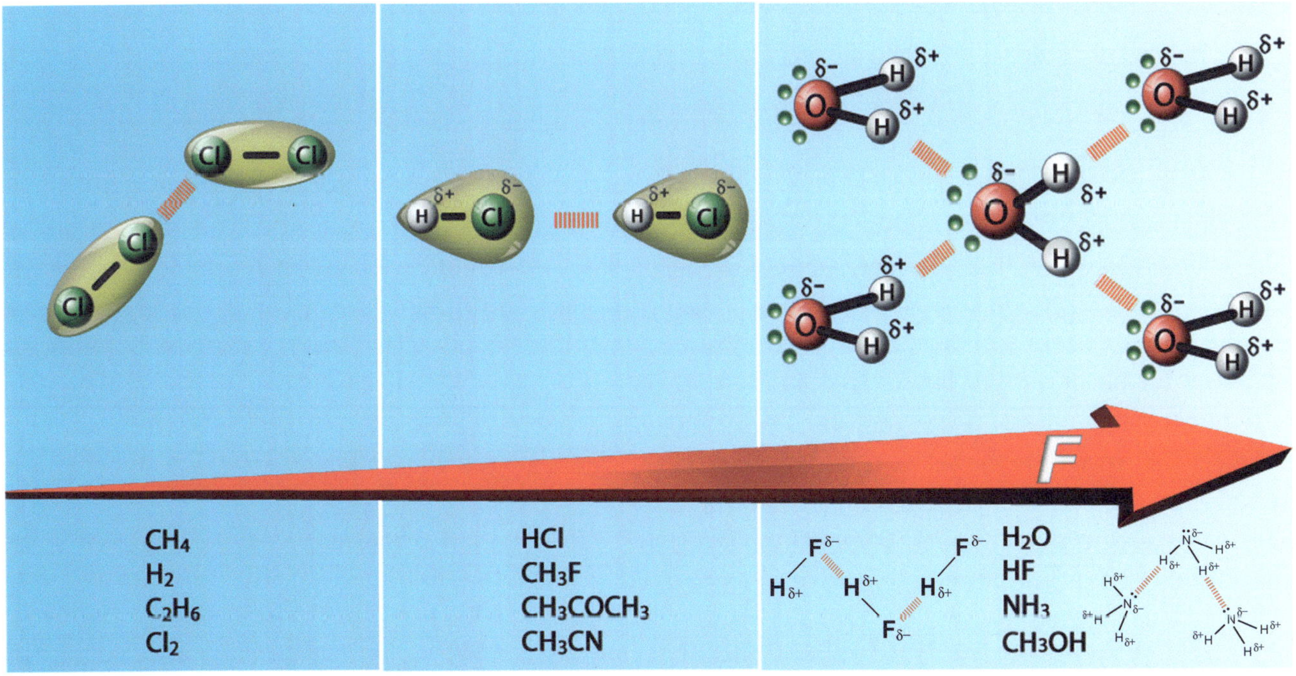

Figure III.A.4.1.2: Intermolecular (*between different molecules*) bonding: Van Der Waal's forces (weak) and hydrogen bonding (strong). London forces between Cl_2 molecules, dipole-dipole forces between HCl molecules and H-bonding between H_2O molecules. Note that a partial negative charge on an atom is indicated by δ^- (delta negative), while a partial positive charge is indicated by δ^+ (delta positive). Notice that one H_2O molecule can potentially form 4 H-bonds with surrounding molecules which is highly efficient. The preceding is one key reason that the boiling point of water is higher than that of ammonia, hydrogen fluoride or methanol.

High-level Importance

such as oxygen (O), nitrogen (N) or fluorine (F), that attract electrons strongly. Because of the differences in electronegativity between H and O or N or F (CHM 2.3, 3.1.1), the electrons that constitute the covalent bond are closer to the O, N or F nucleus than to the H nucleus leaving the latter relatively unshielded. The unshielded proton is strongly attracted to the O, N or F atoms of neighboring molecules since these form the negative end of a strong dipole.

The slightly positive charge of the hydrogen atom will then be strongly attracted to the more electronegative atoms of nearby molecules. These forces are weaker than *intra*molecular bonds (e.g. covalent bonds; CHM 3.2), but are much stronger than the other two types of intermolecular forces. Hydrogen bonding is a special case of dipole-dipole interaction. Hydrogen bonds are characterised by unusually strong interactions and high boiling points due to the vast amount of energy required (*relative to other intermolecular forces*) to break the hydrogen bonds. {Though the H-bonding atoms can be remembered by the mnemonic "Hydrogen is FON!", sulfur is also known to H-bond under certain conditions though far weaker than the more electronegative FON atoms (FON = fluorine, oxygen, nitrogen).}

4.2.1 Viscosity

Viscosity is analogous to friction between moving solids. It may, therefore, be viewed as the resistance to the flow of layers of fluid or liquid past each other. This also means that viscosity, like friction, results in dissipation of mechanical energy. As one layer flows over another, its motion is transmitted to the second layer and causes this layer to be set in motion. Since a mass *m* of the second layer is set in motion and some of the energy of the first layer is lost, there is a transfer of momentum between the layers.

The greater the transfer of this momentum from one layer to another, the more energy that is lost and the slower the layers move.

The viscosity (η) is the measure of the efficiency of transfer of this momentum. Therefore the higher the viscosity coefficient, the greater the transfer of momentum and loss of mechanical energy, and thus loss of velocity. The reverse situation holds for a low viscosity coefficient (*see* PHY 6.1.4, and Physics Chapter 6 GAMSAT-level practice questions).

Consequently, a high viscosity coefficient substance flows slowly (e.g. molasses), and a low viscosity coefficient substance flows relatively fast (e.g. water). Consider the following examples at room temperature and atmospheric pressure, from low to high viscosity: acetone (= nail polish remover, paint thinner) < water < motor oil < maple syrup < honey < molasses < fondue < toothpaste.

Note that the transfer of momentum to adjacent layers is in essence, the exertion of a force upon these layers to set them in motion.

4.3 Solid Phase

Solids have definite volume and shape and are incompressible (*incapable of having its volume squashed!*) under pressure. Intermolecular forces between molecules of molecular solids, and electrostatic (i.e. coulombic or "opposite charges attract") forces between ions of ionic solids, are strong enough to hold them into a relatively rigid structure. A solid may be crystalline (*ordered*) or amorphous (*disordered*).

A crystalline solid ("*crystals*"), such as table salt (NaCl), has a structure with an ordered geometric shape (CHM 3.1.1). Its atoms are arranged geometrically with a repeating pattern. It has a specific melting point. An amorphous solid, such as glass, has a molecular structure with no specific shape. It melts over a wide range of temperatures since the molecules require different amounts of energies to break bonds between them.

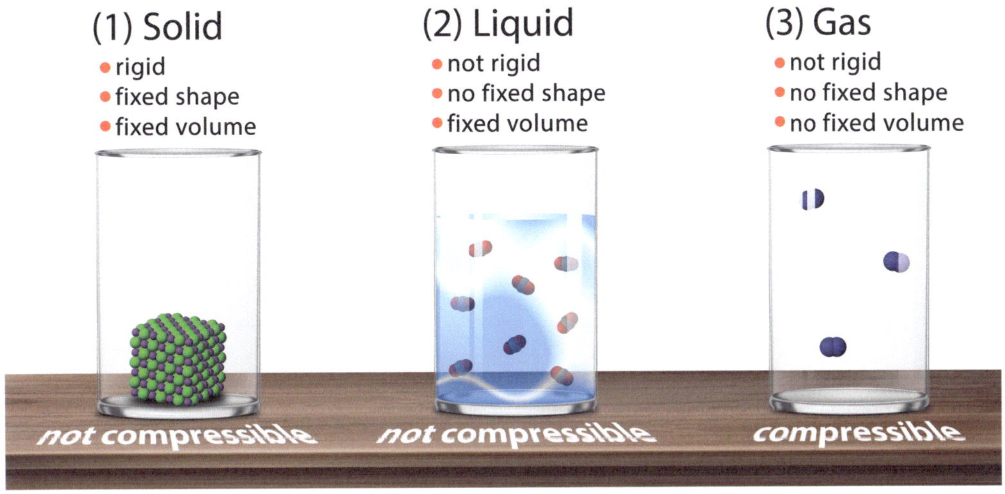

Figure III.A.4.1.3: Phases of matter (*not drawn to scale!*). **(1)** A larger crystal structure of table salt (sodium chloride, NaCl) than the one we saw in CHM 3.1.1; **(2)** CO_2 in liquid water (*a low-calorie carbonated drink!*); **(3)** 78% of the air you are breathing now: N_2. Note that it may be more accurate to deem liquids as *nearly* incompressible.

4.4 Phase Equilibria (Solids, Liquids and Gases)

4.4.1 Phase Changes

Elements and compounds can undergo transitions between the solid, liquid and gaseous states. They can exist in different phases and undergo phase changes which need *not* involve chemical reactions. Phase changes are reversible with an equilibrium existing between each of the phases. A phase is a homogeneous, physically distinct and mechanically separable part of a system. Each phase is separated from other phases by a physical boundary.

High-level Importance

A few examples:

1. Ice/liquid water/water vapor (3 phases)
2. Any number of gases mix in all proportions and therefore constitute just one phase.
3. The system $CaCO_3(s) \rightarrow CaO(s) + CO_2(g)$ (2 phases, i.e. 2 solids: $CaCO_3$ and CaO and a gas: CO_2)
4. A saturated salt solution with a few crystals of NaCl left at the bottom of the container (3 phases: solution, undissolved salt, vapor)

An example of a phase change is the vaporisation of water into its vapor state. A system is considered homogeneous when it is uniform throughout its volume so that its properties are the same in all parts. This does not imply a single molecular species: a solution of sodium chloride is homogeneous provided its concentration is the same throughout.

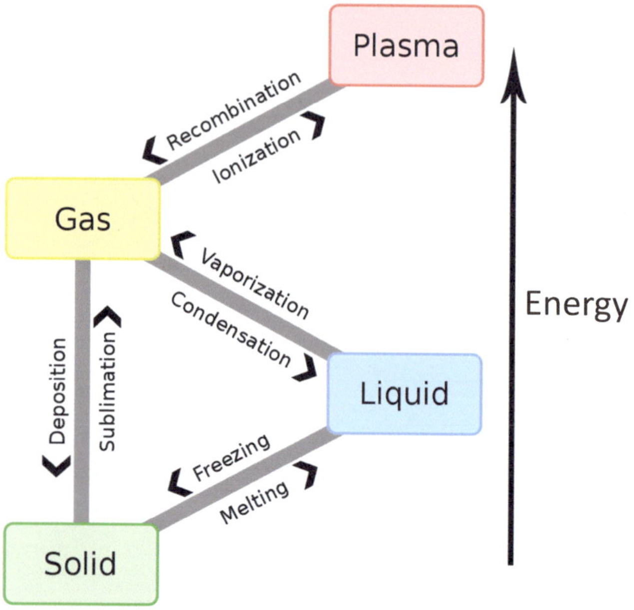

Figure III.A.4.2: Phase changes among the four fundamental states of matter (solid, liquid, gas and plasma). Ionised plasma, to one degree or the other, can be found in neon signs, lightning, the sun and the stars. The chemistry of plasma is beyond the scope of the assumed knowledge for this exam.

4.4.2 Freezing Point, Melting Point, Boiling Point

The conversion of a liquid to a gas is called vaporisation. We can increase the rate of vaporisation of a liquid by: (i) increasing the temperature, (ii) reducing the pressure, or (iii) both. Molecules escape from a liquid because, even though their average kinetic energy is constant, not all of them move at the same speed (*see Figure III.A.4.1*). A fast moving molecule can break away from the attraction of the others and pass into the vapor state. When a tight lid is placed on a vessel containing a liquid, the vapor molecules cannot escape and some revert back to the liquid state. The number of molecules leaving the liquid at any given time equals the number of molecules returning. Equilibrium is reached and the number of molecules in the fixed volume above the liquid remains constant. These molecules exert a constant pressure at a fixed temperature which is called the *vapor pressure* of the liquid. The vapor pressure is the partial pressure exerted by the gas molecules over the liquid formed by evaporation when it is in equilibrium with the gas phase condensing back into the liquid phase. The vapor pressure of any liquid is dependent on the intermolecular forces that are present within the liquid and the temperature. Weak intermolecular forces result in *volatile* substances, whereas strong intermolecular forces result in nonvolatile substances.

Boiling and evaporation are similar processes but they differ as follows: the vapor from a boiling liquid escapes with sufficient pressure to push back any other gas present, rather than diffusing through it. Vapor pressure increases as the temperature increases, as more molecules have sufficient energy to break the attraction between each other to escape into the gas phase. The boiling point is therefore the temperature at which the vapor pressure of the liquid equals the opposing external pressure. Under a lower pressure, the boiling point is reached at a lower temperature. Increased intermolecular interactions (i.e. H_2O *see* CHM 4.2, alcohol *see* ORG 6.1, etc.) will decrease the vapor pressure thus raising the boiling point. Other factors being equal, as a molecule becomes heavier (*increasing molecular weight*), it becomes more difficult to push the molecule into the atmosphere thus the boiling point increases (i.e. alkanes *see* ORG 3.1.1).

The freezing point of a liquid is the temperature at which the vapor pressure of the solid equals the vapor pressure of the liquid. Increases in the prevailing atmospheric pressure decreases the melting point and increases the boiling point.

When a solid is heated, the kinetic energy of the components increases steadily. Finally, the kinetic energy becomes great enough to overcome the forces holding the components together and the solid changes to a liquid. For pure crystalline solids, there is a fixed temperature at which this transition from solid to liquid occurs. This temperature is called the melting point. Pure solids melt completely at one temperature. Impure solids begin to melt at one temperature but become completely liquid at a higher temperature.

4.4.3 Phase Diagrams

Figure III.A.4.3 shows the temperature of ice as heat is added. Temperature increases linearly with heat until the melting point is reached. At this point, the heat energy added does not change the temperature. Instead, it is used to break intermolecular bonds and convert ice into water. There is a mixture of both ice and water at the melting point. After the complete conversion of ice into water, the temperature rises again linearly with heat addition. At the boiling point, the heat added does not change the temperature because the energy is again used to break the intermolecular bonds. After complete conversion of water into gas, the temperature will rise linearly again with heat addition.

Thus, during a phase change, there is no change in temperature. The energy that is added into the system is being used to weaken/break intermolecular forces; in other words, there is an increase in the potential energy of molecules rather than an increase in the average kinetic energy of molecules.

High-level Importance

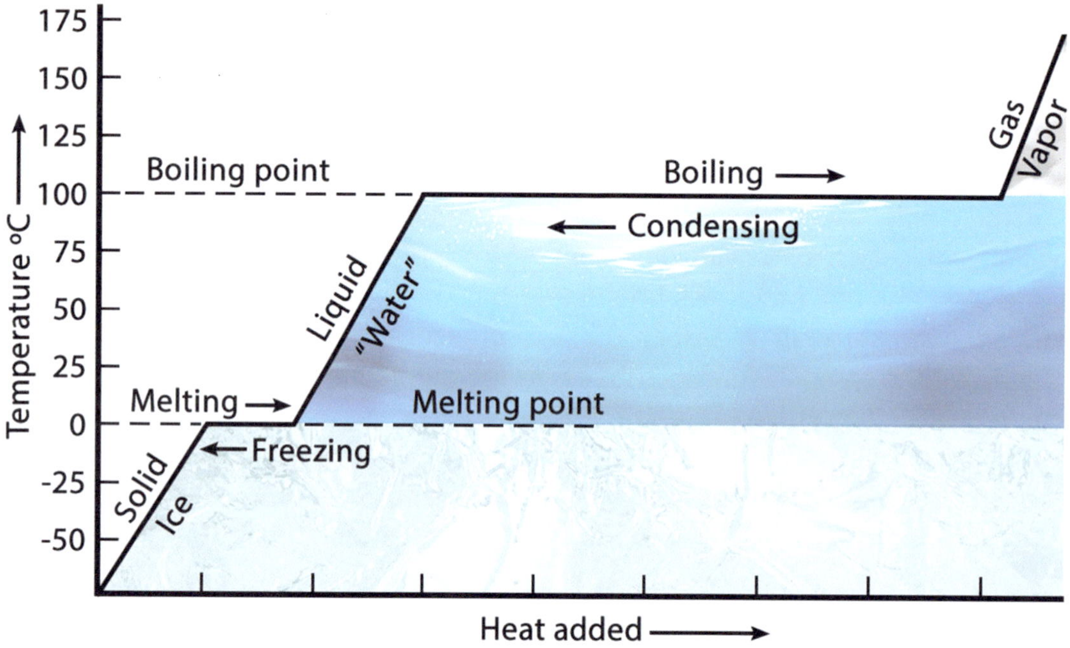

Figure III.A.4.3 Heating curve for H_2O.

The amount of energy to change one mole of substance from solid to liquid or from liquid to gas is called the molar *heat of fusion* and the molar *heat of vaporisation* (CHM 8.7). Each phase has its own specific heat. Enthalpy of vaporisation is greater than that of fusion because more energy is required to break intermolecular bonds (*from liquid phase to gas phase*) than just to weaken intermolecular bonds (*from solid phase to liquid phase*).

The temperatures at which phase transitions occur are functions of the pressure of the system. The behavior of a given substance over a wide range of temperature and pressure can be summarised in a phase diagram, such as the one shown for the water system (Fig.III.A.4.4). The diagram is divided into three areas labeled **solid** (ice), **liquid** (water) and **vapor** in each of which only one phase exists. In these areas, *P* and *T* can be independently varied without a second phase appearing. These areas are bounded by curves AC, AD and AB. Line AB represents sublimation/deposition (*sublimation curve*). Line AC represents evaporation/condensation (*vaporisation curve*) and Line AD represents melting/freezing (*fusion curve*). At triple point A, all three phases coexist in equilibrium. At any point on these curves, two phases are in equilibrium. Thus on AC, at a given T, the saturated vapor pressure of water has a fixed value. The boiling point of water (N) can be found on this curve, 100 °C at 760 mmHg pressure. The curve only extends as far as C, the critical point, where the vapor and liquid are indistinguishable. In general, the gas phase is found at high temperature and low pressure; the solid phase is found at low temperatures and high pressure;

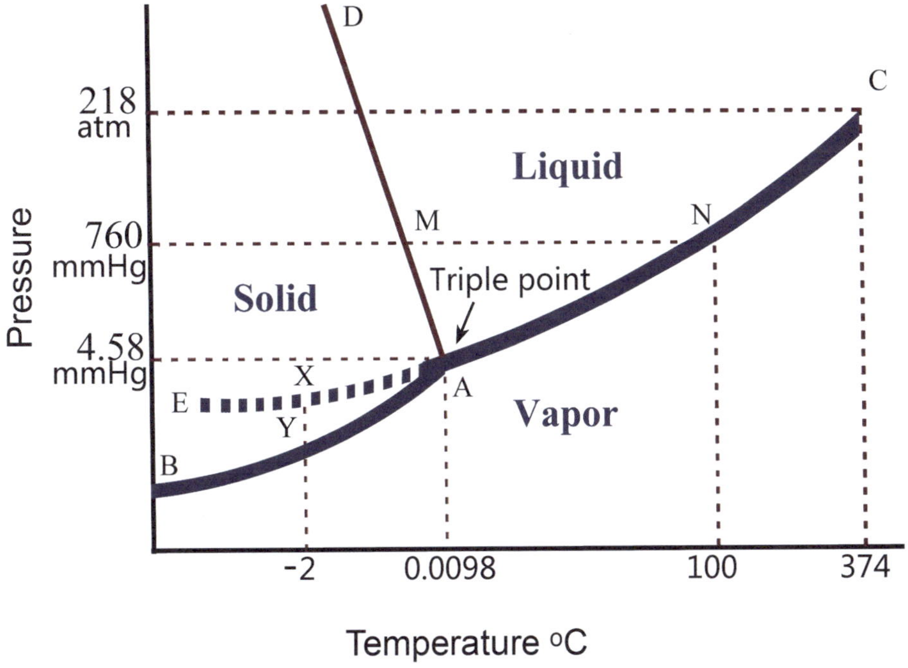

Figure III.A.4.4: Phase diagram for H_2O.

and the liquid phase is found at high temperatures and high pressure. The temperature at which a substance boils when the pressure is 1 atm is called the *normal boiling point*.

The extension of the curve CA to E represents the metastable equilibrium (*meta* = beyond) between supercooled water and its vapor. If the temperature is slightly raised at point X, a little of the liquid will vaporise until a new equilibrium is established at that higher temperature. Curve AB is the vapor pressure curve for ice. Its equilibria are of lower energy than those of AE and thus more stable.

The slope of line AD shows that an increase in P will lower the melting point of ice. This property is almost unique to water. Because of the negative slope of line AD, an isothermal (*same temperature*) increase in pressure will compress the solid (*ice*) into liquid (*water*). Thus H_2O is unique in that its liquid form is denser than its solid form. The high density of liquid water is due mainly to the cohesive nature of the hydrogen-bonded network of water molecules (*see* Figure III.A.4.1.2 in CHM 4.2).

Most substances *increase* their melting points with increased pressure. Thus the line AD slants to the right for almost all substances. Point M represents the true melting point of ice, 0.0023 °C at 760 mmHg of pressure. (The 0 °C standard refers to the freezing point of water saturated with air at 760 mmHg). At point A, solid, liquid and vapor are in equilibrium. At this one temperature, ice and water have the same fixed vapor pressure. This is the triple point, 0.0098 °C at 4.58 mmHg pressure.

High-level Importance

4.5 Manometers: Measuring Gas Pressure

In the GAMSAT Physics Masters Series Chapter 6 (PHY 6.1.2.2), we discussed how pressure is measured with a manometer. This section is either a primer, if you have not read that section, or revision, if you have. And yes, we are setting the table so that some GAMSAT-level practice questions in just a few pages (at the end of this chapter) will become more understandable for you!

When you measure the pressure in your tyres, you are measuring the pressure difference between the tyres and atmospheric pressure, which is the *gauge* (or *gage*) pressure.

Absolute pressure is the pressure of a fluid relative to the pressure in a vacuum. The absolute pressure is then the sum of the gauge pressure, which is what you measure, and the atmospheric pressure.

$$P_{abs} = P_{atm} + P_{gauge}$$

Pressure can be measured in devices in which one or more columns of a liquid (i.e. mercury or water) are used to determine the pressure difference between two points (i.e. U-tube manometer, inclined-tube manometer). Of course, electronic instruments for measurement are used more frequently.

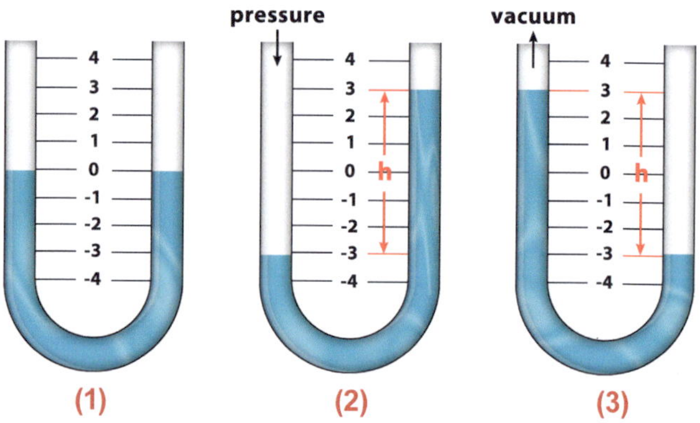

Figure III.A.4.5: Manometers. **(1)** When the U-tube has both ends open to the same pressure, the height of the liquid will be the same in each leg. **(2)** If positive pressure is applied to one leg, it will force a difference in height h. **(3)** When a vacuum (= *no pressure*) is applied to one leg, the liquid rises in that leg and falls in the other.

CHAPTER 4: Phases and Phase Equilibria

GOLD STANDARD FOUNDATIONAL GAMSAT PRACTICE QUESTIONS

1) At a given temperature and pressure, a researcher measured the mass and volume of 4 different samples of nitrogen gas. Which of the samples has the greatest density?

Sample	Mass (mg)	Volume (m^3)
I	1.5	0.50
II	3.0	0.75
III	4.5	1.00
IV	6.0	1.50

A. Sample I
B. Sample II
C. Sample III
D. Sample IV

2) A lab experiment was done which determined that nitrogen gas (N_2) had a density of 1.19 g/L at STP. Which of the following expressions can be used to determine the molar concentration of nitrogen gas in moles/litre?

Note the atomic weight: N = 14 g/mol.

A. (1.19) / (22.4)
B. (1.19) • (14)
C. (1.19) / (28)
D. (1.19) • (28)

3) At STP, the density of a gas was determined to be 2.02 g/L. If the gas is known to be one of the following substances, which one is most likely?

Note that:

- The molar volume at STP is 22.4 L/mol.
- Consider the following values in amu: H = 1.0, C = 12, O = 16.

A. C_3H_8
B. C_2H_2
C. HCHO
D. $CH_3CH_2CH_2CH_2CH_3$

Questions 4–6

The ideal gas law, PV = *n*RT, may be of value for the next 3 questions. {Pressure (P), volume (V), temperature (T), R is constant; and *n* is the number of moles.}

4) Two identical evacuated flasks are filled with different gases to the same pressure and temperature. The first is filled with hydrogen (H_2) and the second with propane. Compared with the first flask, the flask filled with propane ($CH_3CH_2CH_3$) weighs:

{Note the following values in amu: H = 1.0, C = 12.}

A. 11 times more.
B. 22 times more.
C. the same.
D. 44 times more.

5) A basketball with initial pressure P and initial volume V is inflated with air until the pressure becomes 2P and the volume becomes 1.1V. The temperature being kept constant, the weight of air in the ball has increased by a factor of:

A. 2.2
B. 1.1
C. 1.0
D. 2.0

6) Suppose that a gas is kept at constant temperature and the volume is allowed to increase. The pressure of the gas:

A. decreases.
B. stays constant.
C. increases.
D. fluctuates depending on molecular size.

High-level Importance

7) Consider the molecule methanol (CH_3OH).

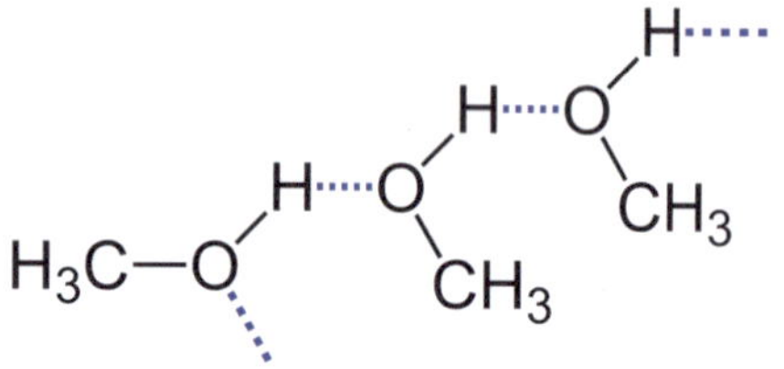

The black lines in the image above represent which of the following?

A. Hydrogen bonds
B. Ionic bonds
C. Covalent bonds
D. Avogadro's bonds

8) Consider the image below.

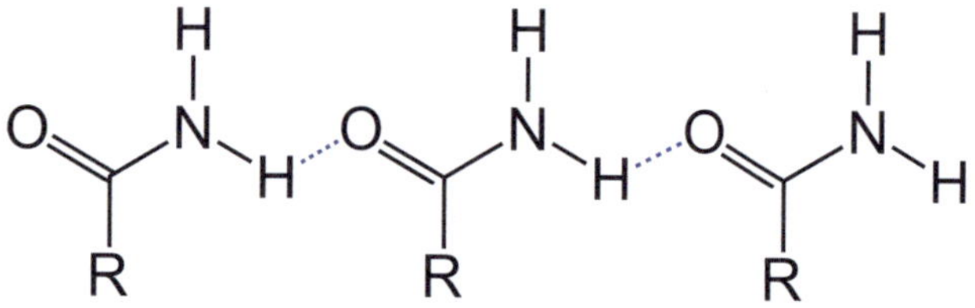

The blue dotted lines likely represent which of the following?

A. Hydrogen bonds
B. Ionic bonds
C. Covalent bonds
D. Covalent bonds with ionic character

9) Consider the phase diagram for water.

Which part of the graph is consistent with the liquid phase?

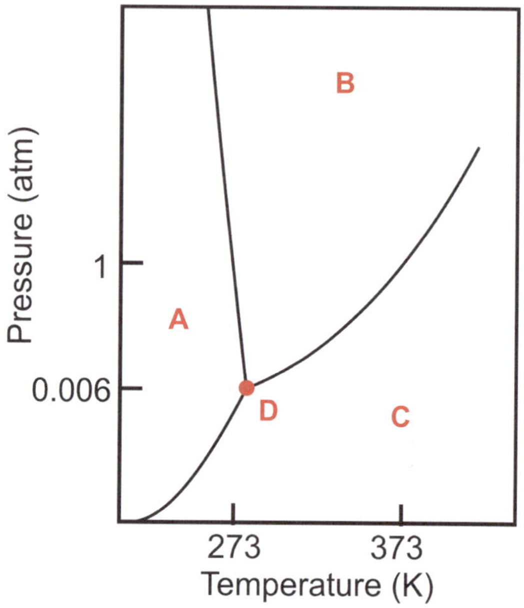

10) Normally, an egg left in boiling water for 10 minutes becomes a firm, "hard boiled" egg. On top of Mount Everest, with a height of 8000 metres, an egg left in boiling water remains soft indefinitely. The egg fails to cook on Mount Everest because:

A. water boils at low temperature when the air pressure is very low.
B. an egg cannot get very hot when gravity is weak.
C. the water is too cold to boil on the mountain.
D. water boils at low temperature when gravity is weak.

GOLD STANDARD GAMSAT-LEVEL PRACTICE QUESTIONS

11) Rockets and satellites are used to measure multiple parameters in the Earth's upper atmosphere (100 to 800 km above the surface of the Earth). Such parameters include fluctuations in temperature as well as total neutral density (i.e. uncharged species) and electron density. These 3 parameters fluctuate during the sun's 11-year activity cycle which is illustrated in Figure 1.

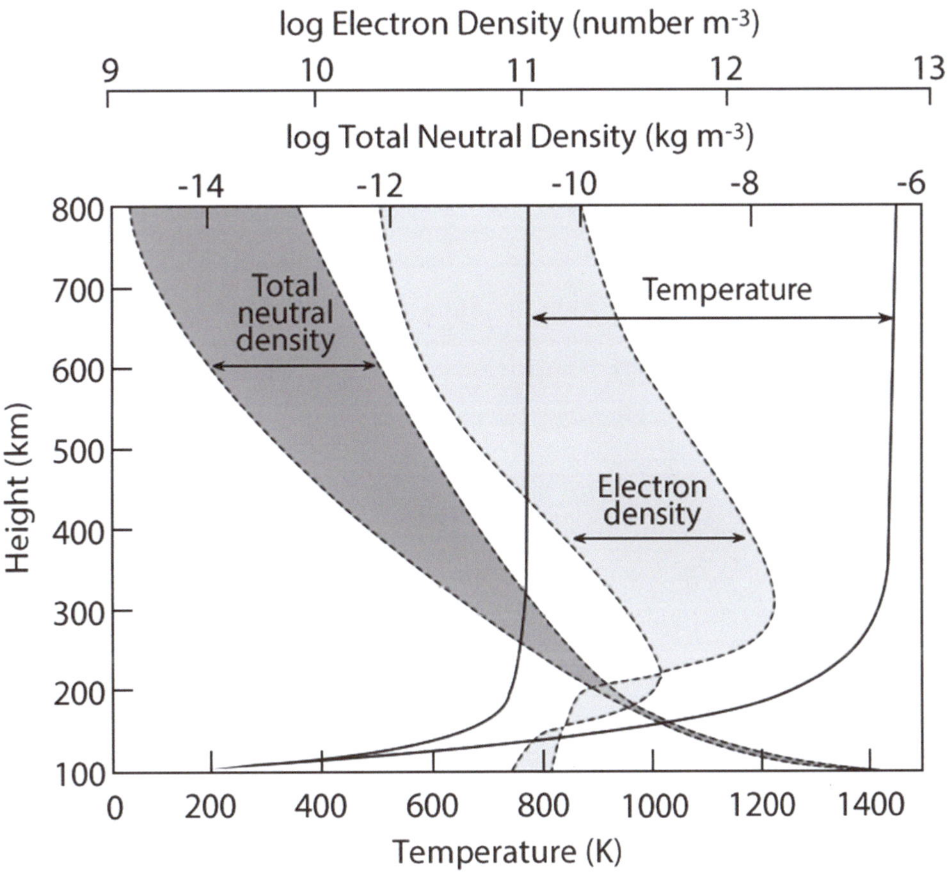

Figure 1

Figure 1 can be used to determine the Fluctuation Factor (FF), as defined as the factor by which the lowest value of a parameter can be multiplied to get its highest value at a specific height. For example, if at a given height, the lowest value of a parameter is *x* and its highest value is 5*x*, then its FF is 5. According to Figure 1, which of the following parameters displays the greatest FF at any height in the upper atmosphere?

A. Total neutral density

B. Electron density

C. Temperature

D. Both **B** and **C** are approximately the highest

12) A phase diagram is a graph that shows the relation between the solid, liquid and gaseous states. Any point in the graph is where 2 phases exist at equilibrium except the triple point where all 3 exist at equilibrium. Solid CO_2 is called "dry ice" because it can go directly from solid to vapour (*sublimation*) at room pressure (i.e. 101.3 kPa). The triple point of CO_2 occurs at 217 K and 515 kPa. A reduction in CO_2 pressure directly correlates with changes in its sublimation, melting and boiling points. Which of the following is a correct representation of the phase diagram for carbon dioxide?

A.

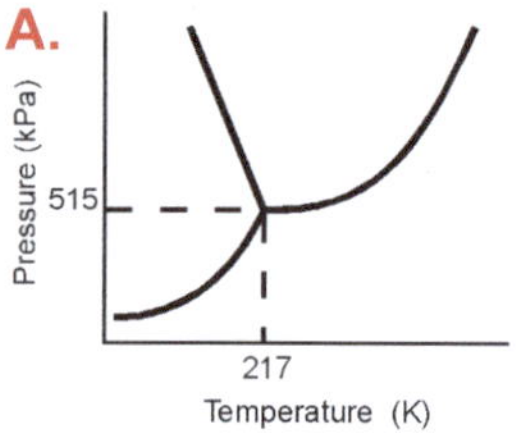

C.

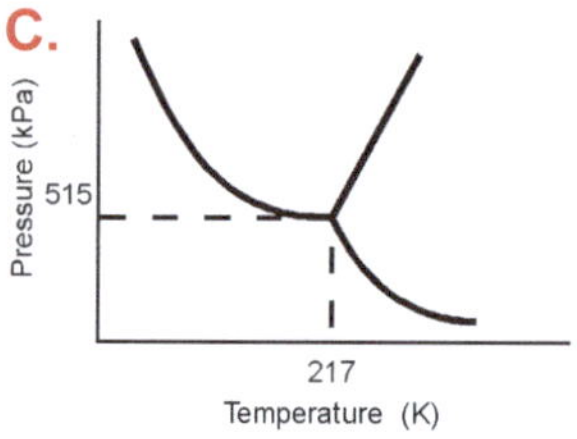

B.

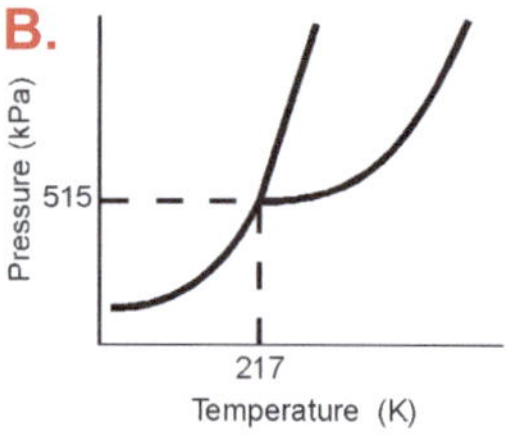

D.

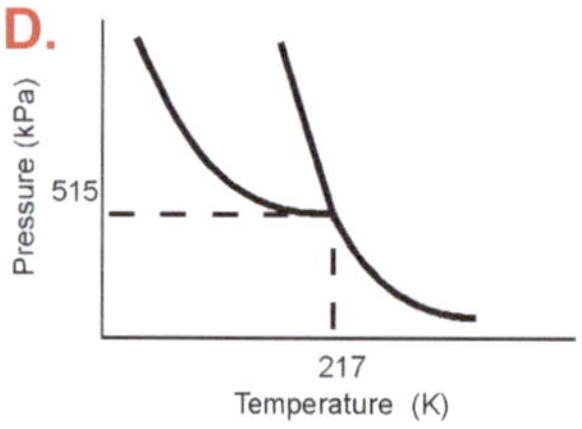

Questions 13–18

In the simple model of a gas as described by the kinetic molecular theory, a gas is pictured as an assembly of particles travelling at high velocities in straight lines in all directions. The particles are constantly colliding, but they are supposed to be perfectly elastic so that no momentum is lost on impact. They are also supposed to be point masses, that is, they have mass but occupy no space. In addition, no attractive or repulsive forces are exerted between particles.

From this theory, and the work of other great scientists like Boyle and Charles, the ideal gas law was devised: PV = nRT where P = pressure of the gas, V = volume of the gas, n = number of moles of gas particles present, T = temperature of the gas in kelvin, and R = universal gas constant.

However, no "real" gas conforms to this "ideal" gas theory, that is, no real gas obeys all of these laws at all temperatures and pressures. These deviations were investigated by the French physicist Amagat, who used pressures up to 320 atmospheres and a range of temperatures to investigate these deviations. The following diagram shows how the PV/nRT value varies with pressure for certain gases at 50 °C.

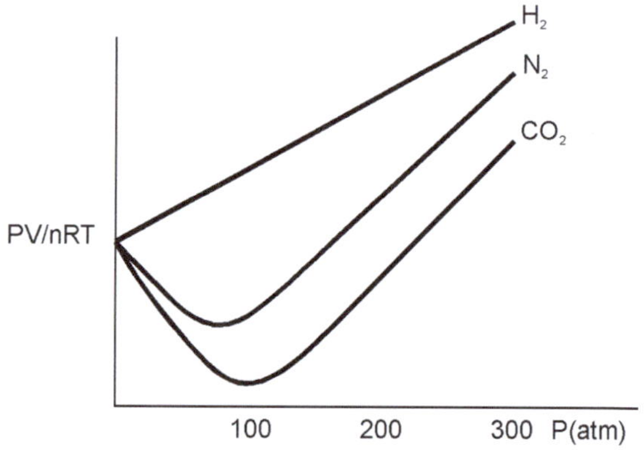

The deviations of real gases from ideality confers a number of properties on the gas which could not be explained by the kinetic molecular theory.

13) What would the PV/nRT versus P graph look like for an ideal gas?

A.

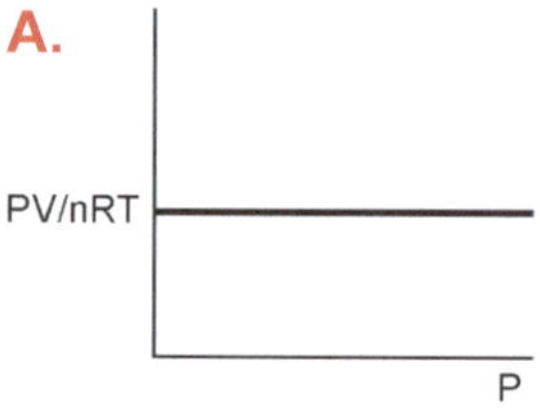

C.

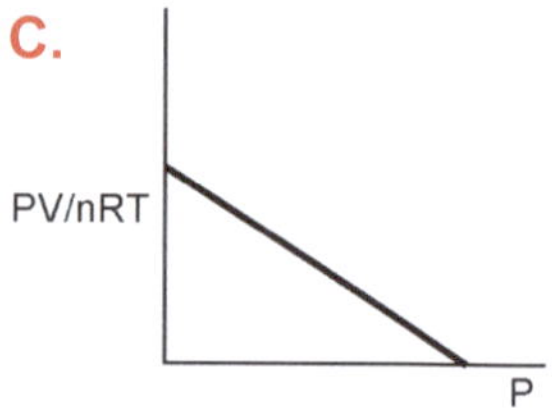

B.

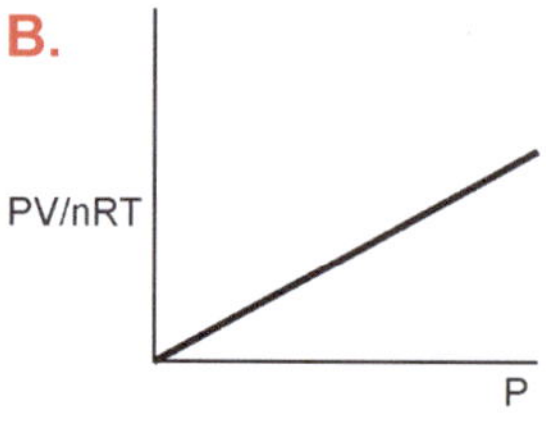

D.

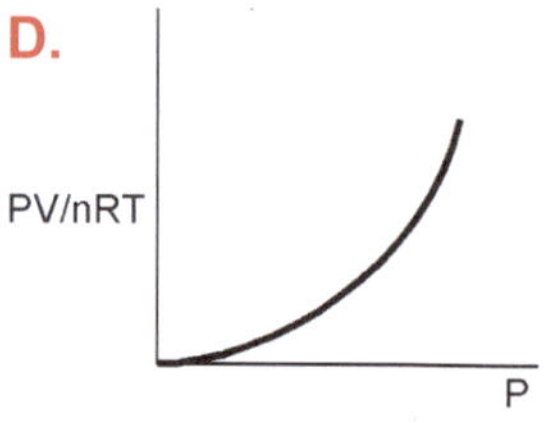

14) Consider the real gas H_2. From the information in the passage, if 1 dm^3 of H_2 gas initially at 50 atmospheres had its pressure increased to 100 atmospheres at a constant temperature, which of the following would be true?

A. Volume = 500 cm^3
B. Volume > 500 cm^3
C. Volume < 500 cm^3
D. The change in volume will depend on the rate of increase of the external pressure.

15) Which of the following does not contribute to the explanation of the deviation of "real" gases from ideality?

A. Gas particles occupy space.
B. Gas particles have an attraction for each other.
C. Gas particles possess mass.
D. Gas particles do not undergo elastic collisions.

16) A sample of N_2, known to contain traces of water, occupied a volume of 200 dm^3 at 25 °C and 1 atm. When passed over solid Na_2SO_4 (drying agent), the increase in mass of the salt was 35.0 grams. What was the partial pressure of the N_2 in the sample? (Assume ideality and molar volume at 25 °C = 24 dm^3)

A. 0.1 atm
B. 0.2 atm
C. 0.4 atm
D. 0.8 atm

17) For a given quantity of an ideal gas, there are state changes in which one of the characteristics of the gas or process remains constant. The processes are defined as follows:

- Isothermal: the temperature remains constant
- Isobaric: the pressure remains constant
- Isochoric: the volume remains constant
- Adiabatic: the heat is not transferred into or out of the system

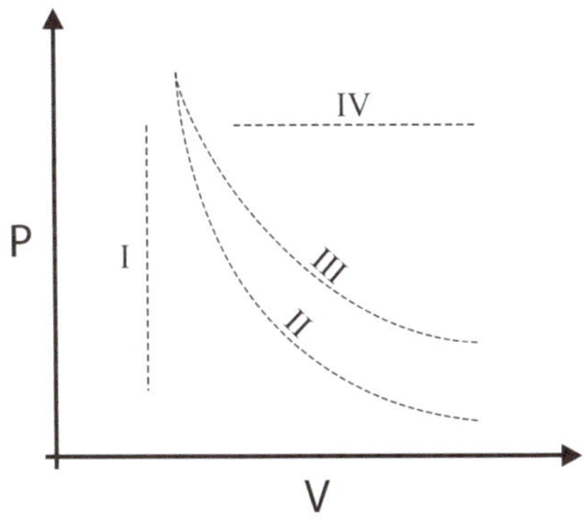

Figure 1: Pressure (P) vs Volume (V) graphs

Which of the following labels in Figure 1 is most consistent with the shape of a graph for the isothermal, isobaric, isochoric and adiabatic processes, respectively?

A. III, IV, I, II
B. III, IV, II, I
C. I, II, IV, III
D. II, IV, III, I

18) Consider the following graph illustrating the evolution of carbon dioxide gas under ideal conditions.

$$CaCO_{3(s)} + 2HCl_{(aq)} \rightarrow CaCl_{2(aq)} + CO_{2(g)} + H_2O_{(l)}$$

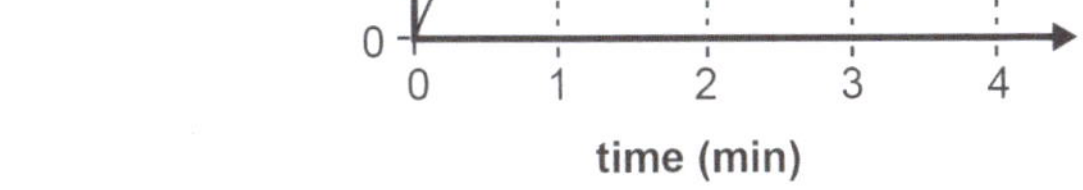

The average rate of reaction is greatest in which of the following time intervals?

A. 0-30 seconds
B. 30-60 seconds
C. 0-1 minute
D. 0-4 minutes

Questions 19–21

The ideal gas law is the equation of state of a hypothetical ideal gas. The state of an amount of gas is determined by its pressure (P), volume (V), and temperature (T) where:

$$PV = nRT$$

R is the Regnault constant, better known as the universal gas constant; and *n* is the number of moles of the substance.

19) Which of the following may be used to determine the molecular weight of an ideal gas from its density, *D*?

A. DP/RT
B. nRT/DP
C. DRT/P
D. P/DRT

20) Given the ideal gas equation, determine which of the following is consistent with the units of the gas constant R.

A. Joules/mole/K
B. (Joules)(mole)/K
C. (Pa)(mole)(K)
D. Pa/mole/K

21) Consider the following form of van der Waal's equation that corrects for the pressure and volume of real gases (*a*, *b* and R are constants, P is pressure, V is volume and T is temperature).

$$\left(P + \frac{a}{V^2}\right)(V - b) = RT$$

In the fundamental quantities of mass (M), length (L) and time (T), the dimensions of the constant *a* would be consistent with which of the following?

A. $M\,L^5\,T^{-2}$
B. $M\,L^{-1}\,T^{-2}$
C. $M\,L^2\,T$
D. L^6

Questions 22–24

Two moles of a diatomic gas P_2 were mixed with four moles of another diatomic gas Q_2 in each of two closed vessels in which the pressure could be altered.

In Experiment 1, which was carried out at 25 °C, all of the P_2 and Q_2 molecules reacted to yield one triatomic product. This took place spontaneously and was associated with an increase in the temperature of the reaction vessel.

In Experiment 2, which was carried out at 0 °C, the reaction vessel was attached to a water manometer: a thin U-tube partially filled with water that allows one to determine the pressure inside the vessel as demonstrated in the figure below.

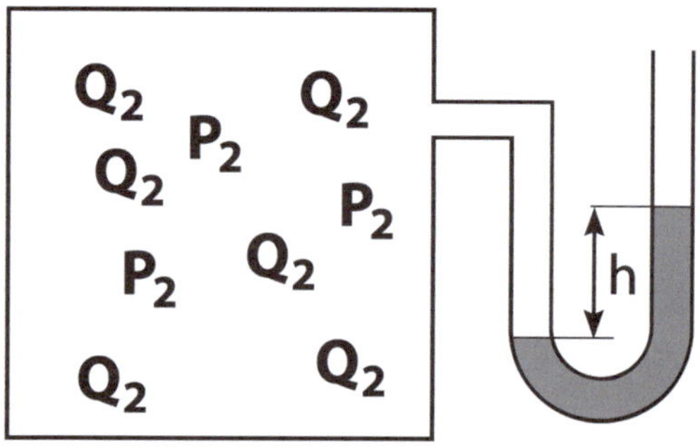

22) Which of the following shows the net reaction between P and Q in Experiment 1?

A. $2P_2 + 4Q_2 \longrightarrow P_4Q_8$
B. $P_2 + 2Q_2 \longrightarrow 2PQ_2$
C. $2P + 4Q \longrightarrow P_2Q_4$
D. $P_2 + Q_4 \longrightarrow P_2Q_4$

23) If the triatomic product is also gaseous, how does the pressure of the vessel before the reaction (= y) compare with the pressure of the vessel after the reaction (= x)?

A. y = (3/2)x
B. y = (2/3)x
C. y = (1/2)x
D. y = (1/3)x

24) The level of water in each arm of the manometer gives the pressure difference between the reaction vessel and the atmosphere. If the water level in the right side is higher, then the reaction vessel is at a higher pressure than the atmosphere and vice-versa. Given that at the start of the reaction, the water levels in both arms of the manometer were equal, all the gases are insoluble, negligible temperature change, and the reaction vessel is half-filled with ether, what did the apparatus look like after the reaction?

A.
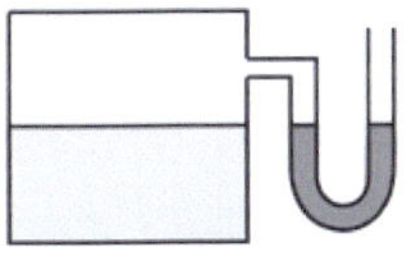

C.
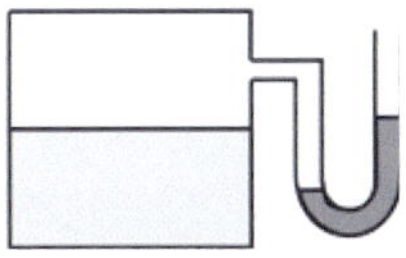

B.
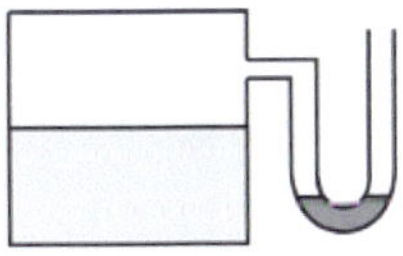

D.
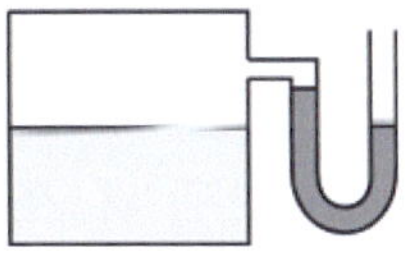

Questions 25–26

Consider the following relationships for ideal gases.

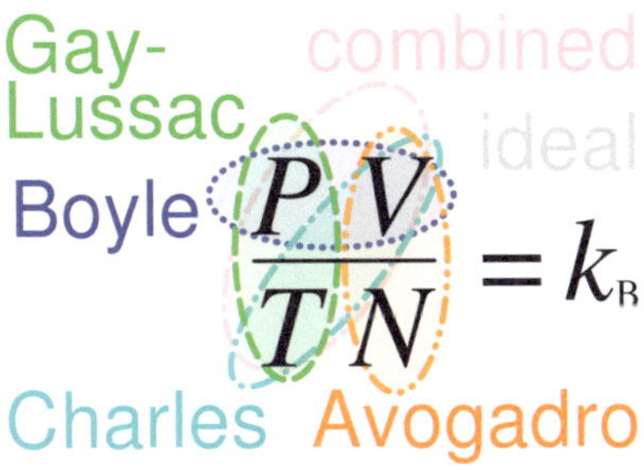

Figure 1: Relationships between Boyle's, Charles's, Gay-Lussac's, Avogadro's, combined and ideal gas laws.
(Cmglee; Wikimedia Commons, 2020)

Note that the representations are pressure (*P*), volume (*V*), temperature (*T*) in kelvin, the number of moles (*N*), and k_B is a constant. For each law, properties circled are variable and properties not circled are held constant. For example, Avogadro's law is V/N = constant.

25) Which of the following graphs best illustrates Gay-Lussac's law?

A.
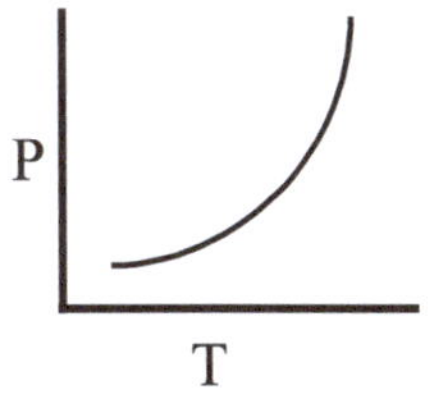

C.
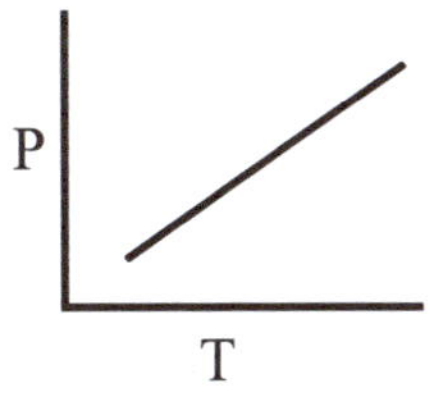

B.
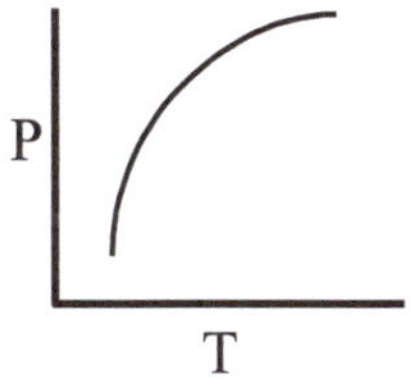

D.
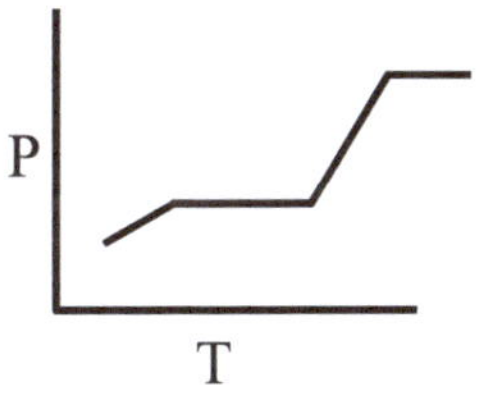

26) Choose one equation from among Boyle's, Charles's, Gay-Lussac's, or Avogadro's law to solve the following problem.

Assume 1 mole of an ideal gas is contained in a cylinder of volume V at a pressure P when the gas is at a temperature of 20 °C. Which of the following represents the gas pressure when the gas is heated to 60 °C? [Note that the absolute temperature in kelvin is 273 above the temperature in Celsius. Also note that the pressure at STP is 1 atm = 760 torr.]

A. 333/293 P
B. 27/67 P
C. P/3
D. 2P

High-level Importance

Questions 27–30

Certain layers of the Earth's atmosphere absorb certain wavelengths of solar radiation while letting others pass through. These types of solar radiation include X-rays, ultraviolet light, visible light, and infrared radiation.

The cross section of Earth's atmosphere in Figure 1 illustrates the altitudes, measured from sea level, at which solar radiation or different ranges of wavelengths are absorbed. Figure 1 also indicates the layers of the atmosphere and how atmospheric density, pressure, and temperature vary with altitude.

Note that:

- 1 Å = 10^{-10} m
- 1 bar = 100 000 Pa

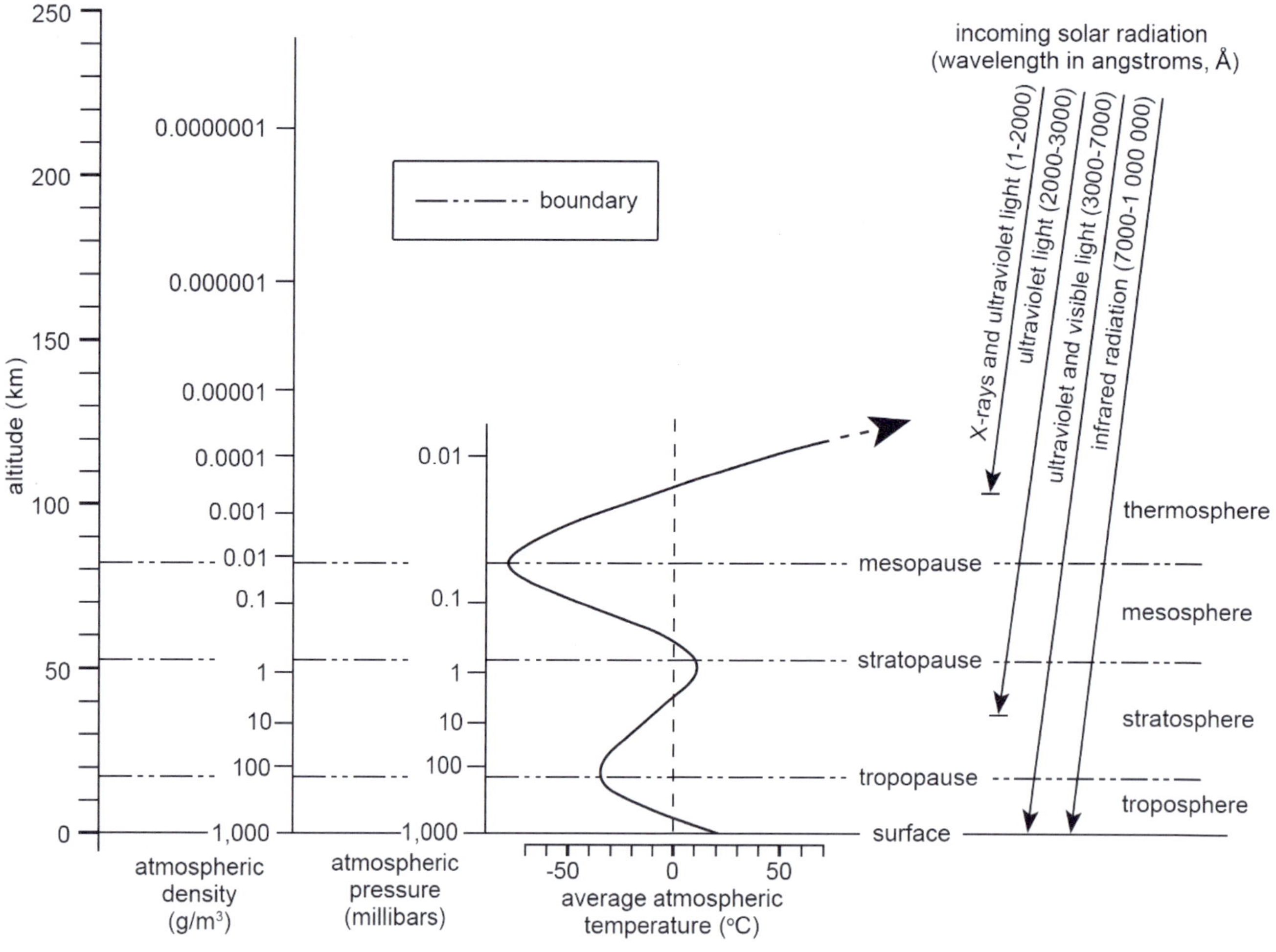

Figure 1

27) Which of the following is **not** consistent with Figure 1?

A. In the mesosphere, temperature decreases as the altitude increases.

B. An atmospheric density of 10^{-4} g/m^3 is unlikely to be affected by X-rays.

C. The coldest naturally occurring place on Earth or in its atmosphere is the mesopause.

D. The pressure drops an average of 4.5 Pa per metre in the first 20 000 metres above sea level.

28) Using the most basic definition, *atmosphere* is the mass of air surrounding the Earth. According to Figure 1, which layer of the atmosphere contains the greatest mass?

A. Mesosphere

B. Stratosphere

C. Troposphere

D. Cannot be determined by the information provided.

29) Although the concentration of the ozone in the ozone layer is very small, it is vitally important to life because it absorbs biologically harmful ultraviolet (UV) radiation coming from the sun. Three categories of UV, based on its wavelength, are referred to as UV-A (400–315 nm), UV-B (315–280 nm), and UV-C (280–100 nm). Which of the following is most consistent with the information provided?

A. Ozone is mostly in the troposphere.

B. Ozone is transparent to UV-A.

C. UV-C reaches the Earth's surface.

D. UV-B is the most dangerous form of UV radiation.

30) A student created a graph of atmospheric pressure vs. altitude using units that are different from Figure 1. Consider the resulting graph:

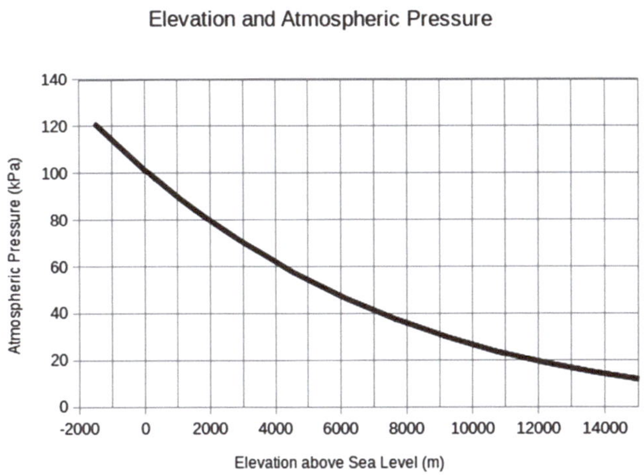

Which of the following conclusions can be made regarding the student's graph in comparison with the actual data illustrated in Figure 1?

A. The data as represented by the student's graph is not consistent with Figure 1.

B. The data is mostly consistent with Figure 1, but the graph should be linear.

C. The shape of the curve is correct but the data is off by orders of magnitude.

D. The data is mostly consistent with Figure 1, and the shape of the curve is correct.

High-level Importance

High-level Importance

SPOILER ALERT

Gold Standard has cross-referenced the content in this chapter to examples from ACER's official GAMSAT practice materials. It is for you to decide when you want to explore these questions since you may want to preserve some of ACER's materials for timed mock-exam practice.

Examples – Intermolecular bonds including H-bonds Q5-9 of 3; equation of state with dimensional analysis Q99-101 of 3; Graham's law (CHM 4.1.3): Q55 and Q106-108 of 3; H-bonds and solubility in water: Q66 of 5; note that Q90-93 of 5: background is H-bonds but not counted because no assumed knowledge based on this chapter. Note that "Q" is followed by the question number, and, for example, "of 1" refers to booklet number 1 which is referenced in the Spoiler Alert table at the end of Chapter 1. The 15 full-length GAMSAT practice tests by Gold Standard, HEAPS-1 through HEAPS-15, contain specific cross-references to this chapter within the worked solutions. Note that the manometer unit is from HEAPS-3; the ideal-gas unit with 6 questions and 4 graphs is from HEAPS-6; and, boil an egg on Mount Everest is from HEAPS-8.

Chapter Checklist

- ☐ Access your online account to view answers, worked solutions and discussion boards.
- ☐ Reassess your 'learning objectives' for this chapter: Go back to the first page of this chapter and re-evaluate the top 3 boxes and the Introduction.
  - ☐ Please be sure that you have completed the *Need for Speed* exercises at the beginning of this chapter.
- ☐ Complete a maximum of 1 page of notes using symbols/abbreviations to represent the entire chapter based on your learning objectives. These are your Gold Notes.
- ☐ Consider your multimedia options based on your optimal way of learning:
  - ☐ Download the free Gold Standard GAMSAT app for your Android device or iPhone.
  - ☐ Create your own, tangible study cards or try the free app: Anki.
  - ☐ Record your voice reading your Gold Notes onto your smartphone (audio files, e.g., *memo* or MP3s) and listen during exercise, transportation, etc.
  - ☐ Try out the Gold Standard GAMSAT online videos at gamsat-prep.com, or you can try other options on YouTube like Khan Academy or Crash Course Chemistry.
- ☐ Reassess your schedule for your full-length GAMSAT practice tests: ACER and/or HEAPS exams. Ensure that you have scheduled one full day to complete a practice test and 1-2 days for a thorough assessment of worked solutions while adding to your abbreviated Gold Notes.
- ☐ Reassess your progress in scheduling and/or evaluating stress reduction techniques such as regular exercise (sports), yoga, meditation and/or mindfulness exercises (*see* YouTube for suggestions).

Chapter 5

Memorise

* Define saturated, supersatured, volatile, nonvolatile
* Common anions and cations in solution
* Units of concentration
* Define electrolytes with examples

Understand

* Colligative properties, Raoult's law
* Phase diagram change due to colligative properties
* Bp elevation, fp depression
* Osmotic press, equation
* Solubility product, common-ion effect
* Solubility rules

Importance

High level: 18% of GAMSAT General Chemistry

questions released by ACER are related to content in this chapter (in our estimation).

* Note that approximately 80% of the questions in GAMSAT General Chemistry are related to just 4 chapters: 4, 5, 6, and 9.

Introduction

A solution is a homogeneous mixture (*uniform*; CHM 1.1) composed of two or more substances. For example, a solute (salt) dissolved in a solvent (water) making a solution (salt water). Solutions can involve gases in liquids (e.g., oxygen in water) or even solids in solids (e.g., alloys). Two substances are *immiscible* if they can't mix to make a solution (e.g., oil and water). Solutions can be distinguished from non-homogeneous (*heterogeneous*) mixtures like colloids and suspensions.

Multimedia Resources at GAMSAT-Prep.com

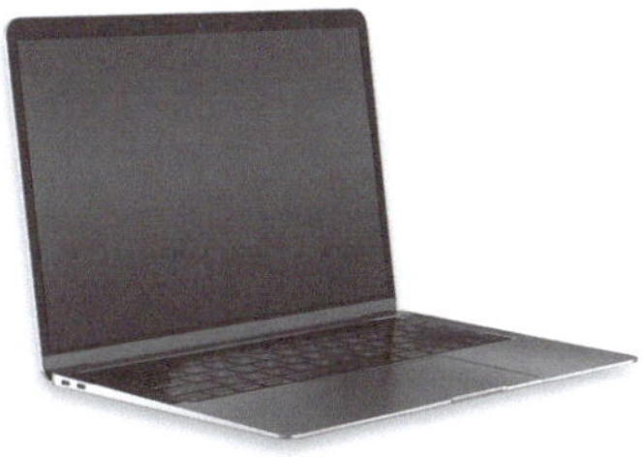

Open Discussion Boards
(*gamsat-prep.com/forum*)

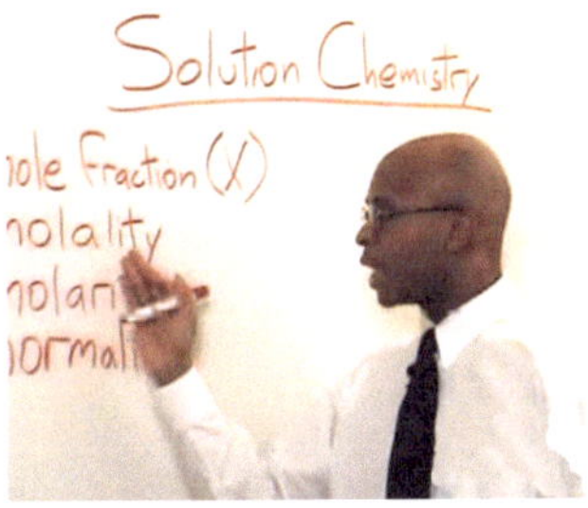

Science Preparation Videos

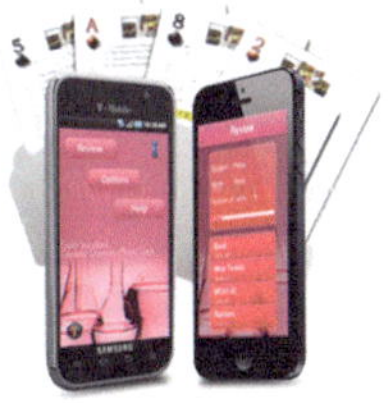

Flashcards

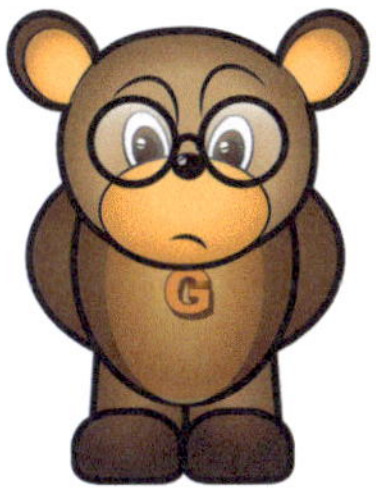

Special Guest

* The real GAMSAT may have advanced-level information presented (i.e. in a passage) but previous knowledge of said information is not required to answer the questions that would follow. Practice questions at the end of this chapter, as well as ACER and GS (HEAPS) practice GAMSATs can help you clarify this point.

5.0 GAMSAT has a *Need for Speed*!

High-level Importance

Section	GAMSAT General Chemistry *Need for Speed* Exercises
5.1	Circle your response. Once the maximum percent of a solute has dissolved in the solvent (*the solubility*), the solution is then which of the following? unsaturated desaturated saturated supersaturated
5.1.2	Consider the phase diagram of water demonstrating the effect of the addition of a solute. In each red box, use one of the following labels: vapor (or gas), solid or liquid. In each blue box, use one of the following labels: **(1)** solution or **(2)** solvent. 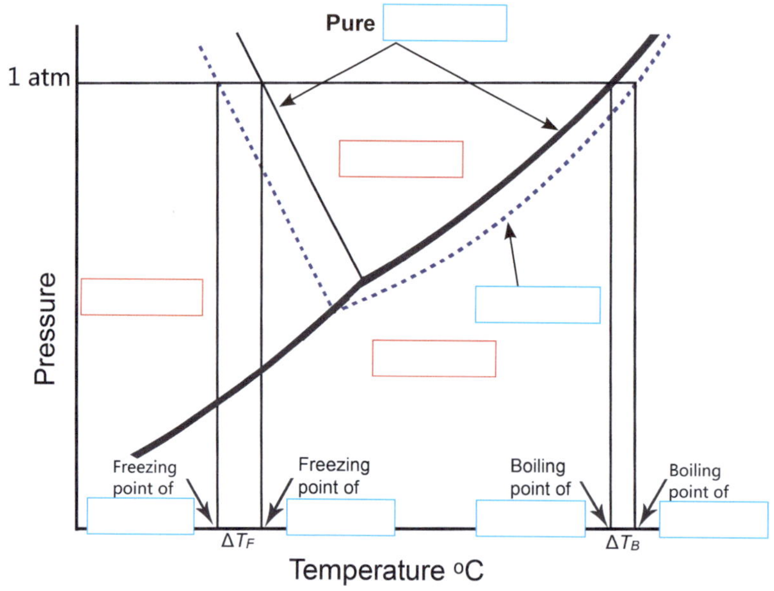
5.2	Complete the missing entries. Note: It is not mandatory to commit these common ions to memory, but it will make understanding chemistry a lot easier.

Common Anions

	Fluoride		Hydroxide	ClO^-	Hypochlorite
	Chloride	NO_3^-	Nitrate	ClO_2^-	Chlorite
	Bromide	NO_2^-	Nitrite	ClO_3^-	Chlorate
	Iodide		Carbonate	ClO_4^-	Perchlorate
O^{2-}	Oxide		Sulfate	SO_3^{2-}	Sulfite
S^{2-}	Sulfide		Phosphate	CN^-	Cyanide
N^{3-}	Nitride	$CH_3CO_2^-$	Acetate	MnO_4^-	Permanganate

5.2	**Common Cations** (table below)

Common Cations

	Sodium		Hydrogen
	Lithium		Calcium
	Potassium		Magnesium
	Ammonium		Iron (II)
	Hydronium	Fe^{3+}	Iron (III)

Use the "drop and swap" technique (*see* CHM 3.1.1, 5.3.4), and the information in the tables for Common Anions and Common Cations, to write the molecular formulas for the compounds below.

For example, sodium chloride: ______NaCl______

Calcium chloride (5.3.1): ________________

Sodium sulfate (5.3.1): ________________

Calcium nitride (5.2): ________________

5.3.1 Define molarity.

Define density.

5.3.2 Generally speaking, as temperature increases, what happens to the solubility of salts?

Generally speaking, as temperature increases, what happens to the solubility of gases?

5.1 Solutions and Colligative Properties

High-level Importance

Water (H_2O) is a universal solvent known as a pure substance (CHM 1.1) or a one-component system. Pure substances are often mixed together to form solutions. A solution is a sample of matter that is homogeneous but, unlike a pure substance, the composition of a solution can vary within relatively wide limits. Ethanol (= ethyl alcohol = "alcohol"; ORG 6.1) and water are each pure substances and each have a fixed composition, C_2H_5OH and H_2O, but mixtures of the two can vary continuously in composition from almost 100% ethanol to almost 100% water. Solutions of sucrose in water, however, are limited to a maximum percentage of sucrose - the solubility - which is 67% at 20 °C, thus the solution is *saturated*. If the solution is heated, a higher concentration of sucrose can be achieved (i.e. 70%). Slowly cooling down to 20 °C creates a *supersaturated* solution which may *precipitate* (turn to solid) with any perturbation.

Intermolecular forces (*see* CHM 4.2), amongst various other parameters, may either promote or may prevent the formation of a solution. The formation of solutions primarily involves the breaking of intermolecular forces between solutes and between solvents, and the subsequent reformation of new intermolecular interactions amongst the solute and solvent. The initial step in solution formation (i.e. the breakage of intermolecular forces amongst the solutes and solvent, separately) is *endothermic* (requires energy) and the second step (i.e. reformation of intermolecular interactions between solute-solvent) is *exothermic* (releases energy). If an overall reaction in solution formation is exothermic, the new intermolecular bonds between solute and solvent are more stable and a solution is formed. {"enthalpy" is a measure of the total energy; *see* CHM 8.1, 8.2.}

In the energetic requirements of solution formation, the solution may result in either an increase or a decrease in the enthalpy of solution depending on the magnitude of interactions between the solute and solvent. Hence, energy changes do occur when a solution forms (i.e. exothermic or endothermic). An increase in enthalpy, a positive heat of solution, results in more energy in a system, thus less stable and weaker bonds. Whereas a decrease in enthalpy, a negative heat of solution, results in less energy in a system, meaning more stable and stronger bonds, and thus the respective drive to the formation of a solution.

Lastly, the formation of a solution always results in an increase in *entropy* or disorder due to the insidious tendency for energy to disperse.

Generally, the component of a solution that is stable in the same phase as the solution is called the solvent. If two components of a solution are in the same phase, the component present in the larger amount is called the solvent and the other is called the solute. Many properties of solutions are dependent only on the relative number of molecules (or ions) of the solute and of the solvent. Properties that depend **only** on the number of particles present and not the kind of particles are called *colligative properties*. For all colligative properties, a factor known as the Van't Hoff factor (i) is essentially required and defined as, the ratio of moles of particles or ions in a solution to the moles of all undissociated formula units (or molecules) within a solution. The factor (i) is therefore incorporated as a multiple of all the colligative properties equations, respectively. Thus, for non-ionic solutions, the factor (i) is essentially equal to 1 as the particles are undissociated, such as for sugar solutions. However, for ionic solutions, the factor (i) is dependent on the number of ions dissociated in solution (i.e., $NaCl = 2$, $CaCl_2 = 3$, etc.). The most important colligative properties can be found in the following sections.

5.1.1 Vapor-Pressure Lowering (Raoult's Law)

Kitchen chemistry: The more I dissolve sugar in my morning coffee, the less steam there is (= *less vapor* = *vapor pressure lowers*; full disclosure: my coffee tastes like syrup!). Now we need to develop a mathematical model to express the coffee experience of future diabetics.

Experimentally, it can be observed that when dissolving a solute which cannot evaporate (= *nonvolatile*) into a solvent, the vapor pressure of the resulting solution is lower than that of the pure solvent. The extent to which the vapor pressure is lowered in an ideal solution is determined by the amount of solute added, which is expressed by the mole fraction of the solvent in solution ($X_{solvent}$):

$$P = P^{\circ} X_{solvent}$$

where P = vapor pressure of solution

P° = vapor pressure of pure solvent (at the same temperature as P).

When rearranged this way, the vapor pressure at the surface of a solution is quantified by: Raoult's law, which states that the lowering of the vapor pressure of the solvent is proportional to the mole fraction of the solvent and independent of the chemical nature of the solute.

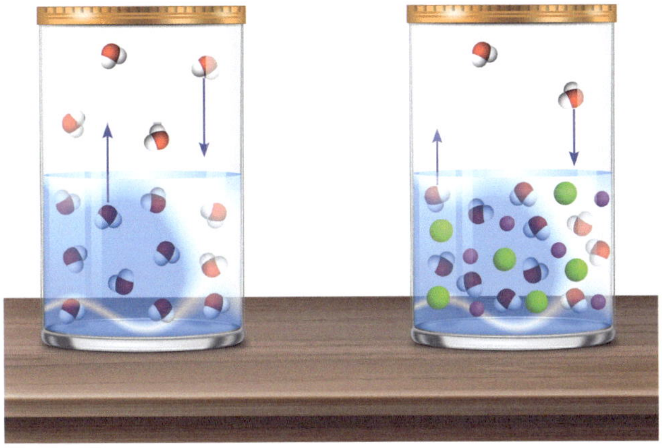

Figure III.A.5.0: Raoult's law. On the left, the most famous solvent in all of the sciences: water. It is in an enclosed container (not unlike a water bottle), and so a *dynamic equilibrium* exists: Some water molecules have enough energy to enter the vapor phase (cf. Maxwell's distribution plot; CHM 4.1.2), while others condense to liquid, but the level of the liquid remains unchanged. On the right, the *solute* salt (NaCl) dissolves in the *solvent* water thereby producing a salt-water *solution*. The salt interferes with the evaporating water, so there is less vapor, thus the vapor pressure is reduced.

5.1.2 Boiling-Point Elevation and Freezing-Point Depression

When the vapor-pressure curve of a dilute solution and the vapor-pressure curve of the pure solvent are plotted on a phase diagram (*see* Figure III.A.5.1), it can be seen that a vapor pressure lowering of a solution occurs at all temperatures and that the freezing point and boiling point of a solution must therefore be different from those of the pure liquid.

The freezing point of a pure solvent (water) is lowered or depressed with the addition of another substance; meaning that a solution (solvent + solute) has a lower freezing point than a pure solvent, and this phenomenon is called a *freezing point depression*. Alternatively, the boiling point of a pure solvent (water) is elevated when another substance is added; meaning that a solution has a higher boiling point than a pure solvent, and this phenomenon is called *boiling point elevation*. The boiling point is therefore higher for the solution than for the pure liquid, and the freezing point is lower for the solution than for the pure liquid. Since the decrease in vapor

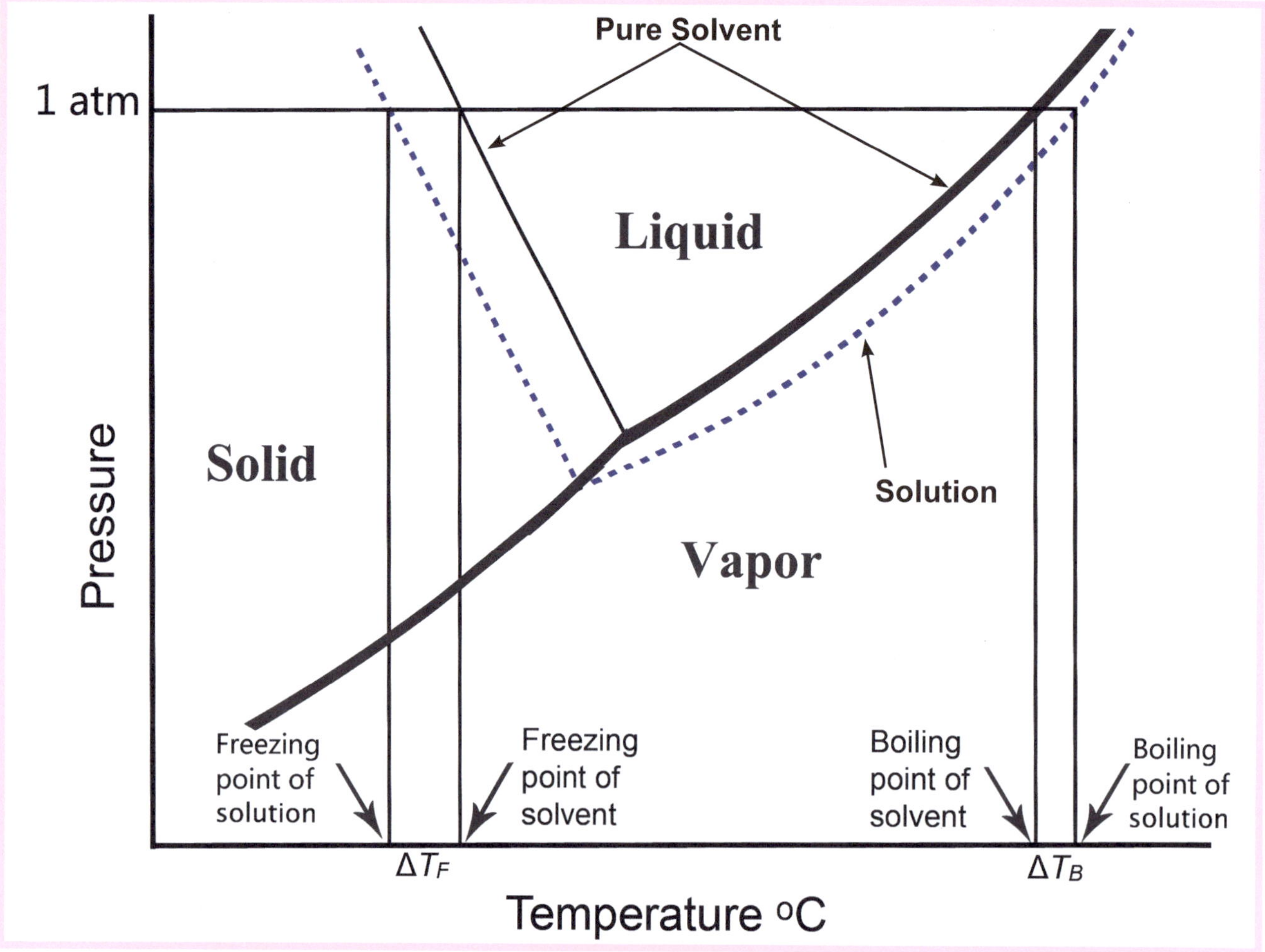

Figure III.A.5.1: Phase diagram of water demonstrating the effect of the addition of a solute.

pressure is proportional to the mole fraction (*see* CHM 5.3.1) of solute, the boiling point elevation (ΔT_B) is also proportional to the mole fraction of solute and:

$$\Delta T_B = i\,K_B'X_B = i\,K_B m$$

where K_B' = boiling point elevation constant for the solvent

X_B = mole fraction of solute

m = *molality* (moles solute per kilogram of solvent; CHM 5.3.1)

i = Van't Hoff factor

K_B is related to K_B' through a change of units.

Similarly, for the freezing point depression (ΔT_F):

$$\Delta T_F = i\,K_F'X_B = i\,K_F m$$

where K_F' = freezing point depression constant for the solvent.

If K_F or K_B is known, it is then possible to determine the molality of a dilute solution simply by measuring the freezing point or the boiling point. These constants can be determined by measuring the freezing point and boiling point of a solution of known molality. If the mass concentration of a solute (in kg solute per kg of solvent) is known and the molality is determined from the freezing point of the solution, the mass of 1 mole of solute can be calculated.

It is important to recall that for a strong electrolyte solution such as NaCl, which dissociates to positive and negative ions, the right-hand side of the equation is multiplied by the Van't Hoff factor (i) equal to the number of ionic species generated per mole of solute. For NaCl, n = 2 but for $MgCl_2$, n = 3. {Remember: colligative properties depend on the **number** of particles present}

5.1.3 Osmotic Pressure

The osmotic pressure (Π) of a solution describes the equilibrium distribution of solvent across semipermeable membranes separated by two compartments. When a solvent and solution are separated by a membrane permeable only to molecules of solvent (a <u>semipermeable</u> membrane), the solvent spontaneously migrates into the solution. The semipermeable membrane allows the solvent to pass but not the solute. Since pure solute cannot pass through the semipermeable membrane into the pure solvent side to equalise the concentrations, the pure solvent begins to then move into the solution side containing the solute. As it does so, the solution level rises and the pressure increases. Eventually a balance is achieved and the increased pressure difference on the solution side is the osmotic pressure. The solvent therefore migrates into the solution across the membrane until a sufficient hydrostatic pressure develops to prevent further migration of solvent. The pressure required to prevent migration of the solvent is there-

High-level Importance

fore the osmotic pressure of the solution and is equal to:

$$\Pi = i\,MRT$$

where R = gas constant per mole
T = temperature in kelvin (K)
M = concentration of solute (mole/litre)
i = Van't Hoff factor

Note: molarity (M) is used in the osmotic pressure formulation in place of molality as is used for the other respective colligative properties as molarity is temperature dependent and molality is not temperature dependent.

Osmosis and osmotic pressure are also discussed in the context of GAMSAT Biology in the following sections: BIO 1.1.1 and 7.5.2.

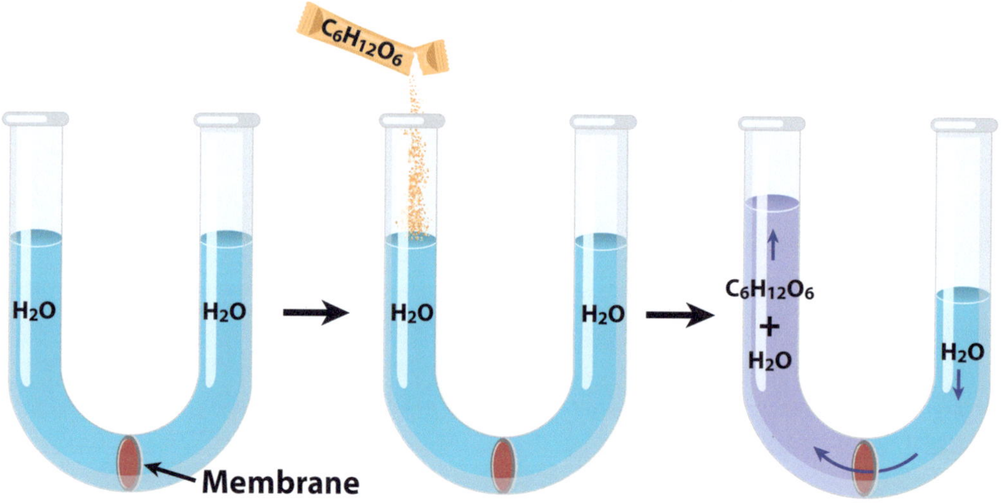

Figure III.A.5.2: Osmosis and osmotic pressure with glucose in water.

5.2 Ions in Solution

An important area of solution chemistry involves aqueous solutions. The word "aqueous" simply means containing or dissolved in water. Water has a particular property that causes many substances to split apart into charged species, that is, to dissociate and form ions. Ions that are positively charged are called cations and negatively charged ions are called anions. {Mnemonic: anions **a**re **n**egative **ions**} As a rule, highly charged species (i.e. $AlPO_4$, Al^{3+}/PO_4^{3-}) have a greater force of attraction, thus are much less soluble in water than species with little charge (i.e. NaCl, Na^+/Cl^-). All the following ions can form in water.

Common Anions					
F^-	Fluoride	OH^-	Hydroxide	ClO^-	Hypochlorite
Cl^-	Chloride	NO_3^-	Nitrate	ClO_2^-	Chlorite
Br^-	Bromide	NO_2^-	Nitrite	ClO_3^-	Chlorate
I^-	Iodide	CO_3^{2-}	Carbonate	ClO_4^-	Perchlorate
O^{2-}	Oxide	SO_4^{2-}	Sulfate	SO_3^{2-}	Sulfite
S^{2-}	Sulfide	PO_4^{3-}	Phosphate	CN^-	Cyanide
N^{3-}	Nitride	$CH_3CO_2^-$	Acetate	MnO_4^-	Permanganate

Common Cations			
Na^+	Sodium	H^+	Hydrogen
Li^+	Lithium	Ca^{2+}	Calcium
K^+	Potassium	Mg^{2+}	Magnesium
NH_4^+	Ammonium	Fe^{2+}	Iron (II)
H_3O^+	Hydronium	Fe^{3+}	Iron (III)

Table III.A.5.1: Common Anions and Cations.

As opposed to Organic Chemistry, the GAMSAT does not normally ask Inorganic Chemistry nomenclature (= *naming*) questions but it may be useful to have some background regarding the International Union of Pure and Applied Chemistry (IUPAC) standard suffixes: **(1)** Single atom anions are named with an *-ide suffix* (i.e. fluoride); **(2)** Oxyanions (*polyatomic* or "many atom" anions containing oxygen) are named with *-ite* or *-ate*, for a lesser or greater quantity of oxygen. For example, NO_2^- is nitrite, while NO_3^- is nitrate. The hypo- and per- prefixes can also indicate less oxygen and more oxygen, respectively (*see* hypochlorite and perchlorate among the Common Anions in Table III.A.5.1). **(3)** -ium is a very common ending of atoms in the periodic table (CHM 2.3), and it is also common among cations; **(4)** Compounds with cations: The name of the compound is simply the cation's name (usually the same as the element's), followed by the anion. For example, NaCl is *sodium chloride* and Ca_3N_2 is *calcium nitride*.

5.3 Solubility

High-level Importance

The solubility of any substance is generally defined as the amount of the substance (solute) known to dissolve into a particular amount of solvent at a given temperature. The solubility of a solute into a solvent is dependent on the entropy change of solubilisation as well as the types of intermolecular forces involved (*see* CHM 4.2 and 5.1). *Solvation* or *dissolution* is the process of interaction between solute and solvent molecules. This process occurs when the intermolecular forces between solute and solvent are stronger than those between solute particles themselves. Generally, ionic and polar solutes are soluble in polar solvents and nonpolar solutes are soluble in nonpolar solvents. Consequently, the expression "like dissolves like" is often used for predicting solubility.

In the following section, the definitions of the various solution concentration units are given with examples.

5.3.1 Units of Concentration

In the sections to follow, where possible, please try to complete the calculations as quickly as possible prior to looking at the solutions (i.e. apply dimensional analysis; GM 2.2).

There are a number of ways in which solution concentrations may be expressed.

Molarity (*M*): A one-molar solution is defined as one mole of substance in each litre of solution: M = moles of solute/litre of solution (solution = solute + solvent).

For example: If 55.0 g of $CaCl_2$ (*calcium chloride*) is mixed with water to make 500.0 mL (0.5 L) of solution, approximate the molarity (*M*) of the solution (note the relative atomic masses, amu: Cl = 35.5, Ca = 40).

55.0 g of $CaCl_2$ = 55.0 g/110 g/mol
= 0.50 mol of $CaCl_2$

Therefore, the molarity = 0.50 mol $CaCl_2$/0.5 L = 1.0 mol $CaCl_2$/L solution. Chemists use square brackets as a symbol for molarity in moles/litre (= mol/L); for $CaCl_2$, [1.0].

Normality (*N*): A one-normal solution contains one equivalent per litre. An equivalent is a mole multiplied by the number of reacting units for each molecule or atom; the equivalent weight is the formula weight divided by the number of reacting units.

# of Equiv. = mass (in g)/eq. wt. (in g/equiv.)
= Normality (in equiv./litre)
× Volume (in litres)

For example, sulfuric acid, H_2SO_4, has two reacting units of protons ($2H^+$; CHM 6.1), that is, there are two equivalents of protons in each mole. Thus:

eq. wt. = 98.08 g/mole/2 equiv./mole
= 49.04 g/equiv.

and the normality of a sulfuric acid solution is twice its molarity. Generally speaking:

$$N = n\,M$$

where *N* is the normality,
M the molarity,
n the number of equivalents per unit formula.

Thus for 1.2 M H_2SO_4:

1.2 moles/L × 2 eq/mole = 2.4 eq/L = 2.4 N.

Molality (*m*): A one-molal solution contains one mole/1000 g of solvent.

m = moles of solute/kg of solvent.

For example: If 20.0 g of NaOH is mixed into 500.0 g (0.50 kg) of water, what is the molality of the solution?

20.0 g of NaOH = 20.0 g/40.0 g/mol
= 0.500 mol of NaOH

Therefore, the molality = 0.500 mol NaOH/0.50 kg water = 1.0 mol NaOH/kg water.

Molal concentrations are not temperature-dependent as molar and normal concentrations are (since the solvent volume is temperature-dependent).

Density (ρ): Mass per unit volume at the specified temperature, usually g/mL or g/cm^3 or g/L. Density of liquid water: approx. 1 g/mL = 1000 kg/m^3.

Osmole (*Osm*): The number of moles of particles (molecules or ions) that contribute to the osmotic pressure of a solution.

Osmolarity: A one-osmolar solution is defined as one osmole in each litre of solution. Osmolarity is measured in osmoles/litre of solution (Osm/L).

For example, a 0.001 *M* solution of sodium chloride has an osmolarity of 0.002 Osm/L (*twice the molarity*), because each NaCl molecule ionises in water to form two ions (Na^+ and Cl^-) that both contribute to the osmotic pressure.

Osmolality: A one-osmolal solution is defined as one osmole in each kilogram of solvent. Osmolality is measured in osmoles/kilogram of solvent (Osm/kg).

For example, the osmolality of a 0.01 molal solution of Na_2SO_4 (*sodium sulfate*) is 0.03 Osm/kg because each molecule of Na_2SO_4 ionises in water to give three ions (2 Na^+ and 1 SO_4^{2-}) that contribute to the osmotic pressure.

Mole Fraction: Is expressed as a mole ratio as the amount of solute (in moles) divided by the total amount of solvent and solute (in moles).

For example: If 110.0 g of $CaCl_2$ is mixed with 72.0 g water, approximate the mole fractions of the two components (note the relative atomic masses, amu: H = 1.0, O = 16.0, Cl = 35.5, Ca − 40).

72.0 g of H_2O = 72.0 g/18.0 g/mol
= 4 mol H_2O

110.0 g of $CaCl_2$ = 110.0 g/110 g/mol
= 1 mol $CaCl_2$

Total mol = 4 mol H_2O + 1 mol $CaCl_2$
= 5 mol (H_2O and $CaCl_2$)

Therefore,
$X(CaCl_2)$ = 1 mol $CaCl_2$/5 mol $CaCl_2$ + H_2O = 0.2
and
X(water) = 4 mol H_2O/5 mol H_2O + $CaCl_2$ = 0.8

Note that mole fractions are dimensionless, and the sum of all mole fractions in a given mixture is always equal to 1 (CHM 4.1.9).

Dilution: When solvent is added to a solution containing a certain concentration of solute, it becomes diluted to produce a solution of a lower solute concentration. The equation representing this is:

$$M_iV_i = M_fV_f$$

Where M = molarity and
V = volume with the initial (i) and final (f) concentrations being measured.

For example: How many mL of a 10.0 mol/L NaOH solution is needed to prepare 500 mL of a 2.00 mol/L NaOH solution?

Given: $M_iV_i = M_fV_f$, where M_i = 10.0 mol/L, M_f = 2.00 mol/L and V_f = 500 mL. Therefore, rearranging the equation gives $V_i = M_f \times V_f/M_i$ and so V_i = (2.00 mol/L)(0.5 L)/(10.0 mol/L) = 100 mL.

5.3.2 Solubility Product Constant, the Equilibrium Expression

Any solute that dissolves in water to give a solution that contains ions, and thus can conduct electricity, is an *electrolyte*. The solid (s) that dissociates into separate ions surrounded by water is hydrated, thus the ions are aqueous (*aq*).

If dissociation is extensive and irreversible (*symbolised below by an arrow pointing in only one direction*), we have a strong electrolyte:

$$NaCl\ (s) \rightarrow Na^+\ (aq) + Cl^-\ (aq)$$

If dissociation is incomplete and reversible (*symbolised below by a double-sided arrow*), we have a weak electrolyte:

$$CH_3COOH\ (aq) \rightleftharpoons CH_3COO^-\ (aq) + H^+\ (aq)$$

If dissociation does not occur, we have a nonelectrolyte:

$C_6H_{12}O_6$ (aq) or glucose (*a 'sugar' or carbohydrate*) does NOT dissociate.

Strong electrolytes: salts (NaCl), strong acids (HCl), strong bases (NaOH).

Weak electrolytes: weak acids (CH_3COOH), weak bases (NH_3), complexes ($Fe[CN]_6$), tap water, certain soluble organic compounds, highly-charged species (CHM 5.2; $AlPO_4$, $BaSO_4$; exception: AgCl as it is a precipitate in aqueous solutions).

Nonelectrolytes: deionised water, soluble organic compounds (sugars).

The solubility of a solute is the maximum amount of solute that can be dissolved in an appropriate solvent at a particular temperature. It can be expressed in units of concentration such as molarity, molality and so on (*see* CHM 5.3.1). When a maximum amount of solute has been dissolved, the solution is in equilibrium and is said to be saturated. As temperature increases, the solubility of most salts generally increases. However, it is the opposite for gases, as the solubility of gases is known to generally decrease as temperature increases. {*Example: A carbonated drink loses its fizz as it warms up.*}

When substances have limited solubility and their solubility is exceeded, the ions of the dissolved portion exist in equilibrium with the solid material. When a compound is referred to as insoluble, it is not completely insoluble, but is slightly soluble. *We will now examine slightly or sparingly soluble compounds.*

For example, if solid silver chloride (AgCl) is added to water, a very small portion will dissolve:

$$AgCl\ (s) \rightleftharpoons Ag^+\ (aq) + Cl^-\ (aq)$$

The precipitate (*the solid component*) will have a definite solubility (i.e. a definite amount in g/litre) or molar solubility (in moles/litre) that will dissolve at a given temperature.

An overall equilibrium constant can be written for the preceding equilibrium, called the solubility product, K_{sp}, given by the following equilibrium expression (note that the square brackets refer to concentration in mol/L):

$$K_{sp} = [Ag^+][Cl^-]$$

In general, each concentration must be raised to the power of that ion's coefficient in the dissolving equation (in our example = 1). A different example would be Ag_2S which would have the following solubility product expression: $K_{sp} = [Ag^+]^2[S^{2-}]$. The calculation of molar solubility s in mol/L for AgCl would simply be: $K_{sp} = [s][s] = s^2$. On the other hand, the expression for Ag_2S would become: $K_{sp} = [2s]^2[s] = 4s^3$.

Knowing K_{sp} at a specified temperature, the molar solubility of compounds can be calculated under various conditions. The amount of slightly soluble salt that dissolves does not depend on the amount of the solid in equilibrium with the solution, as long as there is enough to saturate the solution. Rather, it depends on the volume of solvent. {Note: a low K_{sp} value means little product therefore low solubility and vice-versa}.

The following are examples of problems on solubility product constant and solubility calculations given one or the other.

The molar solubility of $PbCl_2$ in an aqueous solution is 0.0159 M. What is the K_{sp} for $PbCl_2$?

$$PbCl_2(s) \rightleftharpoons Pb^{2+}\ (aq) + 2Cl^-(aq)$$
$$K_{sp} = [Pb^{2+}][Cl^-]^2$$

For every mol of $PbCl_2$ that dissociates, one mol of Pb^{2+} and two mol of Cl^- are produced. Since the molar solubility is 0.0159 M, $[Pb^{2+}] = 0.0159$ M and $[Cl^-] = 0.0159 \times 2 = 0.0318$ M.

Therefore,

$$K_{sp} = [0.0159][0.0318]^2 = 1.61 \times 10^{-5}$$

Another example: What are the concentrations of each of the ions in a saturated solution of Ag_2CrO_4 given that solubility product constant K_{sp} is 1.1×10^{-12}?

$$Ag_2CrO_4(s) \rightleftharpoons 2Ag^+\ (aq) + CrO_4^{2-}\ (aq)$$
$$K_{sp} = [Ag^+]^2\ [CrO_4^{2-}]$$

For every Ag_2CrO_4 that dissociates, two mol of Ag^+ ion and one mol of CrO_4^{2-} ion are produced.

Let x = concentration of CrO_4^{2-}, then 2x = concentration of Ag^+

Therefore,

$$K_{sp} = [2x]^2\,[x]$$
$$1.1 \times 10^{-12} = [2x]^2\,[x]$$

solving for x gives; $x = 6.50 \times 10^{-5}$ M

so,

$$[Ag^+] = 1.3 \times 10^{-4} \text{ M and}$$
$$[CrO_4^{2-}] = 6.5 \times 10^{-5} \text{ M}$$

"If you're not part of the solution, you're part of the precipitate!" :)

5.3.3 Common-ion Effect on Solubility

If there is an excess of one ion over the other, the concentration of the other is suppressed. This is called the common-ion effect. The solubility of the precipitate is decreased and the concentration can still be calculated from the K_{sp}.

For example, Cl^- ion can be precipitated out of a solution of AgCl by adding a slight excess of $AgNO_3$. If a stoichiometric amount of $AgNO_3$ is added, $[Ag^+] = [Cl^-]$. If excess $AgNO_3$ is added, $[Ag^+] > [Cl^-]$ but K_{sp} remains constant. Therefore, $[Cl^-]$ decreases if $[Ag^+]$ is increased. Because the K_{sp} product always holds, precipitation will not take place unless the product of $[Ag^+]$ and $[Cl^-]$ exceeds the K_{sp}. If the product is just equal to K_{sp}, all the Ag^+ and Cl^- ions would remain in solution. Thus, the solubility of an ionic compound in solution containing a common ion is decreased in comparison to the same compound's solubility in water.

As another example, the solubility of CaF_2 in water at 25 °C would be much larger in comparison to the solubility of the same CaF_2 compound in a solution containing a common ion such as NaF. This decrease in solubility of CaF_2 in a solution containing NaF would be due to the common fluoride (F^-) ion effect on the solubility of CaF_2.

5.3.4 Solubility Product Constant (K_{sp}) vs. Reaction Quotient (Q_{sp})

Solubility product constants are used to describe saturated solutions of ionic compounds of relatively low solubility. A saturated solution is in a state of dynamic equilibrium described by the equilibrium constant (K_{sp}).

$$M_xA_y(s) \leftrightarrow x\,M^{y+}(aq) + y\,A^{x-}(aq)$$

The solubility product constant $K_{sp} = [M^{y+}]^x[A^{x-}]^y$ in a solution at equilibrium (saturated solution). Note that "M" is meant to symbolise the metal and "A" represents the anion. Also note how the superscripts in the ions match the subscripts in the reactant (*drop and swap*; CHM 3.1.1).

A reaction quotient is defined by the same formula: $Q_{sp} = [M^{y+}]^x [A^{x-}]^y$ in a solution at any point, not just equilibrium.

K_{sp} therefore represents the ion product at equilibrium while Q_{sp} represents the ion product at any point, not just at equilibrium; and in fact, equilibrium is just a special case of the reaction coefficient as we will see below:

If $Q_{sp} < K_{sp}$, the solution is unsaturated and no precipitate will form.

If $Q_{sp} = K_{sp}$, the solution is saturated and at equilibrium.

If $Q_{sp} > K_{sp}$, the solution is supersaturated and unstable. A solid salt will precipitate until ion product once again equals to K_{sp}.

5.3.5 Solubility Rules

The chemistry of aqueous solutions is such that solubility rules can be established:

1. All salts of alkali metals are soluble.
2. All salts of the ammonium ion are soluble.
3. All chlorides, bromides and iodides are water soluble, with the exception of Ag^+, Pb^{2+}, and Hg_2^{2+}.
4. All salts of the sulfate ion (SO_4^{2-}) are water soluble with the exception of Ca^{2+}, Sr^{2+}, Ba^{2+}, and Pb^{2+}.
5. All metal oxides are insoluble with the exception of the alkali metals and CaO, SrO and BaO.
6. All hydroxides are insoluble with the exception of the alkali metals and Ca^{2+}, Sr^{2+}, Ba^{2+}.
7. All carbonates (CO_3^{2-}), phosphates (PO_4^{3-}), sulfides (S^{2-}) and sulfites (SO_3^{2-}) are insoluble, with the exception of the alkali metals and ammonium.

We do not suggest that you memorise the solubility rules. The rules should, however, confirm what you have been seeing regarding the common substances that have been presented in this chapter like sodium chloride, calcium chloride, sodium sulfate, sodium hydroxide, silver chloride, strong vs. weak electrolytes, etc. It is expected that you are familiar with the solubility of the common substances and, if reminded of the rules during an exam (or practice), that you can apply those rules to more unfamiliar substances.

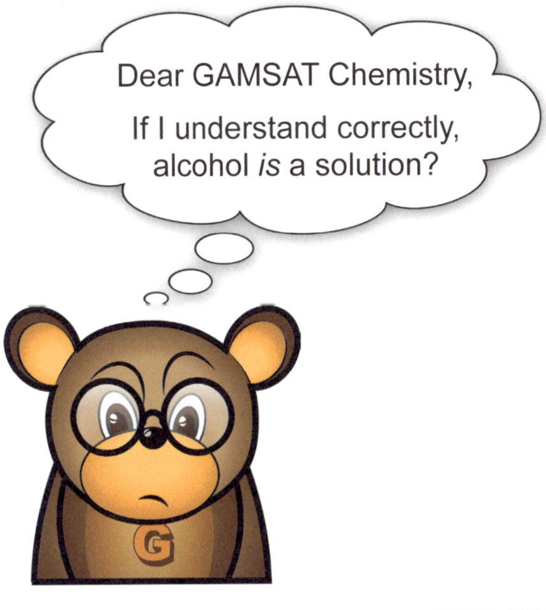

High-level Importance

CHAPTER 5: Solution Chemistry

GOLD STANDARD FOUNDATIONAL GAMSAT PRACTICE QUESTIONS

1) In the water molecule:

A. unequal sharing of electrons results in a polar molecule.
B. the polarity of the molecule causes it to cling to other water molecules.
C. the oxygen molecule is more electronegative than the hydrogens.
D. All of the above are correct.

2) Which solution is the most concentrated?

A. 1 mole of solute dissolved in 1 litre of solution
B. 2 moles of solute dissolved in 3 litres of solution
C. 6 moles of solute dissolved in 4 litres of solution
D. 4 moles of solute dissolved in 8 litres of solution

3) In 0.20 M Na_2CrO_4, the ion concentrations are likely to be which of the following?

	$[Na^+]$	$[CrO_4^{2-}]$
A	0.40 M	0.20 M
B	0.20 M	0.20 M
C	0.20 M	0.40 M
D	0.40 M	0.80 M

4) How are the boiling and freezing points of a sample of water affected when salt is dissolved in the water?

A. The boiling point decreases and the freezing point decreases.
B. The boiling point decreases and the freezing point increases.
C. The boiling point increases and the freezing point decreases.
D. The boiling point increases and the freezing point increases.

5) At constant temperature, what is the effect of an increase in pressure on a liquid-gas equilibrium mixture?

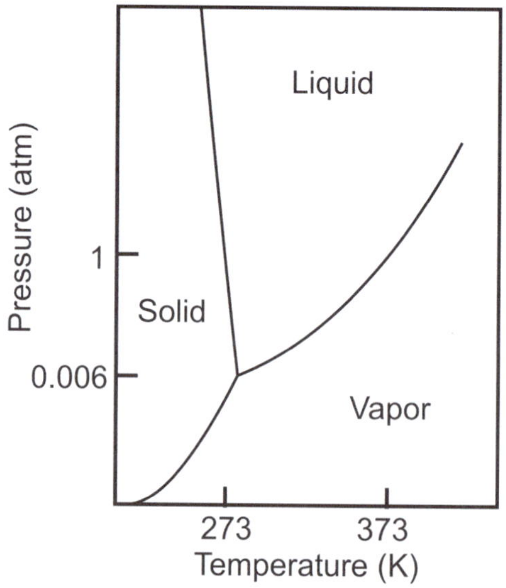

A. Increase in vapor pressure
B. Decrease hydrogen bonding
C. Increase in amount of gas present
D. Increase in amount of liquid present

6) Consider the three beakers labelled I, II and III. Each beaker contains a different volume of a saturated solution of PbI_2 and a different mass of the solid precipitate PbI_2.

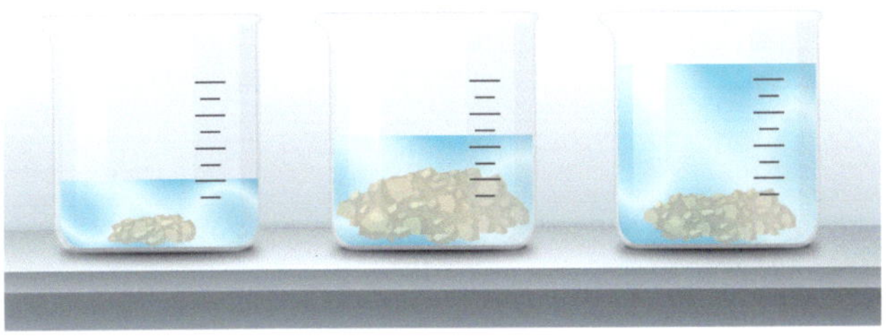

What is the relationship between $[Pb^{2+}]$ in solution in the three beakers?

A. I = II = III
B. I > II > III
C. II > III > I
D. III > II > I

7) The solubility product constants for three zinc compounds are given below. Which of these compounds is LEAST soluble?

$K_{sp}ZnCO_3$	$K_{sp}ZnC_2O_4$	$K_{sp}ZnS$
2.1×10^{-11}	2.5×10^{-9}	8×10^{-25}

A. ZnC_2O_4
B. ZnS
C. $ZnCO_3$
D. Cannot be determined without knowing the concentrations of the solutions involved.

8) Which of the following is the expression for the solubility product constant of the reaction below?

$$H_2CO_3 + H_2O \rightarrow H_3O^+ + HCO_3^-$$

A. $K_{sp} = [HCO_3^-][H_3O^+] / [H_2CO_3]$
B. $K_{sp} = [HCO_3^-][H_3O^+]$
C. $K_{sp} = [H_2CO_3] / [HCO_3^-][H_3O^+]$
D. $K_{sp} = [H_2CO_3] / [H_3O^+]$

9) Magnesium sulfate is added to a solution that is 10^{-4} M in each of the ions F^- and CO_3^{2-} until the Mg^{2+} concentration is also 10^{-4} M. Which of the following salts would be expected to precipitate from the final mixture?

Note that: K_{sp} $MgF_2 = 10^{-8}$; K_{sp} $MgCO_3 = 10^{-5}$

A. $MgCO_3$ only
B. MgF_2 only
C. Neither MgF_2 nor $MgCO_3$
D. Both MgF_2 and $MgCO_3$

10) A 1.0 M solution of sucrose freezes at –1.64 °C. What will be the freezing point of the solution after complete hydrolysis (i.e.: when sucrose is digested, it is hydrolysed to form glucose and fructose)?

A. –0.82 °C
B. –1.64 °C
C. –3.28 °C
D. The freezing point constant for water is needed in order to answer correctly.

High-level Importance

GOLD STANDARD GAMSAT-LEVEL PRACTICE QUESTIONS

11) What would be the expected change in terms of the solubility of a gas when a solution containing the gas is heated, and when a solution containing the gas has the pressure over the solution decreased, respectively?

A. Increase, increase
B. Increase, decrease
C. Decrease, increase
D. Decrease, decrease

12) Hard water is water that has a high mineral content, largely made up of calcium and magnesium carbonates, bicarbonates and sulfates. Consider the following graph of the ionic content of a water sample.

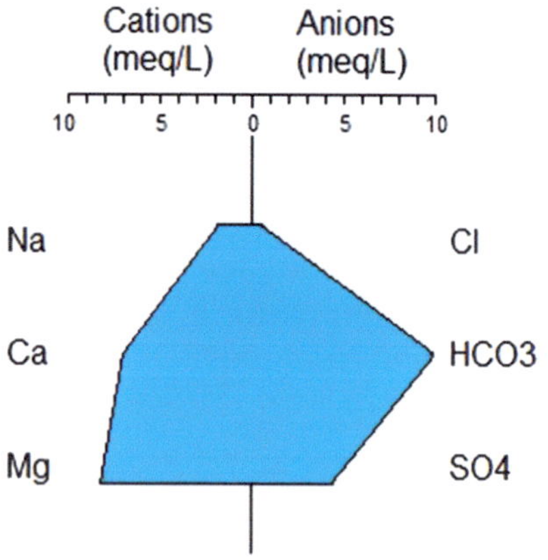

Figure 1: Concentrations of major ions in a water sample

Total hardness (TH) of the water is the sum of the concentration of calcium and magnesium ions. What is the TH of the water sample in Figure 1?

A. Between 5 and 9 meq/L
B. Between 9 and 12 meq/L
C. More than 12 meq/L
D. Exactly equal to the anionic concentration

13) Suppose that the vapor pressure of pure benzene at room temperature is measured as P_B. A nonvolatile substance is dissolved in the benzene, and P_s, the vapor pressure of the solution, is measured. Which of the following is true?

A. $P_B > P_s$
B. Cannot be determined from the information provided.
C. $P_B = P_s$
D. $P_B < P_s$

Questions 14–19

Solubility is the property of a solid, liquid or gaseous chemical substance called the 'solute' to dissolve in a solid, liquid or gaseous substance called the 'solvent' thus forming a 'solution'.

Consider Table 1.

Saturated Solution	A solution with solute that dissolves until it is unable to dissolve anymore, leaving the undissolved substances (the precipitate) - if any - at the bottom.
Unsaturated Solution	A solution (*with less solute than the saturated solution*) that completely dissolves, leaving no remaining substances.
Supersaturated Solution	A solution (*with more solute than the saturated solution*) that contains more dissolved solute than the saturated solution.

Table 1

A curve line drawn on a graph illustrating the relationship between temperature, and the solubility at saturation of the substance at different temperatures, is called a *solubility curve*. Consider the following solubility curves.

Note that the density of liquid water is 1 g/mL.

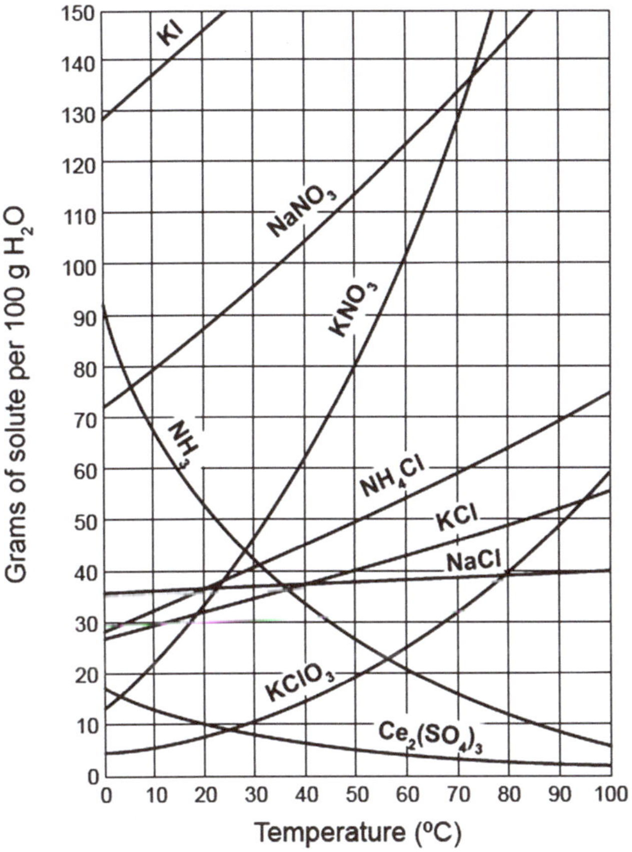

Figure 1

14) A researcher dissolved 30 g of an unknown compound in 50 mL of water at 38 °C to just achieve saturation. Based on Figure 1, which of the following is the most likely candidate for the unknown compound?

A. NH_3
B. KCl
C. KNO_3
D. NaCl

15) A saturated solution of KCl is formed in 250 grams of water. If the saturated solution is cooled from 85 °C to 30 °C, how many grams of KCl precipitate will form?

A. 15 g
B. 37.5 g
C. 42.5 g
D. 87.5 g

16) Which of the following phases dissolved in water can best be inferred to explain the difference in the solubility curves in Figure 1 for ammonia (NH_3) and ammonium chloride (NH_4Cl), respectively?

A. Liquid, solid
B. Solid, liquid
C. Solid, gas
D. Gas, solid

17) Conductivity of a substance relates - in part - to its ability to conduct or transmit electricity. Based on Figure 1, which of the following would result in the greatest increase in conductivity of a saturated solution at 0 °C as compared to a saturated solution at 20 °C?

A. NaCl
B. KI
C. $NaNO_3$
D. KNO_3

18) Which of the following represents an unsaturated solution once thoroughly mixed with 100 g of water?

A. 80 g of KNO_3 at 50 °C
B. 15 g of $KClO_3$ at 31 °C
C. 119 g of $NaNO_3$ at 60 °C
D. Neither **A** nor **B** nor **C** is unsaturated.

19) A solution of 50 grams of KCl in 100 g of H_2O at 85 °C was very slowly cooled to 60 °C without any precipitate formed. The conversion of the original solution to the new solution can best be described as which of the following?

A. Unsaturated to saturated
B. Unsaturated to supersaturated
C. Saturated to unsaturated
D. Saturated to supersaturated

Questions 20–23

A piper plot is often used to visualise the chemistry of a rock, soil, or water samples. There are 3 components: a ternary (or triangular) diagram in the lower left representing the 3 cations, a ternary diagram in the lower right representing the 3 anions, and a diamond plot (or 'trapezoid') in the middle representing a combination of the two. Note that following a line parallel to the outer axis of each ternary diagram, and projecting each point in the ternary diagrams upward until they intersect will create one the associated point in the diamond plot. These three points represent one sample. The procedure is repeated for other samples.

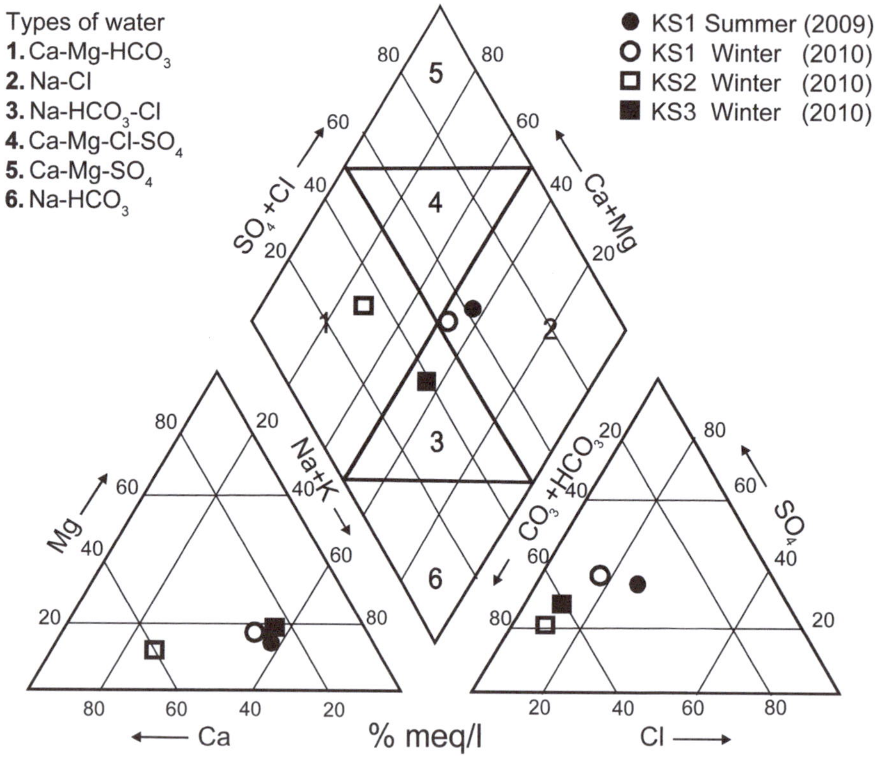

Figure 1: Piper diagram of well-water samples. (Ref. Journal of Water Resource and Protection Vol.4 No.5, 2012, Article ID:19469, 13 pages; DOI:10.4236/jwarp.2012.45032)

Note that:

- The water types are labelled in regions of the diamond-shaped graph as **1**, **2**, **3**, **4**, **5** and **6**.
- The ionic charges of the various species do not have to be taken into account for any of the calculations.
- All percentages refer to: % meq/l.

20) According to Figure 1, what is the approximate percentage of sodium and potassium in KS1 Summer?

A. 20%
B. 55%
C. 65%
D. 80%

21) A KS4 Winter sample was taken that is not shown in Figure 1 with the following results... Ca: 38%, Cl: 32%, SO_4: 59%, Na and K: 35%. Determine the concentration of Mg.

A. 35%
B. 27%
C. 21%
D. 11%

22) The type of water indicated by the number 5 in the legend of Figure 1 would be expected to have less sodium and potassium than all samples except which of the following?

A. KS1 Summer
B. KS1 Winter
C. KS2 Winter
D. KS3 Winter

23) If the highest possible value of a ternary diagram is X, and the 3 component ions are a, b and c, then which of the following represents the relationship between the 4 variables?

A. $b + c = X + a$
B. $c + a = X + b$
C. $X - b - c = a$
D. $X = 2a + b + c$

Questions 24–25

As opposed to solids, gases have decreased solubility with increasing temperature. In fact, when a carbonated drink (soda/pop) is manufactured, water is chilled, optimally to just above freezing, in order to permit the maximum amount of carbon dioxide to dissolve. Then CO_2 is pumped in at high pressure, the pressure is maintained by closing the container (can or bottle), which forces the carbon dioxide to dissolve into the liquid, creating carbonic acid.

It is pressure and temperature that drive the outgassing process. Diving underwater exposes the body to increasing pressure. A diving cylinder (scuba tank) is used to store and transport high pressure breathing gas. As the dive becomes deeper, inhaled gas is absorbed into body tissue in higher concentrations than normal (Henry's Law). Surfacing from a deep dive underwater, unused gases (inert) like nitrogen try to do the same thing in your bloodstream that happens when you open a container of pop. The release of these bubbles (outgassing) produces the symptoms of decompression sickness (= 'the bends') that can be painful or even fatal.

Henry's law relates the molar concentration of a gas C (mol/L), the pressure P of the gas (atm) on the surface of the liquid, with Henry's constant k as follows:

$$C = k \cdot P$$

24) The solubility of pure oxygen in water at 20 °C and 2.00 atm pressure is 2.76×10^{-3} mole/litre. Calculate the concentration of O_2 (mole/litre) at 20 °C and a partial pressure of 0.21 atm.

A. 2.9×10^{-4} mol/L
B. 2.9×10^{-3} mol/L
C. 2.76×10^{-6} mol/L
D. 2.76×10^{-5} mol/L

Question 25 refers to the following additional information.

Oxygen is carried in the blood in two forms: (1) dissolved in plasma and red blood cell water (about 2% of the total) and (2) reversibly bound to hemoglobin (about 98% of the total).

Helium is often used to replace atmospheric nitrogen, to one degree or another, in scuba tanks - both to avoid the narcotic effect of nitrogen outgassing and because less helium than nitrogen dissolves at any given pressure. Trimix is a breathing gas, consisting of oxygen, and the two less soluble gases, helium and nitrogen.

25) Which of the following would be most consistent with the relative values for Henry's constant for helium (k_h), oxygen (k_o) and nitrogen (k_n)?

A. $k_o > k_h > k_n$
B. $k_n > k_h > k_o$
C. $k_h > k_n > k_o$
D. $k_o > k_n > k_h$

Questions 26–28

Qualitative analysis involves the distinguishing of one chemical species from another. This utilises simple techniques such as colour discrimination and complex processes such as flame analysis. Qualitative analysis must not be confused with quantitative analysis which is concerned with the amount of a certain species present. The two techniques are often used in tandem in many scientific experiments.

One of the commonly used reagents in qualitative analysis in hydrogen sulfide. This gas is notorious for being the major component in the odor of rotten eggs. The hydrogen sulfide is added as a saturated solution of hydrogen sulfide in propanone. Many different types of reactions can then occur, and these form the basis for the preliminary distinguishing of cations in solution as shown in Figure 1.

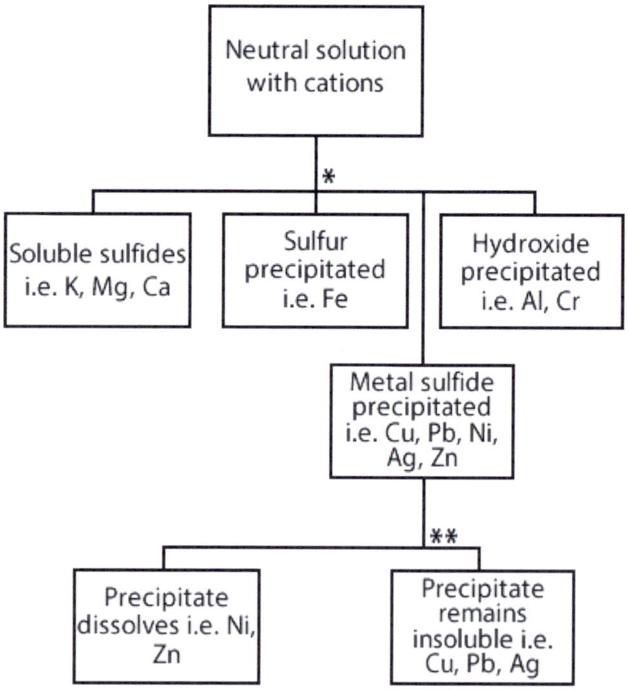

Figure 1: Qualitative analysis of cations.

* Addition of H_2S in propanone.
** Addition of acid.

26) According to Figure 1, the technique described in the passage allows one to differentiate between which of the following pairs of cations?

A. Al^{3+} and Cr^{2+}
B. Pb^{2+} and Ag^{+}
C. K^{+} and Ca^{2+}
D. Zn^{2+} and Mg^{2+}

27) Given that $K_{a1}(H_2S) = 9.1 \times 10^{-8}$, what can be inferred about PbS, CuS, and Ag_2S from Figure 1?

A. They have large solubility products.
B. They have small solubility products.
C. Their K_{sp} values are exactly the same.
D. They will not be precipitated in alkaline solution.

28) Given the following solubility product data, choose the correct order of precipitation (most likely to least likely to precipitate) of the following sulfides.

Sulfides	Solubility Product
ZnS	1.0×10^{-21}
PbS	8.0×10^{-28}
MnS	1.4×10^{-15}

A. PbS, ZnS, then MnS
B. MnS, ZnS, then PbS
C. ZnS, MnS, then PbS
D. PbS, MnS, then ZnS

Questions 29–30

Raoult's law states that the partial pressure of each component of an ideal mixture of liquids is equal to the vapor pressure of the pure component multiplied by its mole fraction in the mixture. Thus, the relative lowering of vapor pressure of a solution of with a nonvolatile solute is equal to the mole fraction of solute in the solution.

Mole fraction of A = X_A = (moles of A)/(total number of moles)

Where two volatile liquids A and B are mixed with each other to form a solution, the vapor phase consists of both components of the solution. Once the components in the solution have reached equilibrium, the total vapor pressure of the solution can be determined by combining Raoult's law with Dalton's law of partial pressures to give:

$$\text{Total } P = P_A + P_B = P_A^{o}X_A + P_B^{o}X_B$$

where P^o is the vapor pressure of the pure component.

If a non-volatile solute (*zero vapor pressure, does not evaporate*) is dissolved into a solvent to form an ideal solution, the vapor pressure of the final solution will be lower than that of the solvent.

Consider Figure 1.

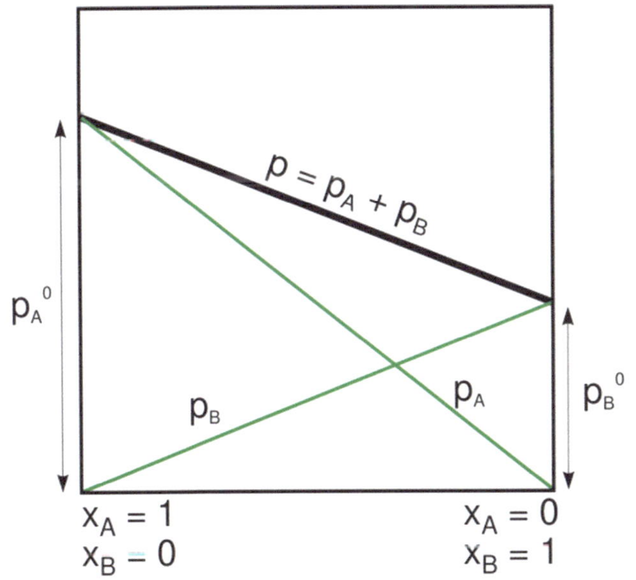

Figure 1: Vapor pressure of a binary solution that obeys Raoult's law. The oblique, black line shows the total vapor pressure, and the two green lines are the partial pressures of the two components A and B.

29) Based on Figure 1, which of the following most accurately represents the components in solution?

- **A.** Components A and B are non-volatile
- **B.** The total vapor pressure at all mole fractions is mostly due to component A.
- **C.** The point at which both components contribute equally to the total vapor pressure, component A is in the greater concentration.
- **D.** Pure component B has a lower vapor pressure than pure component A.

30) Which of the following, if true, is the best example of Raoult's law?

- **A.** Champagne bubbles when opened to the atmosphere.
- **B.** Waxed cars result in rain beading and running off the waxed surfaces.
- **C.** Salt lakes evaporate more slowly than fresh water lakes.
- **D.** Water has a relatively high boiling point due to hydrogen bonding.

High-level Importance

SPOILER ALERT

Gold Standard has cross-referenced the content in this chapter to examples from ACER's official GAMSAT practice materials. It is for you to decide when you want to explore these questions since you may want to preserve some of ACER's materials for timed mock-exam practice.

Examples – Freezing point depression: Q14-15 of 1; molar concentration and molecular weight: Q49-50 of 1; Raoult's law with a simple deviation: Q10-11 of 2; Ksp Q93 of 3; Ksp Q46 of 4; Henry's law Q81-84 of 4; ions in solution (straight drop and swap; CHM 3.1.1, 5.3.4): Q64 of 5; H-bonds and solubility in water: Q66 of 5; note that Q90-93 of 5: background is H-bonds but not counted because no assumed knowledge based on this chapter. Note that "Q" is followed by the question number, and, for example, "of 1" refers to booklet number 1 which is referenced in the Spoiler Alert table at the end of Chapter 1. The 15 full-length GAMSAT practice tests by Gold Standard, HEAPS-1 through HEAPS-15, contain specific cross-references to this chapter within the worked solutions. The flow chart with ions is from HEAPS-3; the gas solubility independent question is from HEAPS-6; the saturation curve unit with 6 questions is from HEAPS-9.

Chapter Checklist

- ☐ Access your online account to view answers, worked solutions and discussion boards.
- ☐ Reassess your 'learning objectives' for this chapter: Go back to the first page of this chapter and re-evaluate the top 3 boxes and the Introduction.
  - ☐ Please be sure that you have completed the *Need for Speed* exercises at the beginning of this chapter.
- ☐ Complete a maximum of 1 page of notes using symbols/abbreviations to represent the entire chapter based on your learning objectives. These are your Gold Notes.
- ☐ Consider your multimedia options based on your optimal way of learning:
  - ☐ Download the free Gold Standard GAMSAT app for your Android device or iPhone.
  - ☐ Create your own, tangible study cards or try the free app: Anki.
  - ☐ Record your voice reading your Gold Notes onto your smartphone (audio files, e.g., *memo* or MP3s) and listen during exercise, transportation, etc.
  - ☐ Try out the Gold Standard GAMSAT online videos at gamsat-prep.com, or you can try other options on YouTube like Khan Academy or Crash Course Chemistry.
- ☐ Reassess your schedule for your full-length GAMSAT practice tests: ACER and/or HEAPS exams. Ensure that you have scheduled one full day to complete a practice test and 1-2 days for a thorough assessment of worked solutions while adding to your abbreviated Gold Notes.
- ☐ Reassess your progress in scheduling and/or evaluating stress reduction techniques such as regular exercise (sports), yoga, meditation and/or mindfulness exercises (*see* YouTube for suggestions).

ACIDS AND BASES

Chapter 6

Memorise

* Define: Bronsted acid, base, pH
* Examples of strong/weak acids/bases
* K_w at STP, neutral H_2O pH, conjugate acid/base, zwitterions
* Equations: K_a, K_b, pK_a, pK_b, K_w, pH, pOH
* Equivalence point, indicator, rules of logarithms

Understand

* Calculation of K_a, K_b, pK_a, pK_b, K_w, pH, pOH
* Calculations involving strong/weak acids/bases
* Salts of weak acids/bases, buffers; indicators
* Fundamentals: Titration curve

Importance

High level: 22% of GAMSAT General Chemistry

questions released by ACER are related to content in this chapter (in our estimation).

* Note that approximately 80% of the questions in GAMSAT General Chemistry are related to just 4 chapters: 4, 5, 6, and 9.

GAMSAT-Prep.com

Introduction

Acids are compounds that, when dissolved in water, give a solution with a hydrogen ion concentration $[H^+]$ greater than that of pure water. Acids turn litmus paper (*an indicator*) red. Examples include acetic acid (*in vinegar*) and sulfuric acid (*in car batteries*). Bases may have $[H^+]$ less than pure water and turn litmus blue. Examples include sodium hydroxide (= *lye, caustic soda*) and ammonia (*used in many cleaning products*).

No one can predict exactly what topics you will see during your GAMSAT exam. Clearly, this chapter presents a traditional GAMSAT topic, and even if you do not have many questions with assumed knowledge from this chapter on your real GAMSAT, the use of logs, algebraic manipulations, and reasoning will apply to many other GAMSAT topics. There are several equations that we recommend that you commit to memory for this chapter. But note that ACER will normally provide these equations in the passage or preamble: however, knowing these equations in advance provides a distinct advantage.

Multimedia Resources at GAMSAT-Prep.com

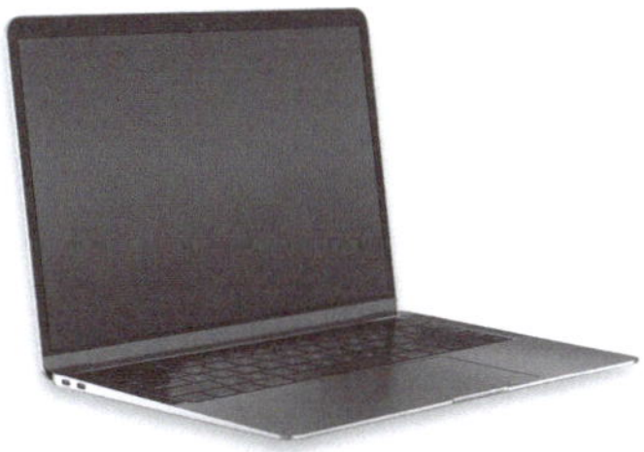

Open Discussion Boards
(*gamsat-prep.com/forum*)

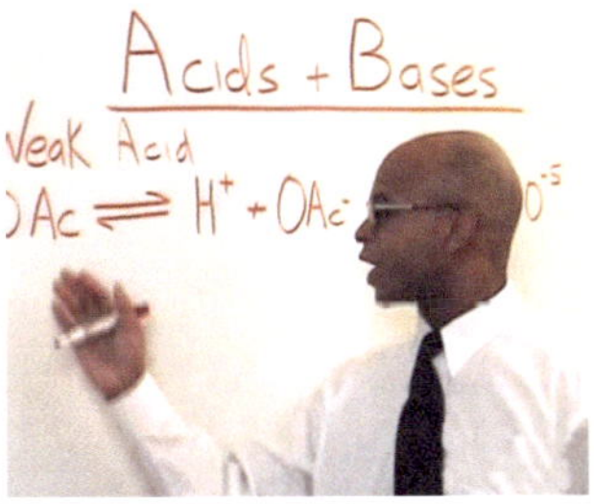

Science Preparation Videos

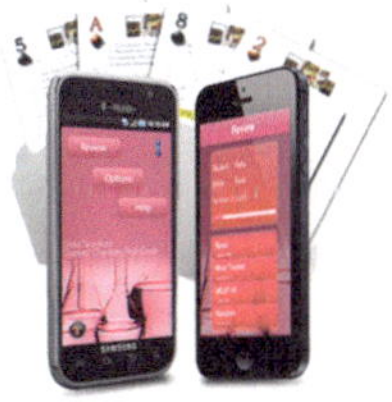

Flashcards

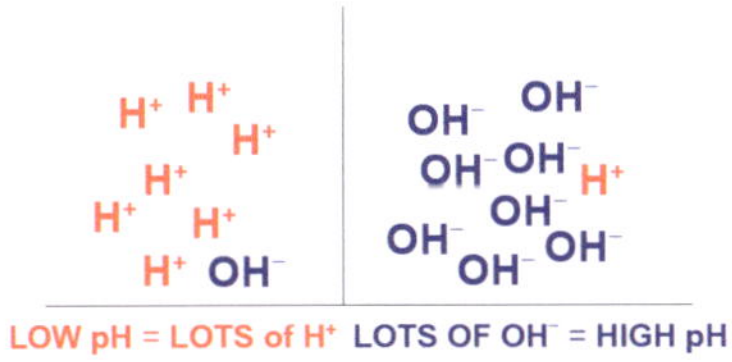

Special Guest

* The real GAMSAT may have advanced-level information presented (i.e. in a passage) but previous knowledge of said information is not required to answer the questions that would follow. Practice questions at the end of this chapter, as well as ACER and GS (HEAPS) practice GAMSATs can help you clarify this point.

6.0 GAMSAT has a *Need for Speed*!

High-level Importance

Section	GAMSAT General Chemistry *Need for Speed* Exercises
6.1	Define: An acid is a ________________
	Complete these 2 chemical equations illustrating the ionisation of acids: $HA + H_2O \rightleftharpoons$ $HCN \rightleftharpoons$
	Consider the following chemical equation. $HA \rightleftharpoons H^+ + A^-$ What is the expression for the K_a? $K_a =$ What is the relationship between pK_a and K_a? $pK_a =$
	Write the molecular formulas for these 'popular' acids.
6.2	Define: A base is a ________________
	Consider the following chemical equation. $B + H_2O \rightleftharpoons HB^+ + OH^-$ What is the expression for the K_b? $K_b =$ What is the relationship between pK_b and K_b? $pK_b =$
	Complete these 2 chemical equations illustrating the ionisation of bases: $NH_3 + H_2O \rightleftharpoons$ $F^- + H_2O \rightleftharpoons$
6.3	Circle either 'stronger' or 'weaker': The larger the dissociation constant (K_a or K_b), the (stronger / weaker) the acid or the base, respectively.

STRONG	WEAK	STRONG	WEAK
Perchloric $HClO_4$	Hydrocyanic HCN	Sulfuric _______	Sulfurous H_2SO_3
Chloric $HClO_3$	Hypochlorous HClO	Hydrobromic HBr	Hydrogen Sulfide H_2S
Nitric HNO_3	Nitrous HNO_2	Hydriodic HI	Phosphoric _______
Hydrochloric ____	Hydrofluoric _____	Hydronium Ion _____	Carboxylic acids: Benzoic, Acetic, etc.

6.3

Consider the conjugate acid-base pairs below. Fill in the missing entries.

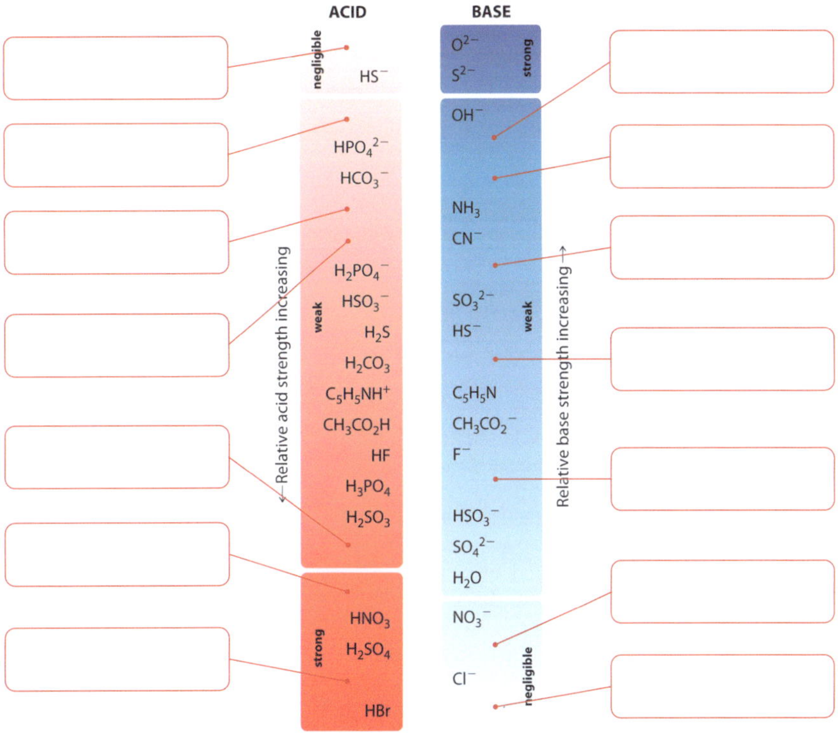

Circle either 'strong' or 'weak':

A strong acid (HCl) has a (strong / weak) conjugate base (Cl^-), and a strong base (NaOH) has a (strong / weak) conjugate acid (H_2O).

6.5

What is the relationship between pH and hydrogen ion concentration?

pH =

What is the relationship between pOH and hydroxide ion concentration?

pOH =

At 25 °C, pH + pOH = ________

Complete the missing information and circle either 'acidic' or 'basic':

At 25 °C, A pH of ___ is neutral. Values of pH that are greater than ___ are (acidic / basic) and values that are lower are (acidic / basic).

6.5.1

What is the pH of 0.001 M HCl?

6.7

Complete the following neutralisation reaction.

HCl(aq) + NaOH(aq) →

6.1 Acids

High-level Importance

A useful definition is given by Bronsted and Lowry: an acid is a proton (i.e. hydrogen ion; H^+) donor (cf. Lewis acids/bases, *see* CHM 3.4). A substance such as HF is an acid because it can donate a proton to a substance capable of accepting it. In aqueous solution, water is always available as a proton acceptor, so that the ionisation of an acid, HA, can be written as:

$$HA + H_2O \rightleftharpoons H_3O^+ + A^-$$

or: $$HA \rightleftharpoons H^+ + A^-$$

The equilibrium constant is (*note the product of the products over the reactant*):

$$K_a = [H^+][A^-]/[HA] \text{ and } pK_a = -\log_{10}K_a$$

Examples of the ionisation of acids are:

$$HCl \rightarrow H^+ + Cl^- \qquad K_a = 1.3 \times 10^6$$

$$HF \rightleftharpoons H^+ + F^- \qquad K_a = 6.7 \times 10^{-4}$$

$$HCN \rightleftharpoons H^+ + CN^- \qquad K_a = 7.2 \times 10^{-10}$$

Acids are generally divided into two categories known as binary acids and oxyacids. The first category is that of acids composed of hydrogen and a nonmetal such as chlorine (HCl). For the halogen containing binary acids, the acid strength increases as a function of the halogen size. Moreover, as the halogen size increases, its bond length increases while its bond strength decreases and as such, its acidity increases. Thus, the acidity of HI > HBr > HCl > HF.

The second category of acids form from oxyanions (anions containing a nonmetal and oxygen such as the hydroxide or nitrate ions, *see* CHM 5.2) are known as the oxyacids. The oxyacids contain a hydrogen atom covalently bonded to an oxygen atom which is bonded to another central atom X (H-O-X-etc). The more oxygen atoms that are bounded to the central atom, the more acidic the oxyacids (e.g. HClO vs $HClO_4$). Some examples of oxyacids are listed in Table III.A.6.1.

Note: a diprotic acid (*two protons*, i.e. H_2SO_4) would have K_a values for each of its two ionisable protons: K_{a1} for the first and K_{a2} for the second. Diprotic or any polyprotic acids are known to ionise in successive steps in which each of the steps contain their own dissociation or ionisation acid constant, K_a. The first ionisation constant (K_{a1}) is typically much larger than the subsequent ionisation constants ($K_{a1} > K_{a2} > K_{a3}$, etc...).

Table III.A.6.1: Examples of acids that dissociate (CHM 5.2) completely (*strong*) and only partially (*weak*).

STRONG	WEAK	STRONG	WEAK
Perchloric $HClO_4$ Chloric $HClO_3$ Nitric HNO_3 Hydrochloric HCl	Hydrocyanic HCN Hypochlorous HClO Nitrous HNO_2 Hydrofluoric HF Carbonic H_2CO_3	Sulfuric H_2SO_4 Hydrobromic HBr Hydriodic HI Hydronium Ion H_3O^+	Sulfurous H_2SO_3 Hydrogen Sulfide H_2S Phosphoric H_3PO_4 Carboxylic acids: Benzoic, Acetic, etc.

A base is defined as a proton acceptor. In aqueous solution, water is always available to donate a proton to a base, so the ionisation of a base B, can be written as:

$$B + H_2O \rightleftharpoons HB^+ + OH^-$$

The equilibrium constant is:

$$K_b = [HB^+][OH^-]/[B] \quad \text{and} \quad pK_b = -\log_{10}K_b$$

Examples of the ionisation of bases are:

$$CN^- + H_2O \rightleftharpoons HCN + OH^- \quad K_b = 1.4 \times 10^{-5}$$

$$NH_3 + H_2O \rightleftharpoons NH_4^+ + OH^- \quad K_b = 1.8 \times 10^{-5}$$

$$F^- + H_2O \rightleftharpoons HF + OH^- \quad K_b = 1.5 \times 10^{-11}$$

Strong bases include any hydroxide of the group 1A and 2A metals (e.g. NaOH, $Ca(OH)_2$). The most common weak bases are ammonia (NH_3) and any organic amine (ORG 11.1.1).

6.3 Conjugate Acid-Base Pairs

The strength of an acid or base is related to the extent that the dissociation proceeds to the right, or to the magnitude of K_a or K_b; the larger the dissociation constant, the stronger the acid or the base. From the preceding K_a values (CHM 6.1), we see that HCl is the strongest acid (almost 100% ionised), followed by HF and HCN. From the K_b's given, NH_3 is the strongest base listed, followed by CN^- and F^-. Clearly, when an acid ionises, it produces a base. The acid, HA, and the base produced when it ionises, A^-, are called a conjugate acid-base pair, so that the couples HF/F^- and HCN/CN^- are conjugate acids and bases.

Thus, an acid that has donated a proton becomes a conjugate base and a base that has accepted a proton becomes a conjugate acid of that base. For example, HCO_3^-/CO_3^{2-} are a conjugate acid/base pair, wherein HCO_3^- is the acid and CO_3^{2-} is the conjugate

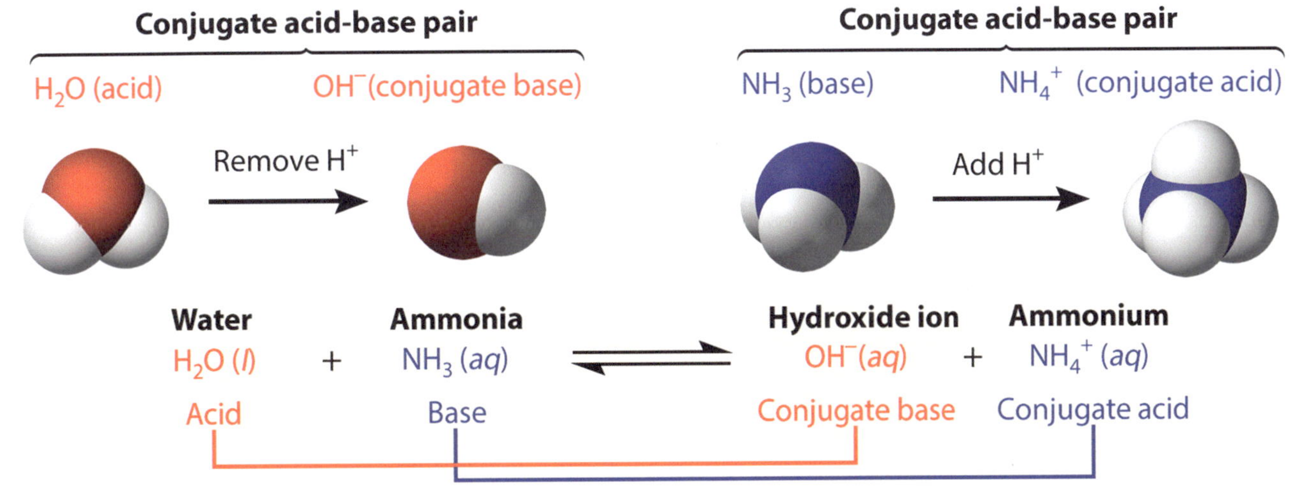

High-level Importance

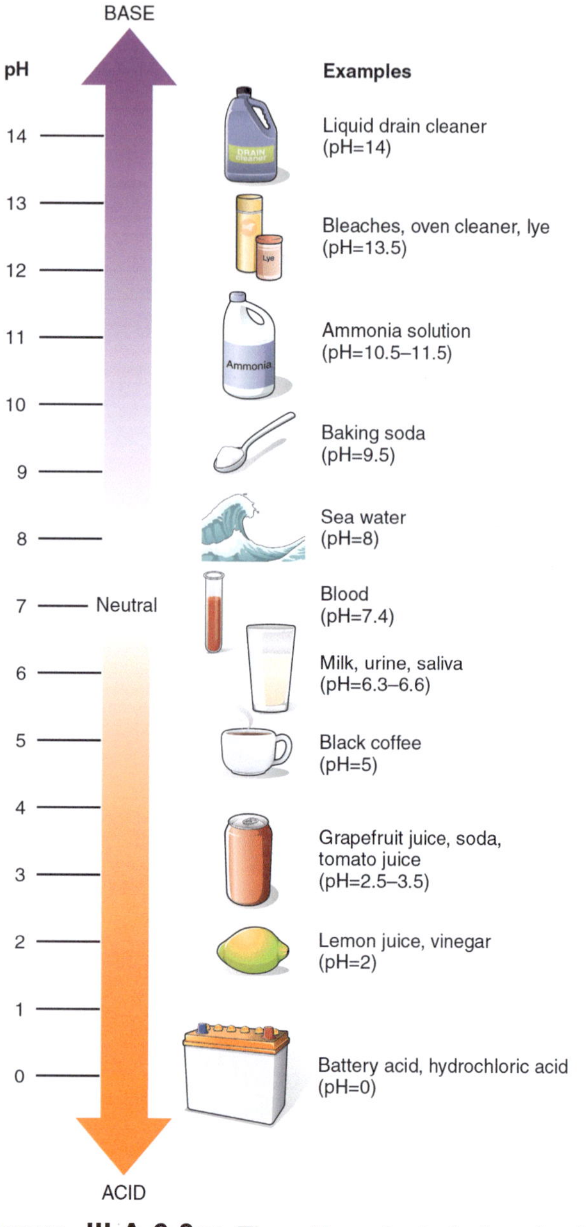

Figure III.A.6.0a: The pH scale including "real-world" examples. Note that near the top of the pH scale is a solution (*lye*) which most commonly refers to sodium hydroxide (NaOH), but historically has also referred to the related base potassium hydroxide (KOH). And at the lower end of the pH scale, though not referenced in the image above, would be *gastric* (stomach) acid. It is generally considered to have a pH of 2, though it ranges from 1.5 to 3.5 (cf. BIO 9.3). (OpenStax CNX; 2020)

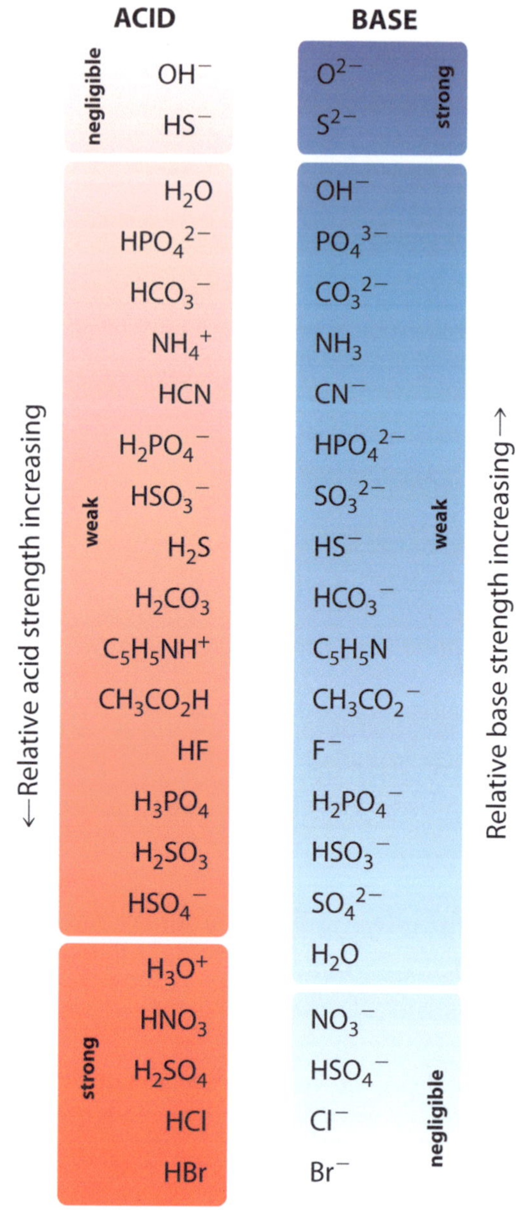

Figure III.A.6.0b: Conjugate acids and conjugate bases. Do not memorise, but notice the trends and relationships. For example, acids release H^+, so notice that in each pair of species on the same line, the base (*in the right column*) has "lost" H^+. Also note that the strongest acids are at the bottom left, and the strongest bases are at the top right. The conjugate base of a strong acid is a very weak base, and, conversely, the conjugate acid of a strong base is a very weak acid. (Lumen; MCC Chemistry, 2021)

base. Both dissociate partially in water and reach equilibrium.

A strong acid (HCl) has a weak conjugate base (Cl^-), and a strong base (NaOH) has a weak conjugate acid (H_2O). {*See* the image showing the reaction of water and ammonia towards the beginning of CHM 6.3; of course, water is neutral, but it may behave like an acid or base depending on its environment, CHM 6.8.}

Another example of conjugate acid-base pairs is amino acids (ORG 12.1). Amino acids bear at least 2 ionisable weak acid groups, a carboxyl (–COOH) and an amino ($-NH_3^+$) which act as follows:

$$R\text{–}COOH \rightleftharpoons R\text{–}COO^- + H^+$$

$$R\text{–}NH_3^+ \rightleftharpoons R\text{–}NH_2 + H^+$$

$R\text{–}COO^-$ and $R\text{–}NH_2$ are the conjugate bases (i.e. proton acceptors) of the corresponding acids. The carboxyl group is thousands of times more acidic than the amino group. Thus in blood plasma (pH ≈ 7.4) the predominant forms are the carboxylate anions ($R\text{–}COO^-$) and the protonated amino group ($R\text{–}NH_3^+$). This form is called a *zwitterion* as demonstrated by the amino acid alanine at a pH near 7:

$CH_3\text{–}CH\text{–}COO^-$ (with NH_3^+ on the central CH)

Alanine

The zwitterion bears no net charge.

A Gold Standard Conjugate Song: Although this does not rhyme, it has its own rhythm and it summarises a string of ideas that often trip up students during the exam. A new mantra or song to sing (context: *this is on a relative basis*): A weak acid has a low K_a, a high pK_a, a low pK_b and high K_b of the conjugate base. And, of course, vice versa in each account: A strong acid has a large K_a, a low pK_a, a high pK_b and low K_b of the conjugate base. Of course, high K_b means that the base is strong, and low K_b means that the base is weak. These relationships have nothing to do with logs, but everything to do with the negative sign in the expressions for pK_a and pK_b, as well as the relationship between those two expressions which we will explore in CHM 6.7.

6.4 Water Dissociation

Water itself can ionise:

$$H_2O + H_2O \rightleftharpoons H_3O^+ + OH^-$$

or:

$$H_2O \rightleftharpoons H^+ + OH^-$$

At STP, $K_w = [H^+][OH^-] = 1.0 \times 10^{-14}$ = ion product constant for water. It increases with temperature and in a neutral solution, $[H^+] = [OH^-] = 10^{-7}$ M. Note that $[H_2O]$ is not included in the equilibrium expression because it is a pure liquid and it is a large constant ($[H_2O]$ is incorporated in K_w). Also note that $pK_w = -\log K_w = -\log 10^{-14} = 14$ at STP.

6.5 The pH Scale

High-level Importance

The pH of a solution is a convenient way of expressing the concentration of hydrogen ions $[H^+]$ in solution, to avoid the use of large negative powers of 10. It is defined as:

$$pH = -\log_{10}[H^+]$$

At 25 °C, the pH of a neutral solution of pure water, where $[H^+] = 10^{-7}$, is 7 (*see* Fig III.A.6.0a).

A similar definition is used for the hydroxyl ion concentration:

$$pOH = -\log_{10}[OH^-]$$

Since, $K_w = [H^+][OH^-]$

And so, $1.0 \times 10^{-14} = [H^+][OH^-]$

And taking the –log of both sides gives $-\log[1.0 \times 10^{-14}] = -\log[H^+][OH^-]$

So, $14.0 = -\log[H^+] + -\log[OH^-]$

Therefore, 14.0 = pH + pOH

Finally, at 25 °C, pH + pOH = 14.0

A pH of 7 is neutral. Values of pH that are greater than 7 are alkaline (*basic*) and values that are lower are acidic.

The pH can be measured precisely with a pH meter (*quantitative*) or globally with an indicator which will have a different colour over different pH ranges (*qualitative*). For example, *litmus paper* (very common) becomes blue in basic solutions and red in acidic solutions; whereas, *phenolphthalein* is colourless in acid and pink in base.

We will see in CHM 6.9 that a weak acid or base can serve as a visual (*qualitative*) indicator of a pH range. Usually, only a small quantity (i.e. drops) of the indicator is added to the solution as to minimise the risk of any side reactions.

6.5.1 Properties of Logarithms

Many GAMSAT problems every year rely on a basic understanding of logarithms (GM 3.7, 3.8) for one or more of: pH problems, reaction rates (CHM 9.5), Gibbs free energy (CHM 9.10), the Nernst equation (CHM 10.3), and decibels/sound (PHY 8.3). Here are the rules you must know:

1) $\log_a a = 1$
2) $\log_a M^k = k \log_a M$
3) $\log_a(MN) = \log_a M + \log_a N$
4) $\log_a(M/N) = \log_a M - \log_a N$
5) $10^{\log_{10} M} = M$

For example, let us calculate the pH of 0.001 M HCl. Since HCl is a strong acid, it will completely dissociate into H^+ and Cl^-, thus:

$$[H^+] = 0.001$$
$$-\log[H^+] = -\log(0.001)$$
$$pH = -\log(10^{-3})$$
$$pH = 3 \log 10 \quad \text{(rule \#2)}$$
$$pH = 3 \quad \text{(rule \#1, a = 10)}$$

6.6 Weak Acids and Bases

Weak acids (HA) and bases (B) partially dissociate in aqueous solutions reaching equilibrium following their dissociation. The following is the generic reaction of any weak acid (HA) dissociation in an aqueous solution.

$$HA + H_2O \rightleftharpoons A^- + H_3O^+$$

Now let us begin by taking a closer look at the development of the acid and base equilibrium constants. Like all equilibrium, acid/base dissociation will have a particular equilibrium constant (K_a or K_b) which will determine the extent of the dissociation (CHM 6.3). Thus, from the preceding equation for any generic acid (HA), the acid dissociation constant $K = [H_3O^+][A^-]/[H_2O][HA]$.

Very little water actually reacts and thus the concentration of water during the reaction is constant and can therefore be excluded from the expression for K. Therefore, this gives rise to the acid dissociation constant known as K_a.

Where, $K_a = K[H_2O] = [H_3O^+][A^-]/[HA]$

Likewise for a weak base dissociation in equilibrium,

$$B + H_2O \rightleftharpoons OH^- + BH^+$$

This gives rise to the base dissociation constant known as K_b.

Where, $K_b = K[H_2O] = [OH^-][BH^+]/[B]$

Weak acids and bases are only partially ionised. The ionisation constant can be used to calculate the amount ionised, and from this, the pH.

Since weak acids are not completely dissociated, one needs to find the $[H^+]$ from the acid dissociation and then use a method known in most textbooks as the "ICE method". ICE is an acronym used in which, I = Initial acid $[H^+]$ concentration, C = Change in acid $[H^+]$ concentration and E = acid $[H^+]$ concentration at equilibrium. Thus, the acid concentration $[H^+]$ also represented as (x) at equilibrium is then used to calculate the pH. NOTE: the equilibrium concentration x is usually very small as the acid (or base) is weak and partially dissociated (or ionised). The following is an example of the application of the ICE method in solving for the $[H^+] = x$ at equilibrium and subsequently determining the pH of a weak acid solution.

Example: Calculate the pH and pOH of a 10^{-2} M solution of acetic acid (HOAc). K_a of acetic acid at 25 °C = 1.75×10^{-5}.

$$HOAc \rightleftharpoons H^+ + OAc^-$$

The concentrations are:

	[HOAc]	$[H^+]$	$[OAc^-]$
Initial	10^{-2}	0	0
Change	$-x$	$+x$	$+x$
Equilibrium	$10^{-2} - x$	x	x

$K_a = [H^+][OAc^-]/[HOAc] = 1.75 \times 10^{-5}$
$= (x)(x)/(10^{-2} - x)$

The solution is a quadratic equation which may be simplified if less than 5% of the acid is ionised by neglecting x compared to the concentration (10^{-2} M in this case). We then have:

$$x^2/10^{-2} = 1.75 \times 10^{-5}$$
$$x^2 = 1.75 \times 10^{-7}$$
$$x^2 = 17.5 \times 10^{-8}$$
$$x = 4.2 \times 10^{-4} = [H^+]$$

And $pH = -\log(4.2 \times 10^{-4}) = 3.4$
$pOH = 14.00 - 3.4 = 10.6$

To confirm the 5% criterion one needs to calculate as follows: $(4.2 \times 10^{-4})/(1.00 \times 10^{-2}) \times 100 = 4.2\%$ which is less than 5% and therefore justifies the usage of the 5% criterion.

Similar calculations hold for weak bases. Note that all the preceding can be estimated without a calculator with basic maths skills. The square root is half of the exponent, thus the root of 10^{-8} is 10^{-4} (GM 1.5). Since the square root of 16 is 4, root 17.5 must be a bit more than 4 (to estimate pH, *see* CHM 6.6.1). If you are struggling with the maths, join the discussion "6.6 Weak Acids and Bases - log calculations" at gamsat-prep.com/forum.

6.6.1 Determining pH with the Quadratic Formula

If you need to calculate pH on the GAMSAT, it is very unlikely that you would need to use the quadratic equation; however, you are expected to be familiar with the different ways to calculate pH and that is why it is presented here.

The solutions of the quadratic equation

$$ax^2 + bx + c = 0$$

are given by the formula (do not memorise):

$$x = [-b \pm (b^2 - 4ac)^{1/2}]/2a$$

The problem in CHM 6.6 can be reduced to

$$K_a = (x)(x)/(10^{-2} - x) = 1.75 \times 10^{-5}$$

or

$$x^2 + (1.75 \times 10^{-5})x + (-1.75 \times 10^{-7}) = 0$$

Using the quadratic equation where $a = 1$, $b = 1.75 \times 10^{-5}$ and $c = -1.75 \times 10^{-7}$, and doing the appropriate multiplications we get:

$$x = [-1.75 \times 10^{-5} \pm (3.06 \times 10^{-10} + 7.0 \times 10^{-7})^{1/2}]/2$$

Thus $x = [-1.75 \times 10^{-5} \pm (7.00 \times 10^{-7})^{1/2}]/2$
$= [-1.75 \times 10^{-5} \pm 8.37 \times 10^{-4}]/2$

Hence the two possible solutions are

$$x = [-1.75 \times 10^{-5} - 8.37 \times 10^{-4}]/2 = -4.27 \times 10^{-4}$$

Or

$$x = [-1.75 \times 10^{-5} + 8.37 \times 10^{-4}]/2 = 4.10 \times 10^{-4}$$

The first solution is a negative number which is physically impossible for $[H^+]$, therefore $pH = -\log(4.10 \times 10^{-4}) = 3.39$.

Our estimate in CHM 6.6 ($pH = 3.38$) was valid as it is less than 1% different from the more precise calculation using the quadratic formula.

Given a multiple choice question with the following choices: 2.5, 3.4, 4.3 and 6.8 – the answer can be easily deduced.

$$-\log(4.10 \times 10^{-4}) = -\log 4.10 - \log 10^{-4}$$
$$= 4 - \log 4.10$$

however

$$0 = \log 10^0 = \log 1 < \log 4.10 << \log 10 = 1$$

Thus a number slightly greater than 0 but significantly less than 1 is subtracted from 4. The answer could only be 3.4.

6.7 Salts of Weak Acids and Bases

A *salt* is an ionic compound in which the anion is not OH^- or O^{2-} and the cation is not H^+.

Acids and bases react with each other, forming a salt and water in a reaction known as a neutralisation reaction. Salts are compounds composed of both a cation and anion (i.e. Na_2SO_4). As salts contain both a cation and anion, salts may therefore form acidic, basic or neutral solutions when dissolved into water. Hence, a salt can react with water to give back an acid or base in a reaction known as salt hydrolysis and thus affect the solution's pH. Moreover, a salt composed of an anion from a weak acid (CH_3COO^-) and a cation from a strong base (Na^+) dissociates and reacts in water to give rise to OH^- ions (a basic solution). Whereas, a salt composed of an anion from a strong acid (Cl^-) and a cation from a weak base (NH_4^+) dissociates and reacts in water to give rise to H^+ (an acidic solution).

Examples:

NaClO dissociates in water:

$$ClO^- + H_2O \rightleftharpoons HClO + OH^- \text{ (Basic)}$$

NH_4NO_3 dissociates in water:

$$NH_4^+ + H_2O \rightleftharpoons H_3O^+ + NH_3 \text{ (Acidic)}$$

The salt of a weak acid is a Bronsted base, which will accept protons. For example,

$$Na^+\,OAc^- + H_2O \rightleftharpoons HOAc + Na^+\,OH^-$$

The HOAc here is undissociated and therefore does not contribute to the pH. Because it hydrolyses, sodium acetate is a weak base (the conjugate base of acetic acid). The ionisation constant is equal to the basicity constant of the salt. The weaker the conjugate acid, the stronger the conjugate base, that is, the more strongly the salt will combine with a proton.

$$K_H = K_b = [HOAc][OH^-]/[OAc^-]$$

K_H is the hydrolysis constant of the salt. The product of K_a of any weak acid and K_b of its conjugate base is always equal to K_w.

$$K_a \times K_b = K_w$$

For any salt of a weak acid, HA, that ionises in water:

$$A^- + H_2O \rightleftharpoons HA + OH^-$$
$$[HA][OH^-]/[A^-] = K_w/K_a.$$

The pH of such a salt is calculated in the same manner as for any other weak base.

Similar equations are derived for the salts of weak bases. They hydrolyse in water as follows:

$$BH^+ + H_2O \rightleftharpoons B + H_3O^+$$

B is undissociated and does not contribute to the pH.

$$K_H = K_a = [B][H_3O^+]/[BH^+]$$

And

$$[B][H_3O^+]/[BH^+] = K_w/K_b.$$

In conclusion, there are four types of salts formed based on the reacting acid and base strengths as follows:

(1) Strong acid + strong base:

$$HCl(aq) + NaOH(aq) \rightarrow NaCl(aq) + H_2O(l)$$

Salts in which the cation and anion are both conjugates of a strong base and a strong acid form neutral solutions. Note the use of a one-sided arrow in the reaction above which implies that the reaction goes to completion (thus only product and no reactant remains). Note the two-sided arrows in the reactions below which imply equilibrium: a point where forward and reverse reactions occur at equal rates (CHM 5.3.2, 9.8).

(2) Strong acid + weak base:

$$HCl(aq) + NH_3(aq) \rightleftharpoons NH_4Cl\ (aq)$$

Salts that are formed based on a strong acid reacting with a weak base form acidic solutions.

(3) Weak acid + strong base:

$$HOAc(aq) + NaOH(aq) \rightleftharpoons NaOAc(aq) + H_2O(l)$$

(note: HOAc = acetic acid = CH_3COOH)

A salt in which the cation is the counterion of a strong base and the anion is the conjugate base of a weak acid results in the formation of basic solutions.

(4) Weak acid + weak base:

$$HOAc(aq) + NH_3(aq) \rightleftharpoons NH_4OAc(aq)$$

A salt in which the cation is a conjugate acid of a weak base and the anion is the anion of a weak acid will form a solution in which the pH will be dependent on the relative strengths of the acid and base.

Note: Using the rules of logarithms (GM 3.7; CHM 6.5.1), we can change

$$K_aK_b = K_w \text{ to } -\log(K_aK_b) = -\log K_w$$

which is the same as

$$(-\log K_a) + (-\log K_b) = -\log K_w.$$

Thus $pK_a + pK_b = pK_w$.

Recall that as STP, $pK_w = 14$ (CHM 6.4, 6.5).

6.8 Buffers

A buffer is defined as a solution that resists change in pH when a small amount of an acid or base is added or when a solution is diluted. A buffer solution consists of a mixture of a weak acid and its salt or of a weak base and its salt.

For example, consider the acetic acid-acetate buffer. The acid equilibrium that governs this system is:

$$HOAc \rightleftharpoons H^+ + OAc^-.$$

Along with the acid equilibrium component of the buffer solution as shown above, the buffer solution must also contain a significant amount of the conjugate base of the acid as a salt. The following equation depicts the conjugate base salt dissociation of the acetic acid-acetate buffer solution:

$$NaOAc \rightarrow Na^+ + OAc^-.$$

Thus, the buffer is made up of two components: **(1)** a weak acid (HOAc) and **(2)** the conjugate base of the weak acid as a salt (NaAOc) so that both components are part of the buffer system in apt concentrations to make for a fully functional buffer.

When a small amount of NaOH base is added to the acetic acid/acetate buffer solution, the OH^- ions from the base will react with the free H^+ ions present in the buffer solution from the acetic acid dissociation. This will shift the equilibrium of the buffer toward the right which means more dissociation of the acid (HOAc). Thus, an increase in $[OH^-]$ from the addition of base to the buffer solution does not change pH significantly due to the reaction of the basic OH^- ions with the free protons (H^+) in solution.

The resistance to pH change is also noted with the addition of an acid (H^+) to the acetic acid/acetate buffer solution. The addition of acidic H^+ from the acid will react with the acetate ions ($HOAc^-$) from the salt dissociation of the buffer and this will also allow for the buffering capacity of the solution. Thus, due to the presence of both a weak acid and a conjugate base from the salt (or common ion), the buffer solution thus is known to maintain a pH within a certain range known as the buffering capacity.

Buffers must contain a significant amount of both a weak acid or weak base and its conjugate salts. A strong acid or strong base would not have any buffering capacity or effect within a buffer system as the dissociation would be irreversible and so the buffer capacity would not be present. In addition, a weak acid or base in itself would also not be able to work as a buffer system regardless of the fact that there is the presence of their conjugates as the concentrations of the conjugate acid or base from the weak acids or bases would not be sufficient to neutralise the addition of acids (H^+) or bases (OH^-). Thus, buffers require the

High-level Importance

addition of a conjugate acid or base as a salt to the weak acid or base component so to increase the salt concentration of the buffer solution.

If we were to add acetate ions into the system (i.e. from the salt), the H^+ ion concentration is no longer equal to the acetate ion concentration. The hydrogen ion concentration is:

$$[H^+] = K_a\ ([HOAc]/[OAc^-])$$

Taking the negative logarithm of each side, where $-\log K_a = pK_a$, yields:

$$pH = pK_a - \log\ ([HOAc]/[OAc^-])$$

or

$$pH = pK_a + \log([OAc^-]/[HOAc])$$

This equation is referred to as the Henderson-Hasselbach equation. It is useful for calculating the pH of a weak acid solution containing its salt. A general form can be written for a weak acid, HA, that dissociates into its salt, A^- and H^+:

$$HA \rightleftharpoons H^+ + A^-$$

$$pH = pK_a + \log([salt]/[acid])$$

The buffering capacity of the solution is determined by the concentrations of HA and A^-. The higher their concentrations, the more acid or base the solution can tolerate. The buffering capacity is also governed by the ratios of HA to A^-. It is maximum when the ratio is equal to 1, i.e. when $pH = pK_a$.

Similar calculations can be made for mixtures of a weak base and its salt:

$$B + H_2O \rightleftharpoons BH^+ + OH^-$$

And

$$pOH = pK_b + \log\ ([salt]/[base])$$

Many biological reactions of interest occur between pH 6 and 8. One useful series of buffers is that of phosphate buffers. By choosing appropriate mixtures of $H_3PO_4/H_2PO_4^-$, $H_2PO_4^-/HPO_4^{2-}$ or HPO_4^{2-}/PO_4^{3-}, buffer solutions covering a wide pH range can be prepared. Another useful clinical buffer is the one prepared from tris(hydroxymethyl)aminomethane and its conjugate acid, abbreviated Tris buffer.

Amphoteric Species: Some substances such as water can act as either an acid or a base (i.e. a dual property). These types of substances are known as amphoteric substances. Water behaves as an acid when reacted with a base (OH^-) and alternatively, water behaves as a base when reacted with an acid (H^+). Many metal oxides and hydroxides are also known to be amphoteric substances. Furthermore, molecules that contain both acidic and basic groups such as amino acids are considered to be amphoteric in nature as well (ORG 12.1.2). The following are examples of the amphoteric nature of HCO_3^- reacting with an acid and a base and water (H_2O) reacting with an acid and base.

In acids: $HCO_3^- + H_3O^+ \rightarrow H_2CO_3 + H_2O$
In bases: $HCO_3^- + OH^- \rightarrow CO_3^{2-} + H_2O$
In acids: $H_2O + HCl \rightarrow H_3O^+ + Cl^-$
In bases: $H_2O + NH_3 \rightarrow NH_4^+ + OH^-$

6.9 Acid-base Titrations

The purpose of a titration is usually the determination of concentration of a given sample of acid or base (the analyte) which is reacted with an equivalent amount of a strong base or acid of known concentration (the titrant). The end point or equivalence point is reached when a stoichiometric amount of titrant has been added. This end point is usually detected with the use of an indicator which changes colour when this point is reached. Note: the end point is not exactly the same as the equivalence point. The equivalence point is where a reaction is theoretically complete whereas an end point is where a physical change in solution such as a colour change is determined by indicators. Regardless, the volume difference between an end point and an equivalence point can usually be ignored.

The end point is determined precisely by measuring the pH at different points of the titration. The curve pH = f(V) where V is the volume of titrant added is called a titration curve. While a strong acid/strong base titration will have an equivalence point at a neutralisation pH of 7, the equivalence point of other titrations do not necessarily occur at pH 7. In fact, a weak acid/strong base titration will result in an equivalence point of a pH > 7 and a strong acid/weak base titration results in an equivalence point of a pH < 7. The differential pH effects at the relative equivalence points are due to the conjugate acids and/or bases formed. An indicator for an acid-base titration is a weak acid or base.

The weak acid and its conjugate base should have two different colours in solution. Most indicators require a pH transition range during the titration of about two pH units. An indicator is chosen so that its pK_a is close to the pH of the equivalence point.

6.9.1 Strong Acid versus Strong Base

In the case of a strong acid versus a strong base, both the titrant and the analyte are completely ionised. For example, the titration of hydrochloric acid with sodium hydroxide:

$$H^+ + Cl^- + Na^+ + OH^- \rightarrow H_2O + Na^+ + Cl^-$$

The H^+ and OH^- combine to form H_2O and the other ions remain unchanged, so the net result is the conversion of the HCl to a neutral solution of NaCl. A typical strong acid-strong base titration curve is shown in Fig. III.A.6.1 (case where the titrant is a base).

If the analyte is an acid, the pH is initially acidic and increases very slowly. When the equivalent volume is reached the pH sharply increases. Midway between this transition jump is the equivalence point. In the case of strong acid-strong base titration the equivalence point corresponds to a neutral pH (because the salt formed does not react with water). If more titrant is added the pH increases and corresponds to the pH of a solution of gradually increasing concentration of the titrant base. This curve is simply reversed if the titrant is an acid.

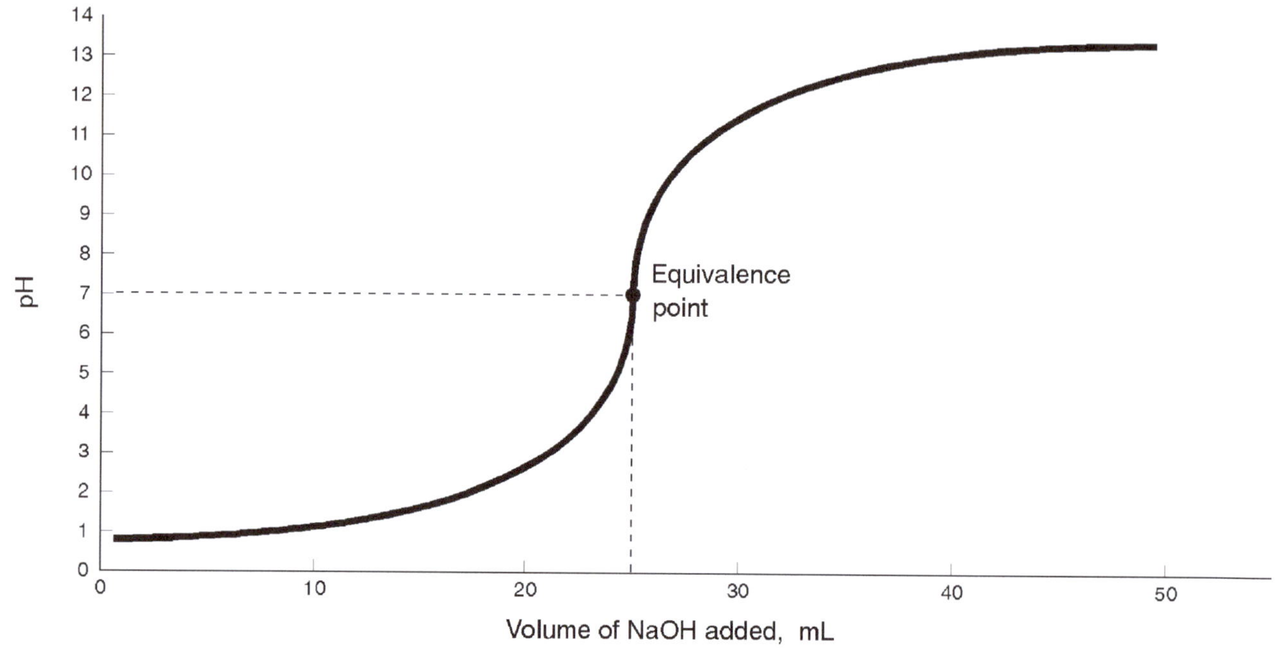

Figure III.A.6.1: The titration curve for a strong acid-strong base is a relatively smooth S-shaped curve with a very steep inclination close to the equivalence point. A small addition in titrant volume near the equivalence point will result in a large change in pH.

6.9.2 Weak Acid versus Strong Base

The titration of acetic acid with sodium hydroxide involves the following reaction:

$$HOAc + Na^+ + OH^- \rightarrow H_2O + Na^+ + OAc^-$$

The acetic acid is only a few percent ionised. It is neutralised to water and an equivalent amount of the salt, sodium acetate. Before the titration is started, the pH is calculated as described for weak acids. As soon as the titration is started, some of the HOAc is converted to NaOAc and a buffer system is set up. As the titration proceeds, the pH slowly increases as the ratio $[OAc^-]/[HOAc]$ changes. Halfway towards the <u>equivalence point</u>, $[OAC^-] = [HOAC]$ and the <u>pH is equal to pK_a</u>. At the equivalence point, we have a solution of NaOAc. Since it hydrolyses, the <u>pH at the</u>

equivalence point will be alkaline. The pH will depend on the concentration of NaOAc. The greater the concentration, the higher the pH. As excess NaOH is added, the ionisation of the base, OAc^-, is suppressed and the pH is determined only by the concentration of excess OH^-. Therefore, the titration curve beyond the equivalence point follows that for the titration of a strong acid. The typical titration curve in this case is illustrated in Figure III.A.6.2.

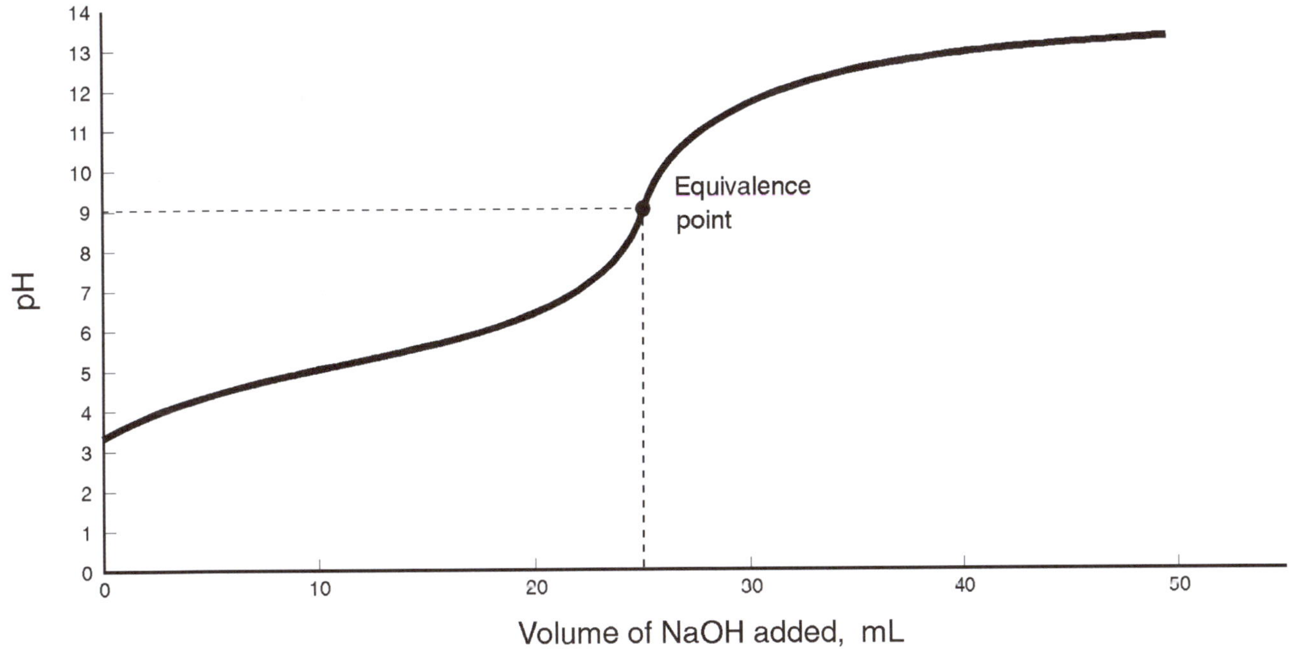

Figure III.A.6.2: The titration curve for a weak acid-strong base or alternatively a strong acid-weak base is somewhat irregular. The pH at the start of the titration prior to base addition is greater than that of a strong acid as the acid is a weak acid. The inclination close to the equivalence point is less significant due to the buffering effect of the solution prior to the equivalence point. A small addition in titrant volume near the equivalence point will therefore result in a small change in pH.

6.9.3 Weak Base versus Strong Acid

The titration of a weak base with a strong acid is analogous to the previous case except that the pH is initially basic and gradually decreases as the acid is added (curve in preceding diagram is reversed). Consider ammonia titrated with hydrochloric acid:

$$NH_3 + H^+ + Cl^- \rightarrow NH_4^+ + Cl^-$$

At the beginning, we have NH_3 and the pH is calculated as for weak bases. As soon as some acid is added, some of the NH_3 is converted to NH_4^+ and we are in the buffer region.

High-level Importance

At the midpoint of the titration, $[NH_4^+] = [NH_3]$ and the pH is equal to (14 – pK_b). At the equivalence point, we have a solution of NH_4Cl, a weak acid which hydrolyses to give an acid solution. Again, the pH will depend on concentration: the greater the concentration, the lower the pH. Beyond the equivalence point, the free H^+ suppresses the ionisation and the pH is determined by the concentration of H^+ added in excess. Therefore, the titration curve beyond the equivalence point will be similar to that of the titration of a strong base. {The midpoint of the titration is considered to be halfway to the equivalence point of the titration curve.}

CHAPTER 6: Acids and Bases

GOLD STANDARD FOUNDATIONAL GAMSAT PRACTICE QUESTIONS

You can refer to any of these key equations in order to solve problems. More often than not, during the real GAMSAT, ACER will provide pH-related equations. However, they have never provided the rules of logarithms. We have provided the log rules to help with your Foundational Practice Questions but they will not be provided for the GAMSAT-level Practice Questions which will follow. All practice questions are at standard temperature and pressure (STP) unless specified otherwise.

- Acids

$$K_a = [H^+][A^-]/[HA]$$

$pK_a = -\log K_a$

- Water Dissociation

$$K_w = [H^+][OH^-] = 1.0 \times 10^{-14}$$

- Salts of Weak Acids and Bases

$$K_a \times K_b = K_w$$

- Buffers

$$pH = pK_a + \log([salt]/[acid])$$

$$pOH = pK_b + \log([salt]/[base])$$

- Bases

$$K_b = [HB^+][OH^-]/[B]$$

$pK_b = -\log K_b$

- The pH Scale

$$pH = -\log_{10}[H^+]$$

$$pOH = -\log_{10}[OH^-]$$

at 25 °C, pH + pOH = 14.0

- Properties of Logarithms

1. $\log_a a = 1$
2. $\log_a M^k = k \log_a M$
3. $\log_a(MN) = \log_a M + \log_a N$
4. $\log_a(M/N) = \log_a M - \log_a N$
5. $10^{\log_{10}(M)} = M$

1) What does a change in pH from 3 to 2 represent in terms of the new H^+ ion concentration of the solution?

A. a decrease × 10
B. an increase × 10
C. a decrease × 1000
D. an increase × 1000

2) What does a change in pH from 3 to 6 represent in terms of the new H^+ ion concentration of the solution?

A. A decrease × 3
B. An increase × 3
C. A decrease × 1000
D. An increase × 1000

3) A base can be defined as a substance that:

A. acts as a proton donor.
B. accepts hydrogen gas.
C. acts as a proton acceptor.
D. increases $[H^+]$ when placed in water.

4) An acid with a large pK_a will normally be expected to have?

A. A strong conjugate base
B. A weak conjugate base
C. A neutral conjugate base
D. No conjugate base

5) For the following reaction, identify the conjugate acid-base pair.

$$H_2PO_4^- (aq) + NH_3 (aq) \rightleftharpoons HPO_4^{2-} (aq) + NH_4^+ (aq)$$

A. H_2PO_4 and NH_3
B. HPO_4^{2-} and NH_4^+
C. $H_2PO_4^-$ and HPO_4^{2-}
D. NH_4^+ and $H_2PO_4^-$

6) Which of the following species can react either as a Bronsted acid or as a Bronsted base?

A. NH_4^+
B. $H_2PO_4^-$
C. SO_4^{-2}
D. PO_4^{-3}

7) In the following reaction, which is a Bronsted base?

$$HC_2O_4^-(aq) + H_2O(\ell) \rightleftharpoons H_3O^+(aq) + C_2O_4^{2-}(aq)$$

A. $HC_2O_4^-$
B. H_2O
C. H_3O^+
D. None of the above

8) What is the conjugate base of HCO_3^-?

A. OH^-
B. H_2CO_3
C. HCO_3^+
D. CO_3^{2-}

9) What is the pH of a 0.001 M HCl solution?

A. 11
B. 1
C. 0.001
D. 3

10) Urine has a pH of approximately 6.0. What is the hydroxide ion concentration of urine?

A. 0.6 M
B. 10^{-6} M
C. 10^{-8} M
D. 0.06 M

GOLD STANDARD GAMSAT-LEVEL PRACTICE QUESTIONS

Questions 11–17

Polyprotic acids are those capable of dissociating more than one ionisable hydrogen. Carbonic acid, H_2CO_3, is an example of a polyprotic acid. It is formed when carbon dioxide dissolves in water. The solubility of CO_2 in water is quite sensitive to pH.

Reaction I: $CO_2 + H_2O \leftrightarrow H_2CO_3$

Carbonic acid has two ionisation equilibria with each having a distinct acid dissociation constant (K_a):

Reaction II: $H_2CO_3 + H_2O \leftrightarrow H_3O^+ + HCO_3^-$

Reaction III: $HCO_3^- + H_2O \leftrightarrow H_3O^+ + CO_3^{2-}$

Note that: The Henderson-Hasselbalch equation links the pH and pK_a of an acid (AH) and its conjugate base (A^-) according to: $pH = pK_a + \log([A^-]/[AH])$.

Carbon dioxide diffuses out of cells and is transported in blood in a few different ways: less than 10% dissolves in the blood plasma, about 20% binds to hemoglobin, while about 70% is converted to carbonic acid to be carried to the lungs.

Carbonic anhydrase is an enzyme present in red blood cells (RBCs) containing zinc coordinated with histidine at the active site that catalyses the reversible hydration of carbon dioxide. Binding of the substrate carbon dioxide occurs at a hydrophobic pocket. The mechanism at the active site can be summarised below.

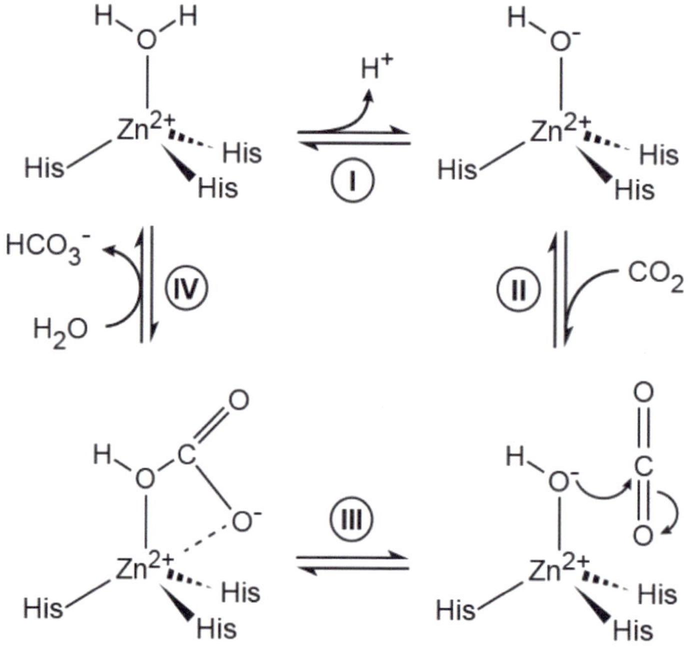

11) It can be assumed that Reaction III is the rate-limiting step of the net reaction of Reactions II and III. What best accounts for this assumption?

A. H_2CO_3 is a stronger acid than HCO_3^-.
B. Reaction II has a slower rate of reaction than Reaction III.
C. Reaction II has a smaller equilibrium constant.
D. HCO_3^- is a weaker base than CO_3^{2-}.

12) As shown in Reaction II and Reaction III, carbonic acid ionises in a stepwise manner. Consequently, two equilibrium expressions (K_{a1} and K_{a2}) can be written for the two ionisation steps. The first ionisation K_{a1} is much larger than the second ionisation constant K_{a2}. Which of the following statements would correctly explain why the value of K_{a1} is much larger than that of K_{a2} for carbonic acid?

A. Carbonic acid is a weak acid and so is completely ionised resulting in a large K_{a1}.
B. It is much easier to remove H^+ from the first ionisation step of carbonic acid as it is uncharged.
C. There really should not be a great difference between the two ionisation constants (K_{a1} and K_{a2}) as both released H^+ ions are from carbonic acid.
D. As the concentration of H^+ released from the first ionisation is much larger than the second ionisation, this will increase the possibility of the second ionisation concentration to be large.

13) If Reaction I had a relatively large equilibrium constant, which of the following proportions might one expect when Reaction I is at equilibrium?

A. 80% CO_2, 20% H_2CO_3
B. 20% CO_2, 80% H_2CO_3
C. 50% CO_2, 50% H_2CO_3
D. 0% CO_2, 100% H_2CO_3

14) From Reaction II of the passage, which of the following would be regarded as an appropriate conjugate acid/base pair, respectively?

A. H_2O / H_3O^+
B. H_2O / HCO_3^-
C. H_2CO_3 / HCO_3^-
D. H_2CO_3 / H_3O^+

15) Which of the following is likely true about the activity of carbonic anhydrase in RBCs?

I. Carbonic anhydrase increases the rate of Reaction I by bringing the reactants into close proximity.
II. The higher the pH, the greater the activity of carbonic anhydrase in the hydration of carbon dioxide.
III. The activity of carbonic anhydrase leads to increased carbon dioxide in RBCs in the lungs.

A I only
B II only
C I and III only
D I, II and III

16) The pK_a of acetic acid is 5. What is the pH at which the concentration of acetic acid will be 10^3 that of its conjugate base?

A. 2
B. 3
C. 5
D. 7

17) The pK_a of acetic acid is 5. What is the pH at which the concentration of acetic acid will be 10^{-6} that of its conjugate base?

A. –1
B. 1
C. 7
D. 11

Questions 18–22

Acid-base indicators such as methyl-orange, phenolphthalein and bromothymol blue are substances which change colour according to the hydrogen ion concentration of the solution to which they are added.

Most indicators are weak acids (or more rarely weak bases) in which the undissociated and dissociated forms have different, distinct colours. If methyl-orange is used as the example and the undissociated form is written as HMe, then the dissociation occurs as shown in Reaction I.

Reaction I

$$\underset{\text{Red}}{HMe} \longleftrightarrow \underset{\text{Colourless}}{H^+} + \underset{\text{Yellow}}{Me^-}$$

The indicator should have a colour change coinciding with the equivalence point of the titration. Usually, the colour change of the indicator occurs over a range of about two pH units. It should be noted that the eye cannot detect the exact end point of the titration. The pK_a of the indicator should be near the pH of the solution at the equivalence point.

Note that: The observed colour is orange if there is a mixture of red and yellow; and the observed colour is green with a mixture of blue and yellow.

18) Hydrogen ion concentration must change by at least what factor such that methyl-orange in solution turns from yellow to red?

A. 2
B. 10
C. 100
D. 200

19) Which of the following is true?

A. The conjugate base of a strong acid is a stronger base.
B. As pK_a increases, acidity decreases.
C. The conjugate acid of a weak base is a very weak acid.
D. As pK_a increases, acidity increases.

20) A titration between equimolar concentrations of hydrochloric acid and sodium hydroxide has an equivalence point with a pH of 7. Given the following information, which indicator is most suitable for detecting the end point of this titration?

Indicator	K_a
Bromothymol blue	3.16×10^{-7}
Cresol red	7.00×10^{-9}
Bromophenol blue	1.58×10^{-4}
p-Xylenol blue	1.10×10^{-2}

A. Bromothymol blue
B. Cresol red
C. Bromophenol blue
D. p-Xylenol blue

21) Given that the K_a (methyl-orange) = 2.0×10^{-4}, a solution of pH = 2 containing the indicator would likely be which of the following?

A. Orange
B. Yellow
C. Colourless
D. Red

22) A solution with a pH = 3.5 containing the methyl-orange indicator would likely be which of the following?

A. Orange
B. Yellow
C. Colourless
D. Red

Questions 23–25

In an aqueous solution, the general form of the equilibrium reaction for the dissociation of an acid is:

$$HA + H_2O \rightleftharpoons A^- + H_3O^+$$

Thus the equilibrium constant for the dissociation of an acid can be represented by:

$$K_a = [A^-][H_3O^+] / [HA]$$

23) What is the $[A^-]/[HA]$ ratio when a weak acid is in a solution one pH unit below its pK_a?

A. 1:1
B. 1:10
C. 10:1
D. 2:1

24) Which of the following can be derived from the acid dissociation constant?

A. $pH = pK_a + \log\left(\frac{[A^-]}{[HA]}\right)$

B. $pH = pK_a + \left(\frac{[A^-]}{[HA]}\right)$

C. $pH = pK_a + \log\left(\frac{[HA]}{[A^-]}\right)$

D. $pK_a = pH + \log\left(\frac{[A^-]}{[HA]}\right)$

25) Which of the following is a conjugate acid-base pair, respectively?

A. H_3PO_4 and PO_4^{-3}
B. $H_2PO_4^-$ and H_3PO_4
C. HPO_4^{-2} and $H_2PO_4^-$
D. $H_2PO_4^-$ and HPO_4^{-2}

26) Which of the following solutions would be expected to have the greatest change in hydrogen ion concentration in moles/L?

A. A pH change from 3 to 2
B. A pH change from 9 to 4
C. A pH change from 13 to 11
D. A pH change from 14 to 10

27) The isoelectric point (pI), is the pH at which a particular molecule carries no net electrical charge in the statistical mean. Consider Figure 1.

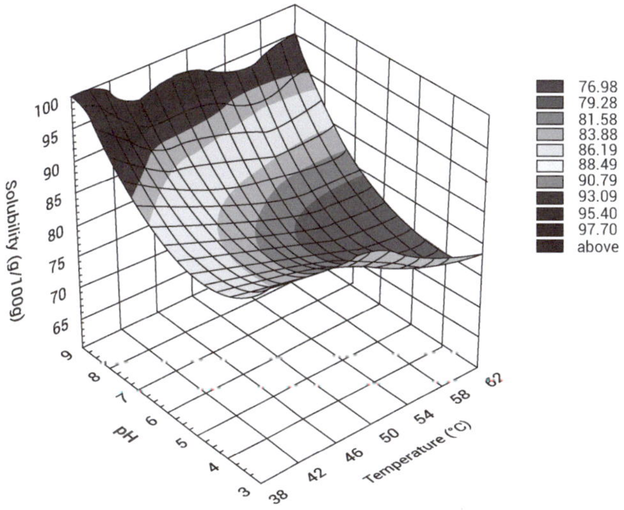

Figure 1: Three-dimensional plot generated for whey protein solubility in water as a function of temperature and pH (ref: Food Science and Technology 38(1):77-80 · February 2005)

Which of the following is consistent with Figure 1?

A. Whey proteins have a net positive charge at a pH of 9.
B. Whey proteins have their lowest solubility below 70 g/100 g.
C. Whey proteins demonstrate increased solubility with increasing temperature.
D. Whey proteins have a pI below pH = 6.

High-level Importance

Questions 28–29

In aqueous solution, water is always available as a proton acceptor, so that the ionisation of an acid, HA, can be written as:

$$HA + H_2O \rightleftharpoons H_3O^+ + A^-$$

or: $$HA \rightleftharpoons H^+ + A^-$$

The equilibrium constant is:

$$K_a = [H^+][A^-]/[HA] \quad \text{and} \quad pK_a = -\log_{10}K_a$$

The biologically active form of phosphorus in water is phosphate. The dissociation of phosphate into its various forms (*speciation*) is pH dependent. At STP:

$$H_3PO_4 \rightleftharpoons H_2PO_4^- \rightleftharpoons HPO_4^{2-} \rightleftharpoons PO_4^{3-}$$

Consider Figure 1

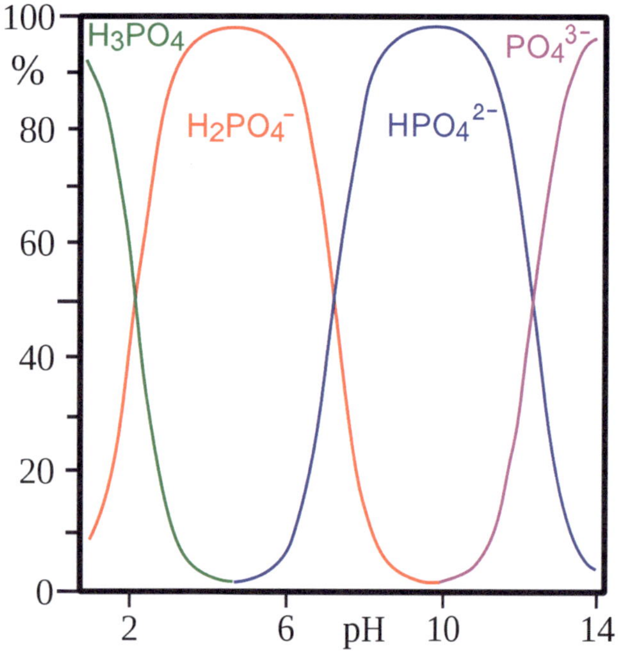

Figure 1

28) Based on Figure 1, which of the following is least likely to represent a pK_a value for phosphate and its various forms?

A. 2.12
B. 7.21
C. 9.42
D. 12.44

29) Consider $H_2PO_4^-$ and HPO_4^{2-}. According to Figure 1, if the protonated form is 10× greater than the deprotonated form, which of the following most accurately predicts the pH of the solution?

A. 6
B. 7
C. 8
D. 9

30) Sulfuric acid, H_2SO_4, is a diprotic acid. Consider the following solutions of sulfuric acid and/or its sodium salts.

Solution I: 0.50 M H_2SO_4
Solution II: 0.50 M $NaHSO_4$
Solution III: 0.50 M Na_2SO_4
Solution IV: A mixture of equal volumes of I and II

Which solution has the highest pH?

A. Solution I
B. Solution II
C. Solution III
D. Solution IV

SPOILER ALERT

Gold Standard has cross-referenced the content in this chapter to examples from ACER's official GAMSAT practice materials. It is for you to decide when you want to explore these questions since you may want to preserve some of ACER's materials for timed mock-exam practice.

Examples – Acid/base and pK_a: Q6-8 of 1; pK_a: Q48 of 1; challenge with acid/base indicators with pK_a: Q36-38 of 2; pK_a/pK_b: Q51 of 2; simple pH calculation Q56 of 2; conjugate base: Q92 of 3; pH and bases: Q33-36 of 4; buffer solutions: Q104-107 of 4; polyprotic-acid unit with 3 pK_a values (*sounds familiar?*): Q8-10 of 5; it looks like K_b and pK_b, but it is really just manipulating logs (GM 3.7): Q109-110 of 5. Note that "Q" is followed by the question number, and, for example, "of 1" refers to booklet number 1 which is referenced in the Spoiler Alert table at the end of Chapter 1. The 15 full-length GAMSAT practice tests by Gold Standard, HEAPS-1 through HEAPS-15, contain specific cross-references to this chapter within the worked solutions. Note that the unit describing polyprotic acids and carbonic anhydrase is a rare visitor from HEAPS-1; the acid/base indicator unit with methyl-orange comes from HEAPS-5.

Chapter Checklist

- ☐ Access your online account to view answers, worked solutions and discussion boards.
- ☐ Reassess your 'learning objectives' for this chapter: Go back to the first page of this chapter and re-evaluate the top 3 boxes and the Introduction.
  - ☐ Please be sure that you have completed the *Need for Speed* exercises at the beginning of this chapter.
- ☐ Complete a maximum of 1 page of notes using symbols/abbreviations to represent the entire chapter based on your learning objectives. These are your Gold Notes.
- ☐ Consider your multimedia options based on your optimal way of learning:
  - ☐ Download the free Gold Standard GAMSAT app for your Android device or iPhone.
  - ☐ Create your own, tangible study cards or try the free app: Anki.
  - ☐ Record your voice reading your Gold Notes onto your smartphone (audio files, e.g., *memo* or MP3s) and listen during exercise, transportation, etc.
  - ☐ Try out the Gold Standard GAMSAT online videos at gamsat-prep.com, or you can try other options on YouTube like Khan Academy or Crash Course Chemistry.
- ☐ Reassess your schedule for your full-length GAMSAT practice tests: ACER and/or HEAPS exams. Ensure that you have scheduled one full day to complete a practice test and 1-2 days for a thorough assessment of worked solutions while adding to your abbreviated Gold Notes.
- ☐ Reassess your progress in scheduling and/or evaluating stress reduction techniques such as regular exercise (sports), yoga, meditation and/or mindfulness exercises (*see* YouTube for suggestions).

THERMODYNAMICS

Chapter 7

Memorise

* Conversion between degrees Celsius (+ 273) and the Kelvin scale**

Understand

* System vs. surroundings
* Law of conservation of energy
* Heat transfer
* Conduction, convection, radiation
* Unit conversions

Importance

Low level: 0% of GAMSAT General Chemistry questions released by ACER are related to content in this chapter (in our estimation).

* Note that approximately 80% of the questions in GAMSAT General Chemistry are related to just 4 chapters: 4, 5, 6, and 9.

GAMSAT-Prep.com

Introduction

Thermodynamics, in chemistry, refers to the relationship of heat with chemical reactions or with the physical state. Thermodynamic processes can be analysed by studying energy and additional topics that we will be examining in the next chapter (Chapter 8) including entropy, volume, temperature and pressure.

Just a reminder: 'Importance Level' does not apply to the multiple-choice questions (MCQs) at the end of the chapter, since they will help you practice reasoning skills that apply to all of GAMSAT Sciences. However, due to the Importance Level for assumed knowledge, there will be no *Need for Speed* exercises for this chapter. The minimum that you should consider is to look at the pretty pictures (!!) in this chapter, observe captions and equations, and then practice. Conversions, application of equations, and a gorgeous graph that demands analysis, await you!

**The reason will be explained in the Spoiler Alert section at the end of this chapter.

Multimedia Resources at GAMSAT-Prep.com

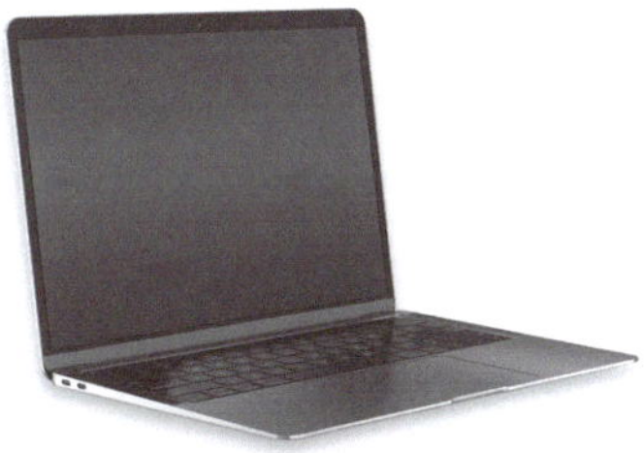

Open Discussion Boards
(gamsat-prep.com/forum)

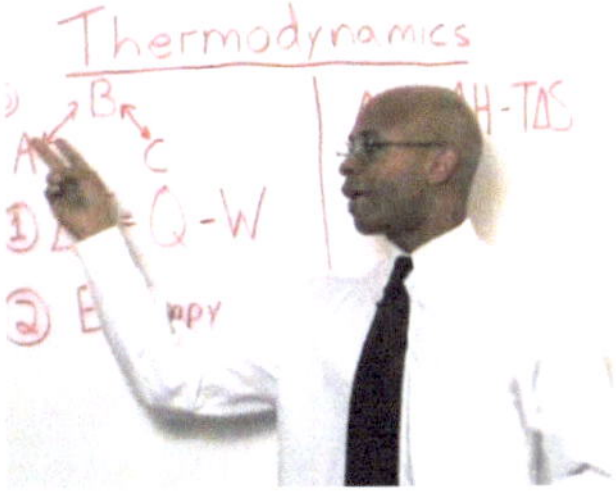

Science Preparation Videos

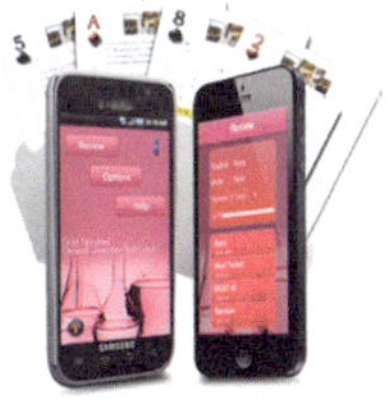

Flashcards

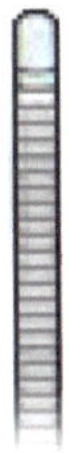

Special Guest

* The real GAMSAT may have advanced-level information presented (i.e. in a passage) but previous knowledge of said information is not required to answer the questions that would follow. Practice questions at the end of this chapter, as well as ACER and GS (HEAPS) practice GAMSATs can help you clarify this point.

7.1 Thermodynamic Transformations: System vs Surroundings

Thermodynamics deals with fundamental questions concerning energy transfers. One difficulty you will have to overcome is the terminology used. For instance, remember that heat and temperature have more specific meanings than the ones attributed to them in every day life.

A thermodynamic transformation can be as simple as a gas leaking out of a tank or a piece of metal melting at high temperature or as complicated as the synthesis of proteins by a biological cell. To solve some problems in thermodynamics we need to define a "system" and its "surroundings." The system is simply the object experiencing the thermodynamic transformation. The gas would be considered as the system in the first example of transformations. Once the system is defined any part of the universe in direct contact with the system is considered as its surroundings. For instance, if the piece of metal is melted in a high temperature oven: the system is the piece of metal and the oven constitutes its surroundings.

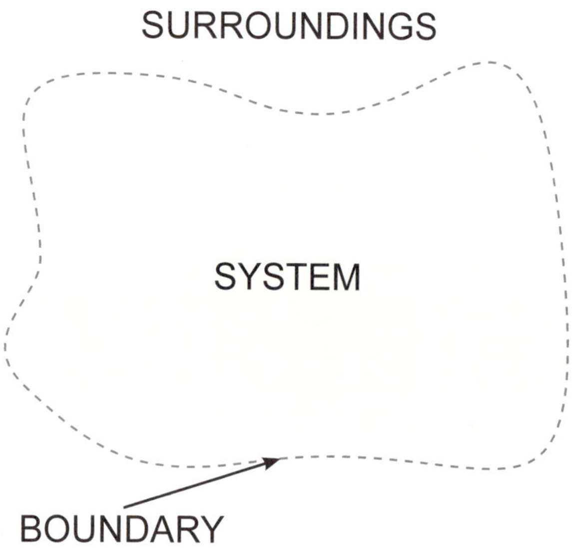

In other instances, the limit between the system and its surroundings is more arbitrary, for example if one considers the energy exchanges when an ice cube melts in a thermos bottle filled with orange juice; the inside walls of the thermos bottle could be considered as part of "the system" or as part of the surroundings. In the first case, one would carry out all calculations as though the entire system (ice cube + orange juice + inside walls) is isolated from its surroundings (rest of the universe) and all the energy exchanges take place within the system. In the second case, the system (ice cube + orange juice) is not isolated from the surroundings (walls) unless we consider that the heat exchanges with the walls are negligible. There is also no need to include any other part of the universe in the latter case since all exchanges take place within the system or between the system and the inside walls of the thermos bottle.

Some systems may exchange both matter and energy with the surroundings. This is called an "open system". Alternatively, some systems may exchange energy only but not matter with the surroundings. This is called a "closed system". Finally, some systems do not exchange matter or energy with their surroundings. This is called an "isolated system". An isolated system therefore does not interact with its surroundings in any way.

Low-level Importance

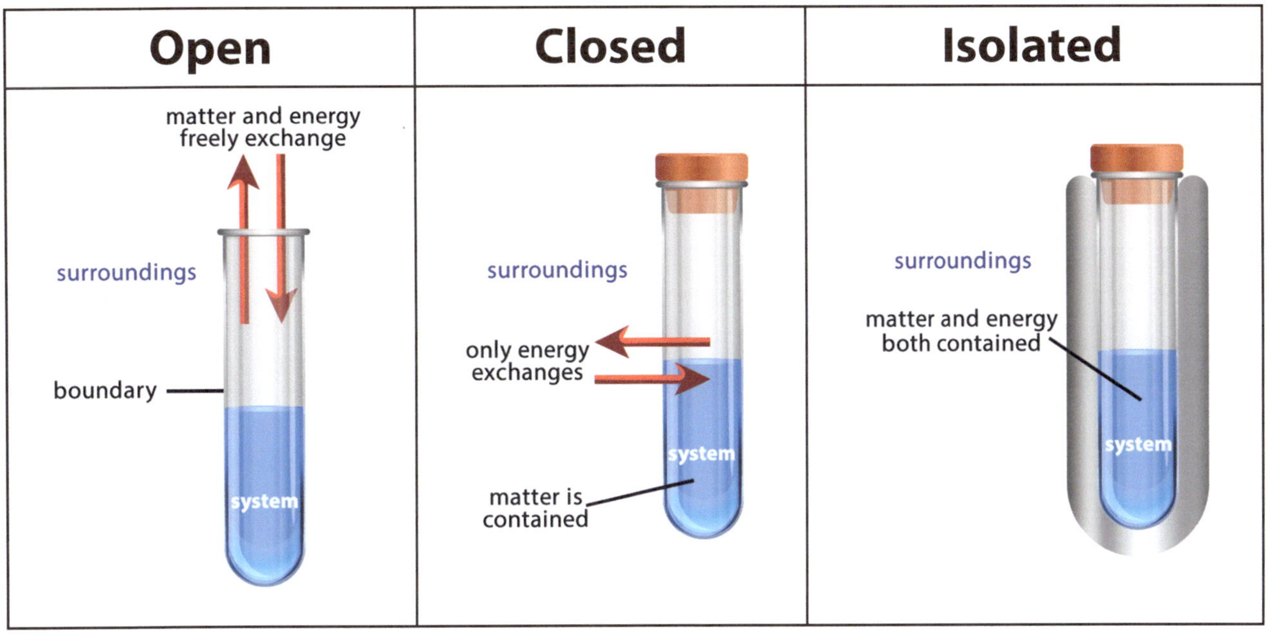

Figure III.A.7.1: System vs. surroundings.

7.2 The First Law of Thermodynamics

Heat, internal energy and work are the first concepts introduced in thermodynamics. Heat is thermal energy (a dynamic property defined during a transformation only), it is not to be confused with temperature (a static property defined for each state of the system). Internal energy is basically the average total mechanical energy (kinetic + potential) of the particles that make up the system. The first law of thermodynamics is often expressed as follows: when a system absorbs an amount of heat Q from the surroundings and does a quantity of work W on the same surroundings its internal energy changes by the amount:

$$\Delta E = Q - W$$

This law is basically the law of conservation of energy for an isolated system. Indeed, it states that if a system does not exchange any energy with its surroundings, its internal energy should not vary. If on the other hand a system does exchange energy with its surroundings, its internal energy should change by an amount corresponding to the energy it takes in from the surroundings.

The sign convention related to the previous mathematical expression of the first law of thermodynamics is:

- heat absorbed by the system: $Q > 0$
- heat released by the system: $Q < 0$
- work done by the system on its surroundings: $W > 0$

Low-level Importance

- work done by the surroundings on the system: $W < 0$

Caution: Some textbooks prefer a different sign convention: any energy (Q or W) flowing from the system to the surroundings (lost by the system) is negative and any energy flowing from the surroundings to the system (gained by the system) is positive. Within such a sign convention the first law is expressed as:

$$\Delta E = Q + W$$

i.e. the negative sign in the previous equation is incorporated in W.

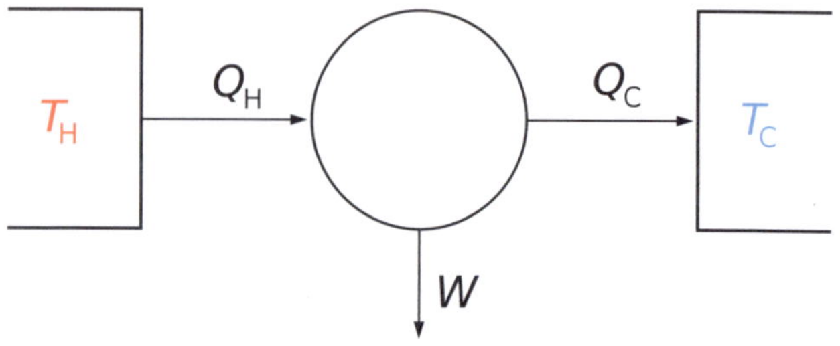

Figure III.A.7.2: The first law of thermodynamics. An amount of heat Q_H (subscript H = hot, C = cold) flows from a high temperature T_H furnace through the fluid of the "working body" (i.e. the system or *working substance*) and the remaining heat Q_C flows into the cold sink T_C, thus forcing the working substance to do mechanical work W on the surroundings. The work could be cycles of contractions and expansions as in the prototypical "Carnot engine" (CHM 8.1.1).

7.3 Equivalence of Mechanical, Chemical and Thermal Energy Units

The previous equation does more than express mathematically the law of conservation of energy, it establishes a relationship between thermal energy and mechanical energy. Historically, thermal energy was expressed in calories (abbreviated as cal.) defined as the amount of thermal energy required to raise the temperature of 1 g of water by 1 degree Celsius. The standard unit used for mechanical work is the joule (J). This unit eventually became the standard unit for any form of energy. The conversion factor between the two units is:

$$1 \text{ cal} = 4.184 \text{ J}$$

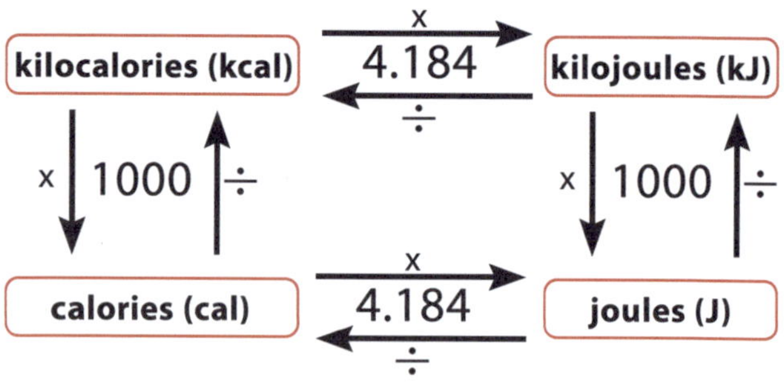

Chemists often refer to the amount of energies exchanged between the system and its surroundings to the mole, i.e., quantities of energy are expressed in J/mol (SI) or cal/mol. To obtain the energy per particle (atom or molecule), you should divide the energy expressed in J or cal by Avogadro's number.

Low-level Importance

There are three temperature scales in use in science textbooks: the Celsius scale, the absolute temperature or Kelvin scale (SI), and the Fahrenheit scale. In **the Celsius scale** the freezing point and the boiling point of water are arbitrarily defined as 0°C and 100 °C, respectively. The scale is then divided into equal 1/100th intervals to define the degree Celsius or centigrade (from latin centi = 100).

The absolute temperature or Kelvin scale is derived from the centigrade scale, i.e., an interval of 1 degree Celsius is equal to an interval of 1 kelvin (note that the Kelvin scale is not technically a degree and thus does not possess the degree ° symbol; small 'k' kelvin has the symbol: K).

The difference between the two scales is in their definitions of the zero point:

$$0\text{ K} = -273.15\ ^\circ\text{C}.$$

Theoretically, this temperature can be approached but never achieved (= *the 'absolute zero'*), it corresponds to the point where all motion is frozen. Experimentally, gases appear to contract indefinitely as temperature decreases. Consistent with the ideal gas law (CHM 4.1.8), an ideal gas at constant pressure must reach zero volume at the absolute zero (T = 0 K). Any real gas actually condenses to a liquid or a solid at some temperature higher than absolute zero. Therefore, the ideal gas law is only an approximation of real gas behavior. All molecular motion does **not** cease at absolute zero but no energy from molecular motion (i.e. heat energy) is available for transfer to other systems, and thus the energy at absolute zero is minimal.

The Fahrenheit scale has the disadvantage of not being divided into 100 degrees between its two reference points: the freezing point of water is 32 °F and its boiling point is 212 °F. To convert Fahrenheit degrees into Celsius degrees you have to perform the following transformation:

$$(X\ ^\circ\text{F} - 32) \times 5/9 = Y\ ^\circ\text{C}$$

or

$$^\circ\text{F} = 9/5\ ^\circ\text{C} + 32.$$

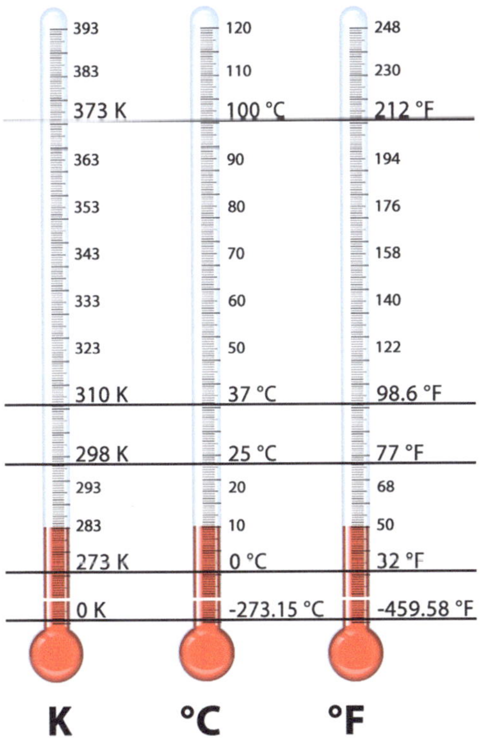

Figure III.A.7.3: Three main temperature scales.

Low-level Importance

7.5 Heat Transfer

There are three ways in which heat can be transferred between the system and its surroundings:

(a) heat transfer by conduction

(b) heat transfer by convection

(c) heat transfer by radiation

In the first case (a) there is an intimate contact between the system and its surroundings and heat propagates through the entire system from the heated part to the unheated parts. A good example is the heating of a metal rod on a flame. Heat is initially transmitted directly from the flame to the rod through the contact between the metal and the flame. When carrying out such an experiment you would notice at some point that the part of the rod which is not in direct contact with the flame becomes hot as well (please do not attempt!). Note that air molecules are too far apart to disperse heat energy efficiently, and thus air is a poor conductor of heat.

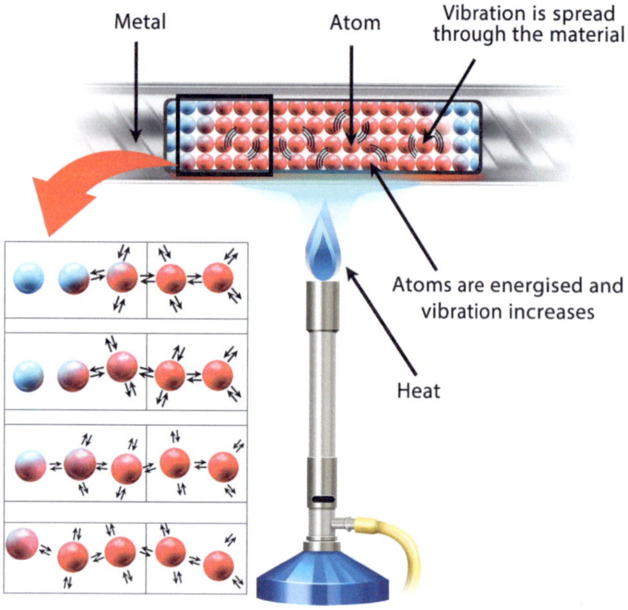

Figure III.A.7.4: Conduction. Note that conduction creates a "domino effect" (*chain reaction*) of particles with increased heat energy.

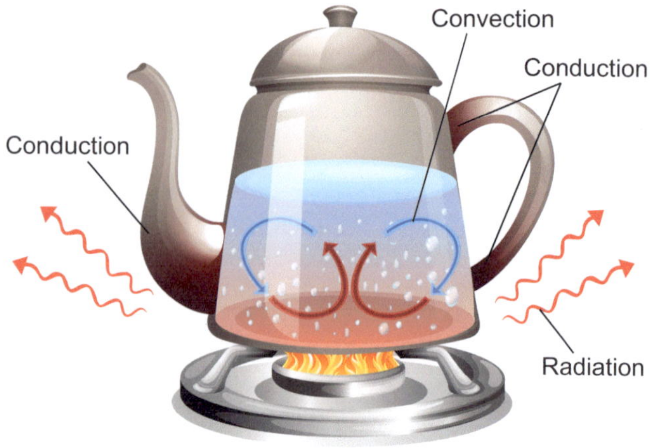

Figure III.A.7.5: Heat transfer methods.

In the second case (b), heat is transferred to the entire system by the circulation of a hot liquid or a gas through it. The difference between this mode of transfer and the previous one, is that the entire system or a major part of it is heated up directly by the surroundings and not by propagation of the thermal energy from the parts of the system which are in direct contact with the heating source and the parts which are not.

In the third case (c) there is no contact between the heating source and the system. Heat is transported by radiation. The perfect example is the microwave oven where the water inside the food is heated by the microwave source.

Low-level Importance

Most heat transfers are carried out by at least two of the three heat-transfer processes at the same time.

Note that when a metal is heated it expands at a rate which is proportional to the change in temperature it experiences. {For a definition of the coefficient of expansion, *see* PHY 6.3.}

Thermal energy will always transfer from an object with more energy to an object with less energy. Heat travels from object to object, cold does not. When you put ice in a drink, cold does not transfer from the ice to the drink, heat travels from the drink into the ice.

7.6 State Functions

As previously mentioned, the first law of thermodynamics introduces three fundamental energy functions, i.e., the internal energy *E*, heat *Q*, and work *W*. Let us consider a transformation that takes the system from an initial state (I) to a final state (F) (which can differ by a number of variables such as temperature, pressure and volume).

The change in the internal energy during this transformation depends only on the properties of the initial state (I) and the final state (F). In other words, suppose that to go from (I) to (F) the system is first subjected to an intermediate transformation that temporarily takes it from state (I) to an intermediate state (Int.) and then to another transformation that brings it from (Int.) to (F), the change in internal energy between the initial state (I) and the final state (F) are independent of the properties of the intermediate state (Int.).

The internal energy is said to be a path-independent function or a state function. This is not the case for *W* and *Q*. In fact, this is quite conceivable since the amount of *W* or Q can be imposed by the external operator who subjects the system to a given transformation from (I) to (F). For instance, *Q* can be fixed at zero if the operator uses an appropriate thermal insulator between the system and its surroundings. In which case the change in the internal energy is due entirely to the work w ($\Delta E = -w$). It is easy to understand that the same result [transformation from (I) to (F)] could be achieved by supplying a small quantity of heat q while letting the system do more work *W* on the surroundings so that $q - W$ is equal to $-w$.

	Work	Heat	Change in internal energy
1st transf.	w	0	$-w$
2nd transf.	$W = w + q$	q	$-w$

Low-level Importance

W and *Q* are not state functions. They depend on the path taken to go from (I) to (F). If you remember the exact definition of the internal energy you will understand that a system changes its internal energy to respond to an input of *Q* and *W*. In other words, contrary to *Q* and *W*, the internal energy cannot be directly imposed on the system.

The fact that the internal energy is a state function can be used in three other equivalent ways:

(i) If the changes in the internal energy during the intermediate transformation are known, they can be used to calculate the change for the entire process from (I) to (F): the latter is equal to the sum of the changes in the internal energy for all the intermediate steps.

(ii) If the change in the internal energy to go from a state (I) to a state (F) is $E_{I \to F}$ the change in the internal energy for an opposite transformation that would take the system from (F) to (I) is:

$$\Delta E_{F \to I} = - \Delta E_{I \to F}$$

(iii) If we start from (I) and go back to (I) through a series of intermediate transformations the change in the internal energy for the entire process is zero.

<u>*W* can be determined experimentally by calculating the area under a pressure-volume curve</u>. The mathematical relation is presented in CHM 8.1.

CHAPTER 7: Thermodynamics

GOLD STANDARD FOUNDATIONAL GAMSAT PRACTICE QUESTIONS

Questions 1–2

To convert between the most commonly used temperature scales (Celsius, Kelvin and Fahrenheit), consider the following transformations.

$$0\ K = -273.13\ °C$$

and

$$(X\ °F - 32) \times 5/9 = Y\ °C$$

or

$$°F = 9/5\ °C + 32.$$

1) Which of the following is the warmest?

- **A.** 20 °C
- **B.** 20 °F
- **C.** 20 K
- **D.** They all represent the same temperature.

2) What is 322 K in degrees Fahrenheit?

- **A.** 112 °F
- **B.** 120 °F
- **C.** 124 °F
- **D.** 128 °F

3) Historically, thermal energy was expressed in calories. A calorie is defined as the amount of thermal energy required to raise the temperature of 1 g of water by 1 degree Celcius (or one kelvin). The standard unit used for mechanical work and energy is the "joule" (J). The conversion factor between the two units is:

$$1 \text{ cal} = 4.184 \text{ J}$$

The "food calorie" or Calorie is actually a kilocalorie and it is most widely used in nutrition. Consider a typical Western diet composed of 2000 Calories per day. Approximately, how many joules does that represent?

A. 8.4 kJ
B. 84 kJ
C. 840 kJ
D. 8.4×10^3 kJ

4) Metal foil would aid in preventing heat gain via which of the following processes?

A. Reflecting radiant energy
B. Conduction
C. Convection
D. Radiation and conduction

5) Down-filled winter clothing reduces heat loss by incorporating pockets of air into the material. Which type of heat transfer process do the air pockets limit?

A. Radiation
B. Conduction
C. Convection
D. Conduction and convection

Questions 6–7

The first law of thermodynamics introduces three fundamental energy functions, i.e., the internal energy E, heat Q, and work W. The internal energy is said to be a path-independent function or a state function.

W and Q are not state functions. They depend on the path taken to go from the initial circumstance to the final circumstance.

6) Beaker A has a 100 g sample of water maintained at 25 °C and 1 atm for 24 hours. Beaker B has 100 g of water that was heated to 100 °C from 0 °C over 23 hours and then cooled to 25 °C at 1 atm by the 24th hour. Which of the following is true?

A. Beaker A has more internal energy than Beaker B.
B. Beaker B has less internal energy than Beaker A.
C. Both beakers have the same internal energy.
D. None of the above.

7) If a system loses 25 kJ of heat at the same time that it is doing 50 kJ of work, what is the change in the internal energy of the system?

A. –25 kJ
B. +25 kJ
C. –75 kJ
D. +75 kJ

High-level Importance

GOLD STANDARD GAMSAT-LEVEL PRACTICE QUESTIONS

Questions 8–10

The human body can gain or lose heat by conduction, convection or radiation. The body maintains a thermal balance by controlling heat loss and heat gain. The six major factors that affect comfort are: 1) air temperature; 2) mean radiant temperature; 3) air speed; 4) the relative humidity; 5) clothing; and 6) level of activity.

A helpful tool for the design of indoor spaces is the effective temperature. This is a fictitious temperature to which combinations of temperature, humidity and air speed correspond. Such combinations should give the same feeling of comfort.

Normal values to maintain comfort indoors:

- An effective temperature in the range of 16-28 degrees Celsius
- Difference between globe and wet bulb temperatures must not be less than 5 degrees Celsius
- Air speed below 0.1 m/s comes with a feeling of stuffiness; 0.1-1.0 m/s is comfortable; above 1.0 m/s: discomfort.

Note that if the person is outdoors, an air speed over 5 m/s causes discomfort.

Consider Figure 1 and its caption on the opposite page.

8) Consider a 25 °C globe temperature, a 20 °C wet bulb temperature, and an effective temperature of 15 °C. According to Figure 1, what is the air speed?

A. 0.1 m/s
B. 1.0 m/s
C. 3.0 m/s
D. 5.0 m/s

9) Consider a 35 °C globe temperature, a 15 °C wet bulb temperature, and an air speed of 1.0 m/s. According to Figure 1, what would be the predicted effective temperature?

A. 18 °C
B. 20 °C
C. 22 °C
D. 24 °C

10) Given the data from the previous question (Question 9), and the information provided in the passage, would the person likely be comfortable indoors?

A. Yes
B. No
C. There is a 50-50 chance.
D. Comfort only depends on the air speed.

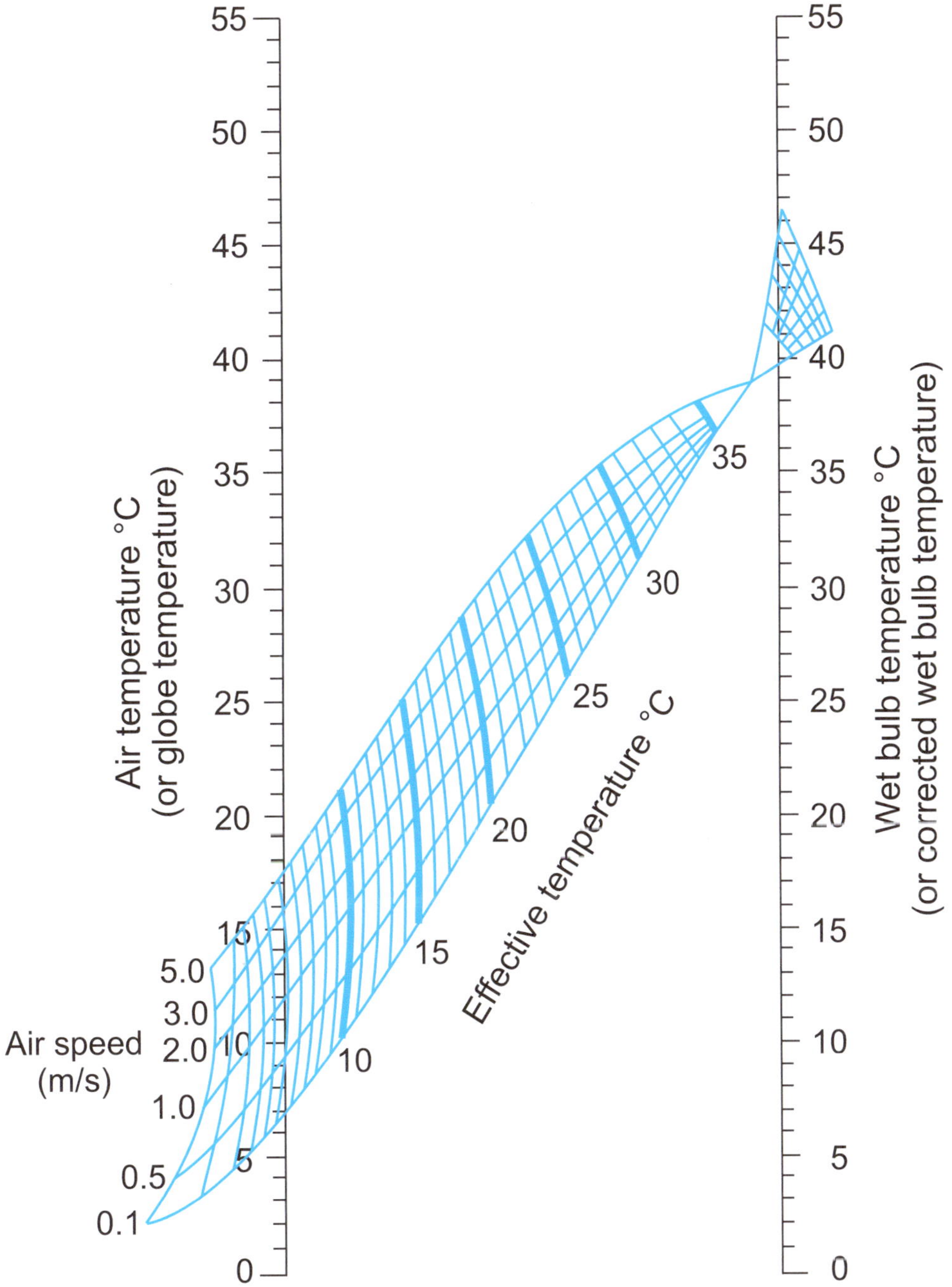

Figure 1: The cooling capacity of air with effective temperatures. There are four parameters: globe temperature, wet bulb temperature, air speed, and effective temperature. Knowing any three of these parameters, permits the determination of the fourth from the graph. Typically, a line is made between the globe and wet bulb temperatures, and then having either the air speed or the effective temperature provides a point of intersection in the blue portion of the graph which reveals the missing parameter.

High-level Importance

SPOILER ALERT

Gold Standard has cross-referenced the content in this chapter to examples from ACER's official GAMSAT practice materials. It is for you to decide when you want to explore these questions since you may want to preserve some of ACER's materials for timed mock-exam practice.

Examples – One! Out of 440 GAMSAT Sciences multiple-choice official practice questions, one strange one! Question 50 from ACER's *GAMSAT Practice Test* (the first one; AKA the Green Booklet) requires the knowledge of the interconversion of degrees Celsius (+ 273) to kelvin in order to solve the problem. Otherwise, that question is really about activation energy and the Arrhenius equation. We will handle all of the preceding in Chapter 8 including testing your memory on that one point (*temperature conversion*) in context with the GAMSAT-level practice questions. Back to Chapter 7: We presented a nomogram in this chapter (Questions 8-10), and ACER has 2 units based on nomograms with no assumed knowledge, and both are in ACER's *GAMSAT Practice Test 3* (the Pink booklet): The ternary diagram (Questions 14-17), and the 'angle of bank' nomogram (Questions 67-68). Note that you have already seen ternary diagrams twice in this book (Chapters 1 and 5), and multiple ternary diagrams and nomograms in the Masters Series Maths and Physics book.

Chapter Checklist

- ☐ Access your online account to view answers, worked solutions and discussion boards.
- ☐ Reassess your 'learning objectives' for this chapter: Go back to the first page of this chapter and re-evaluate the top 3 boxes and the Introduction.
- ☐ Complete a maximum of 1 page of notes using symbols/abbreviations to represent the entire chapter based on your learning objectives. These are your Gold Notes.
- ☐ Consider your multimedia options based on your optimal way of learning:
  - ☐ Download the free Gold Standard GAMSAT app for your Android device or iPhone.
  - ☐ Create your own, tangible study cards or try the free app: Anki.
  - ☐ Record your voice reading your Gold Notes onto your smartphone (audio files, e.g., *memo* or MP3s) and listen during exercise, transportation, etc.
  - ☐ Try out the Gold Standard GAMSAT online videos at gamsat-prep.com, or you can try other options on YouTube like Khan Academy or Crash Course Chemistry.
- ☐ Reassess your schedule for your full-length GAMSAT practice tests: ACER and/or HEAPS exams. Ensure that you have scheduled one full day to complete a practice test and 1-2 days for a thorough assessment of worked solutions while adding to your abbreviated Gold Notes.
- ☐ Reassess your progress in scheduling and/or evaluating stress reduction techniques such as regular exercise (sports), yoga, meditation and/or mindfulness exercises (*see* YouTube for suggestions).

ENTHALPY AND THERMOCHEMISTRY
Chapter 8

Memorise

* Define: endo/exothermic
* Positive, negative or zero: The meaning for Gibbs free energy, enthalpy, entropy, and absolute temperature (always positive!)

Understand

* Area under curve: PV diagram
* Equations for enthalpy, Hess's law, free energy
* Calculation: Hess, calorimetry, bond dissociation energy
* Second law of thermodynamics
* Entropy, free energy and spontaneity

Importance

Medium level: 6% of GAMSAT General Chemistry

questions released by ACER are related to content in this chapter (in our estimation).

* Note that approximately 80% of the questions in GAMSAT General Chemistry are related to just 4 chapters: 4, 5, 6, and 9.

Introduction

Thermochemistry is the study of energy absorbed or released in chemical reactions or in any physical transformation (i.e. phase change like melting and boiling). Thermochemistry for the GAMSAT includes understanding and/or calculating quantities such as enthalpy, heat capacity, heat of combustion, heat of formation, and, in particular, problems related to Gibbs free energy. The latter is used to determine if a chemical reaction would be spontaneous, at equilibrium, or not spontaneous.

Multimedia Resources at GAMSAT-Prep.com

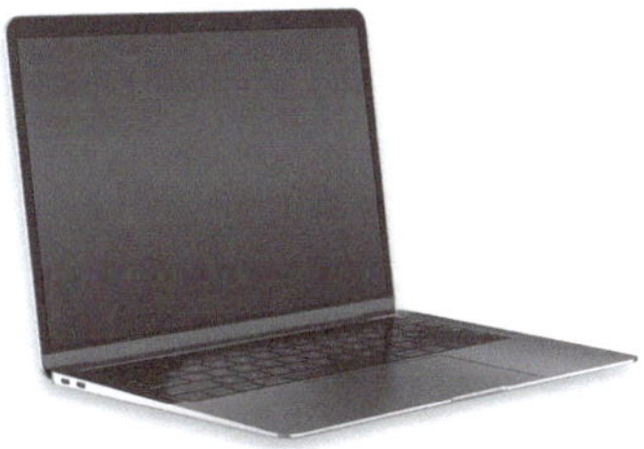

Open Discussion Boards
(gamsat-prep.com/forum)

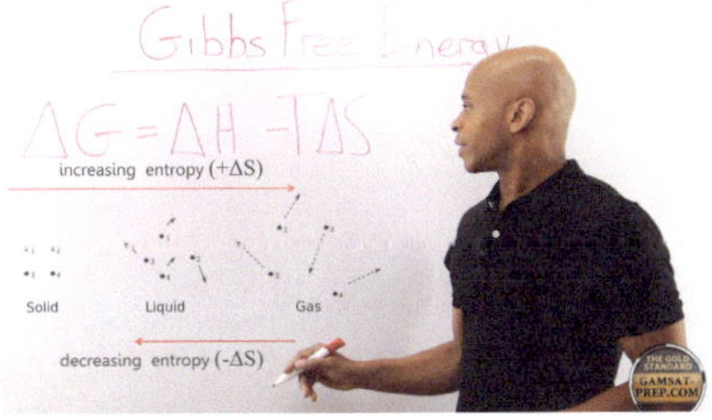

Science Preparation Videos

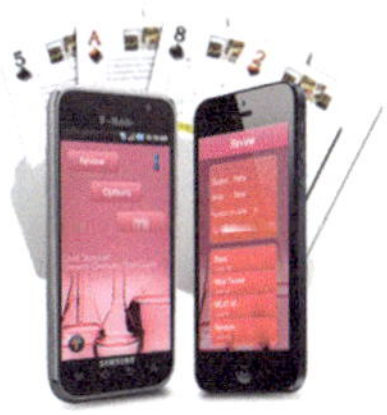

Flashcards

$\Delta G = \Delta H - T\Delta S$

Special Guest

* The real GAMSAT may have advanced-level information presented (i.e. in a passage) but previous knowledge of said information is not required to answer the questions that would follow. Practice questions at the end of this chapter, as well as ACER and GS (HEAPS) practice GAMSATs can help you clarify this point.

8.0 GAMSAT has a *Need for Speed*!

Section	GAMSAT General Chemistry *Need for Speed* Exercises
8.1.1	Consider the following pressure-volume (PV) diagram. 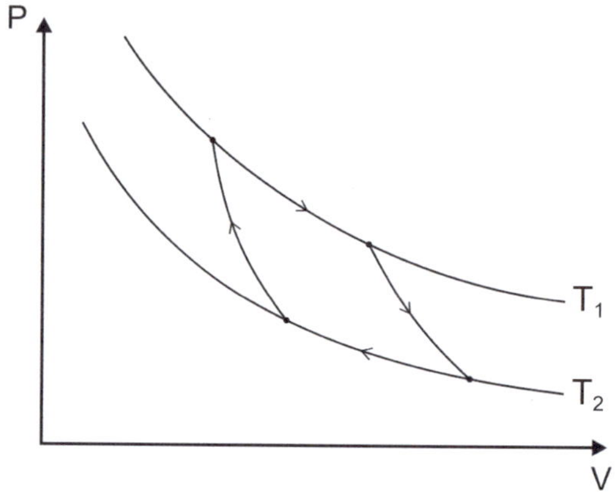 Based on the PV diagram: 1) Circle one of the following relationships which must be true (T: temperature). $T_1 = T_2$ $T_1 > T_2$ $T_1 < T_2$ 2) How can one determine the work done from the PV diagram above?
8.2	Complete the following statements. A chemical reaction during which heat is released is said to be _____________ (and the sign of ΔH is ___________). If a chemical reaction requires the supply of heat, it is said to be _______________ (and the sign of ΔH is ____________).
	Consider the following two chemical reactions and then complete the entry for the overall reaction. reaction 1: $A + B \rightarrow C$ reaction 2: $C \rightarrow D$ overall reaction:
	Enthalpy (H) is a state function. Add one of the following 4 symbols to the blue box: +, −, ×, or ÷. $\Delta H^\circ_{reaction} = \sum \Delta H_f^\circ{}_{(products)}$ ☐ $\sum \Delta H_f^\circ{}_{(reactants)}$

8.9	Entropy (S) is a state function. Add one of the following 4 symbols to the blue box: +, −, ×, or ÷. $\Delta S^\circ_{reaction} = \Delta S^\circ_{products}$ ☐ $\Delta S^\circ_{reactants}$
	Circle either positive or negative below. In a chemical reaction, if the products have more entropy (*randomness*) than the reactants, the ΔS of the reaction is (positive / negative). If the products have less entropy (*randomness*) than the reactants, then the ΔS of the reaction is (positive / negative).
8.9.1	Regarding the **change in entropy**: For each of the 3 chemical reactions below, write (*besides the equation*) either: positive or negative. $2\ NH_4NO_3(s) \rightarrow 2\ N_2(g) + O_2(g) + 4\ H_2O(g)$ $n\ P_4O_{10}(s) + 2n\ H_2O(g) \rightarrow 4\ (HPO_3)_n(s)$ $2\ Cu(s) + O_2(g) \rightarrow 2\ CuO(s)$
8.10	Can the temperature (K) be negative? Yes / No
	Complete the missing entries with one of the following: 0, positive, or negative.

	Spontaneous	Not spontaneous	Equilibrium
Gibbs free energy (ΔG)			

Gibbs free energy is given by:

$$\Delta G = \Delta H - T\Delta S$$

Given the equation for Gibbs free energy (i.e. *not based on rote learning*), complete the 4 missing entries.

Enthalpy change	**Entropy change**	**Gibbs free energy**	**Spontaneity**
positive	positive	depends on T, may be + or −	yes, if the temperature is high enough
negative	positive		
negative	negative	depends on T, may be + or −	yes, if the temperature is low enough
positive	negative		

Medium-level Importance

8.1 Enthalpy as a Measure of Heat

Medium-level Importance

The application of the general laws of thermodynamics to chemistry lead to some simplifications and adaptations because of the specificities of the problems that are dealt within this field. For instance, in chemistry it is critical, if only for safety reasons, to know in advance what amounts of heat are going to be generated or absorbed during a reaction. In contrast, chemists are generally not interested in generating mechanical work, and thus they tend to carry out most of their chemical reactions at constant pressure. For these reasons, although internal energy is a fundamental function, its use is not very adequate in thermochemistry. Instead, chemists prefer to use another function derived from the internal energy: the enthalpy (*H*). This function is mathematically defined as:

$$\Delta H = \Delta E + P \times (\Delta V)$$

where *P* and *V* are, respectively, the pressure and the volume of the system. Hence, the enthalpy change (ΔH) of any system is the sum of the change in its internal energy (ΔE) and the product of its pressure (P) and volume change (ΔV). As the three components, internal energy, pressure and volume are all state functions, the enthalpy (H) or enthalpy change (ΔH) of a system is therefore also a state function. Thus, enthalpy change depends only on the enthalpies of the initial and final states (ΔH) and not on the path and therefore it is an example of a state function itself. The enthalpy change of a reaction is defined by the following equation $\Delta H = H_{final} - H_{initial}$; where ΔH is the enthalpy change, H_{final} is the enthalpy of the products of a reaction, and $H_{initial}$ is the enthalpy of the reactants of a reaction. A positive enthalpy change ($+\Delta H$) would indicate the flow of heat into a system as a reaction occurs and is called an *endothermic reaction*. A cold pack on an arm swelling would be an example of an endothermic reaction. A negative enthalpy change ($-\Delta H$) would be called an *exothermic reaction* which essentially gives heat energy off from a system into its surroundings. A bunsen burner flame (= *a small adjustable gas burner used in chemistry labs; the heat source in* Fig. III.A.7.4, CHM 7.5) would be an example of an exothermic reaction.

You may wonder about the use of artificially introducing another energy function when internal energy is well defined and directly related to kinetic and potential energy of the particles that make up the system. To answer this legitimate question you need to consider the case of the majority of the chemical reactions where P is constant and where the only type of work that can possibly be done by the system is of a mechanical nature. In this case, since a change in internal energy (ΔE) occurring during a chemical reaction is basically a measure of all the system's energy as heat and work (Q + W) exchange with the system's surroundings, therefore, $\Delta E = Q + W$ and since, $W = -P\Delta V$, then, the change in enthalpy during a chemical reaction reduces to: $\Delta H = \Delta E + P \times V = (Q + W) + P \times V = Q + W - W = Q$ In other words, the change in enthalpy during a chemical reaction reduces to:

$$\Delta H = \Delta E + P \times V = (Q + W) + P \times V = Q$$

To summarise: the change of enthalpy is a direct measure of the heat that evolves or is absorbed during a reaction carried out at constant pressure.

8.1.1 Enthalpy Drives Your Car: The Heat Engine and the PV Diagram

We put a liquid that some call 'gas' into a solid and drive, drive, drive! For over a century, the controlling of the combustion (*burning*) of fuel through little explosions has been transferred into real work. The chemistry involves the input of energy and the release of even more energy which permits the harnessing of the expansion of gas and heat to do work. Petrol is a working substance. The discussion of this internal combustion or *heat engine* will lead us to a very 'famous' pressure vs. volume curve (*the PV diagram*) which can also show up in GAMSAT Physics or Biology.

Petrol (*or gasoline*) is the most widely used liquid fuel. It is volatile (*evaporates quickly, lacks hydrogen bonds*), flammable (*easy to set on fire*), and is composed of hydrocarbon molecules, which are compounds that contain hydrogen and carbon only (ORG Chapters 3, 4 and 5).

Unsurprisingly, an internal combustion engine is an engine in which combustion, or the burning of fuel, occurs on the inside. Liquid petrol itself is not actually burned, but its fumes ignite, causing the remaining liquid to evaporate and then burn. The gas expands and the pressure pushes a rod which is attached to a wheel. The rod pushes the wheel and makes it spin around. The spinning wheel is attached to other wheels, such as four car wheels, with a belt or a chain, which permit the wheels to spin and the car to move.

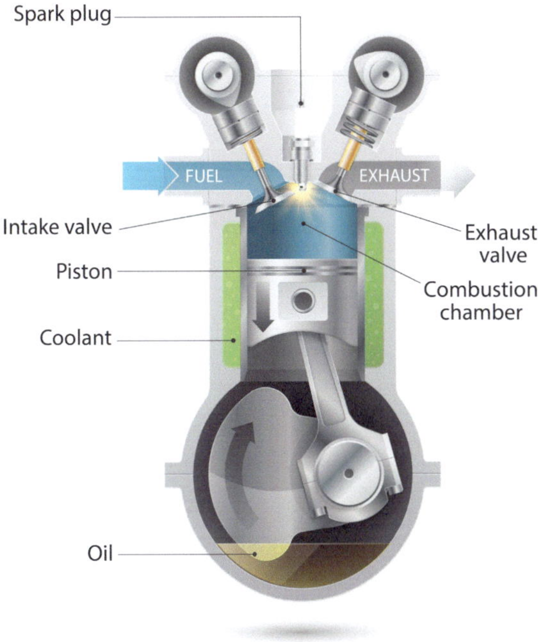

Figure III.A.8.1: Internal combustion engine. The diagram illustrates one of the many cylinders that an engine block may have. Most cars have 4, 6 or 8 cylinders.

Heat engines, such as automobile engines, operate in a cyclic manner: adding energy in the form of heat in one part of the cycle, using that energy to do useful work in another part of the cycle, and then the engine exhausts the heat which cannot be used to do work (*yes, the exhaust pipe at the back of vehicles*).

Thermodynamics is the study of the relationships between heat and work. The first law (CHM 7.2) and second law (CHM 8.8) of thermodynamics dictate the operation of a heat engine. The first law is the application

Medium-level Importance

of the conservation of energy to the system, and the second law sets limits on the possible efficiency of the machine and determines the direction of energy flow.

We have previously seen the ideal gas law (CHM 4.1.8) with chapter-ending practice questions to understand the interplay between P, V and T (pressure, volume and temperature, respectively). We will now examine those same parameters in action as related to a working ideal heat engine described by the Carnot cycle. The process is summarised by the PV diagram, and that is summarised by a diagram that you have seen before in Chapter 7 showing the production of work W by harnessing heat Q (*as the temperature goes from hot to cold*).

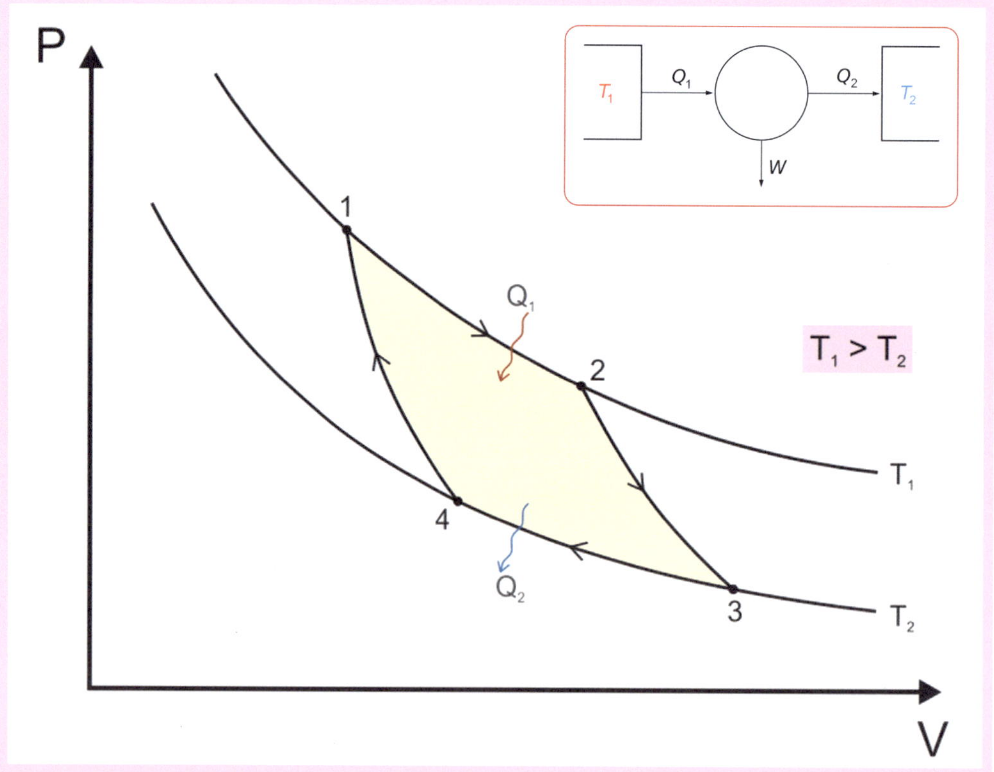

Figure III.A.8.2: Pressure-volume (PV) diagram and the Carnot cycle. From 4 to 1: heat is added (*the spark of the spark plug = ignition → combustion*); from 1 to 2: the gas absorbs heat Q_1, expands (*explosion!*) and does work (e.g. *pushes on a piston*) at constant temperature; from 2 to 3: heat is extracted (*exhaust*) as the gas continues to expand and do work; from 3 to 4: work is done on the gas by adding pressure at constant temperature as heat Q_2 is lost. For a cyclic heat engine process, the PV diagram produces a closed loop. The area inside the loop is a representation of the amount of work done (*shaded area in the diagram*) during a cycle (Spoiler Alert: There might be an artificial lung model based on the same relationships that you might see among the practice questions at the end of this chapter!). Inset: Carnot engine diagram, modified from Chapter 7, where heat Q_1 flows from a high temperature T_1 through the working substance, and the remaining heat Q_2 flows into the cold sink T_2 (*exhaust*), thus forcing the working substance to do mechanical work W on the surroundings, via cycles of contractions and expansions.

8.1.2 The Standard Enthalpy of Formation or Standard Heat of Formation ($\Delta H_f°$)

The standard enthalpy of formation, $\Delta H_f°$, is defined as the change of enthalpy that would occur when one mole of a substance is formed from its constituent elements in a standard state reaction. All elements in their standard states (oxygen gas, solid carbon as graphite, etc., at 1 atm and 25 °C) have a standard enthalpy of formation of zero, as there is no change involved in their formation. The calculated standard enthalpy of various compounds can then be used to find the standard enthalpy of a reaction. For example, the standard enthalpy of formation for methane (CH_4) gas at 25 °C would be the enthalpy of the following reaction:

$$C(s,graphite) + 2H_2(g) \rightarrow CH_4(g),$$

where $\Delta H_f° = -74.6$ KJ/mol. Thus, the chemical equation for the enthalpy of formation of any compound is always written with respect to the formation of 1 mole of the studied compound.

The standard enthalpy change for a reaction denoted as $\Delta H°_{rxn}$, is the change of enthalpy that would occur if one mole of matter is transformed by a chemical reaction with all reactants and products under standard state. It can be expressed as follows:

$$\Delta H°_{rxn} = (\text{sum of } n_f\Delta H°_f \text{ of products}) - (\text{sum of } n_r\Delta H°_f \text{ of reactants}),$$

where n_r represents the stoichiometric coefficients of the reactants and n_f the stoichiometric coefficients of the products. The $\Delta H°_f$ represents the standard enthalpies of formation.

Medium-level Importance

8.2 Heat of Reaction: Basic Principles

As discussed, a chemical reaction during which heat is released is said to be *exothermic* (ΔH is negative). If a chemical reaction requires the supply of heat, it is *endothermic* (ΔH is positive).

Besides the basic principle behind the introduction of enthalpy, there is a more fundamental advantage for the use of this function in thermochemistry: it is a state function. This is a very practical property. For instance, consider two chemical reactions related in the following way:

reaction 1:	$A + B \rightarrow C$
reaction 2:	$C \rightarrow D$

Add reaction 1 and 2, then cancel C from both sides. Thus, if these two reactions are carried out consecutively they lead to the same result as the following reaction:

overall reaction: $A + B \rightarrow D$

Because H is a state function we can apply the same arguments here as the ones we previously used for E. The initial state (I) corresponding to A + B , the intermediate state (Int.) to C, and the final state (F) to the final product D. If we know the changes in the enthalpy of the system for reactions 1 and 2, the change in the enthalpy during the overall reaction is:

$$\Delta H_{OVERALL} = \Delta H_1 + \Delta H_2$$

This is known as Hess's law. Remember that Hess's law is a simple application of the fact that H is a state function.

Thus, since the enthalpy change of a reaction is dependant only on the initial and final states, and not on the pathway that a reaction may follow, the sum of all the reaction step enthalpy changes must therefore be equivalent to the overall reaction enthalpy change (ΔH). The enthalpy change for a reaction can then be calculated without any direct measurement by using previously determined enthalpies of formation values for each reaction step of an overall equation. Consequently, if the overall enthalpy change is determined to be negative ($\Delta H_{net} < 0$), the reaction is exothermic and is most likely to be of a spontaneous type of reaction and a positive ΔH value would correspond to an endothermic reaction. Thus, Hess's law claims that enthalpy changes are additive and thus the ΔH for any single reaction can be calculated from the difference between the heat of formation of the products and the heat of formation of the reactants as follows:

$$\Delta H^\circ_{reaction} = \sum \Delta H_f^\circ{}_{(products)} - \sum \Delta H_f^\circ{}_{(reactants)}$$

where the ° superscript indicates standard state values.

Medium-level Importance

8.3 Hess's Law

Hess's law can be applied in several equivalent ways which we will illustrate with examples...

Example - Assume that we know the following enthalpy changes:

$$2H_2(g) + O_2(g) \rightarrow 2H_2O(l) \qquad \Delta H_1 = -136.6 \text{ kcal} : R1$$

$$Ca(OH)_2(s) \rightarrow CaO(s) + H_2O(l) \qquad \Delta H_2 = 15.3 \text{ kcal} : R2$$

$$2CaO(s) \rightarrow 2\,Ca(s) + O_2(g) \qquad \Delta H_3 = +303.6 \text{ kcal} : R3$$

and are asked to compute the enthalpy change for the following reaction:

$$Ca(s) + H_2(g) + O_2(g) \rightarrow Ca(OH)_2(s) : R$$

It is easy to see that reaction (R) can be obtained by the combination of reactions (R1), (R2) and (R3) in the following way:

$$\begin{array}{lr} -\ 1/2\ (R3): & Ca(s) + 1/2\ O_2(g) \rightarrow CaO(s) \\ +\ 1/2\ (R1): & H_2(g) + 1/2\ O_2(g) \rightarrow H_2O(l) \\ -\quad (R2): & CaO(s) + H_2O(l) \rightarrow Ca(OH)_2(s) \\ \hline & Ca(s) + H_2(g) + O_2(g) \rightarrow Ca(OH)_2(s) \end{array}$$

As we previously explained, since H is a state function the enthalpy change for (R) will be given by:

$$\Delta H = -1/2\Delta H_3 + 1/2\Delta H_1 - \Delta H_2$$

Example - Assume that we have the following enthalpy changes as shown below:

R1: $B_2O_3\ (s) + 3H_2O\ (g) \rightarrow 3O_2\ (g) + B_2H_6\ (g)$ $(\Delta H_1 = 2035\ kJ/mol)$

R2: $H_2O\ (l) \rightarrow H_2O\ (g)$ $(\Delta H_2 = 44\ kJ/mol)$

R3: $H_2\ (g) + (1/2)O_2\ (g) \rightarrow H_2O\ (l)$ $(\Delta H_3 = -286\ kJ/mol)$

R4: $2B\ (s) + 3H_2\ (g) \rightarrow B_2H_6\ (g)$ $(\Delta H_4 = 36\ kJ/mol)$

and are then asked to find the enthalpy change or ΔH_f of the following reaction (R):

R: $2B\ (s) + (3/2)O_2\ (g) \rightarrow B_2O_3\ (s)$ $(\Delta H_f - ?)$

After the required multiplication and rearrangements of all step equations (and their respective enthalpy changes), the result is as follows:

$(-1) \times (R1)$ $B_2H_6\ (g) + 3O_2\ (g) \rightarrow B_2O_3\ (s) + 3H_2O\ (g)$ $(\Delta H_1 = -2035\ kJ/mol)$

$(-3) \times (R2)$ $3H_2O\ (g) \rightarrow 3H_2O\ (l)$ $(\Delta H_2 = -132\ kJ/mol)$

$(-3) \times (R3)$ $3H_2O\ (l) \rightarrow 3H_2\ (g) + (3/2)O_2\ (g)$ $(\Delta H_3 = 858\ kJ/mol)$

$(+1) \times (R4)$ $2B\ (s) + 3H_2\ (g) \rightarrow B_2H_6\ (g)$ $(\Delta H_4 = 36\ kJ/mol)$

adding the equations while canceling out all common terms, we finally obtain:

$2B\ (s) + (3/2)O_2\ (g) \rightarrow B_2O_3\ (s)$ $(\Delta H_f = -1273\ kJ/mol)$

As noted in the initial example, it is shown that the enthalpy change (ΔH_f) for the final reaction is given by the following:

$$\Delta H_f = (-1)\Delta H_1 + (-3)\Delta H_2 + (-3)\Delta H_3 + (1)\Delta H_4$$

There are no general rules that would allow you to determine which reaction to use first and by what factor it needs to be multiplied. It is important to proceed systematically and follow some simple ground rules:

(i) For instance, you could start by writing the overall reaction that you want to obtain through a series of reaction additions.

(ii) Number all your reactions.

(iii) Keep in mind as you go along that the reactants of the overall reaction should always appear on the left-hand side and that the products should always appear on the right-hand side.

(iv) Circle or underline the first reactant of the overall reaction. Find a reaction in your list that involves this reactant (as a reactant or a product). Use that reaction first and write it in such a way that this reactant appears on the left-hand side with the appropriate stoichiometric coefficient (i.e., *if this reactant appears as a product of a reaction on your list you should reverse the reaction*).

(v) Suppose that in (iv) you had to use the second reaction on your list and that you had to reverse and multiply this reaction

Medium-level Importance

by a factor of 3 to satisfy the preceding rule. In your addition, next to this reaction or on top of the arrow write $-3 \times \Delta H_2$.

(vi) Repeat the process for the other reactants and products of the overall reaction until your addition yields the overall reaction. As you continue this process, make sure to cross out the compounds that appear on the right and left-hand sides at the same time.

8.4 Standard Enthalpies

Hess's law has a very practical use in chemistry. Indeed, the enthalpy change for a given chemical reaction can be computed from simple combinations of known enthalpy changes of other reactions. Because enthalpy changes depend on the conditions under which reactions are carried out it is important to define standard conditions:

(i) Standard pressure: 100 kPa (SI unit: 100 000 Pa), which is 1 bar, or approximately 1 atmosphere (atm).

(ii) Standard temperature for the purposes of the calculation of the standard enthalpy change: generally 25 °C (298 K). The convention is that if the temperature of the standard state is not mentioned then it is assumed to be 25 °C, the standard temperature needs to be specified in all other instances.

(iii) Standard physical state of an element: it is defined as the "natural" physical state of an element under the above standard pressure and temperature. For instance, the standard physical state of water under the standard temperature and pressure of 1 atm and 25 °C is the liquid state. Under the same conditions oxygen is a gas.

Naturally, the standard enthalpy change (notation: $\Delta H°$) for a given reaction is defined as the enthalpy change that accompanies the reaction when it is carried out under standard pressure and temperature with all reactants and products in their standard physical state.

Note: The standard temperature defined here is <u>different from the standard temperature for an ideal gas</u> which is: 0 °C (CHM 4.1.1).

8.5 Enthalpies of Formation

The enthalpy of formation of a given compound is defined as the enthalpy change that accompanies the formation of the compound from its constituting elements. For instance, the enthalpy of formation of water is the $\Delta H_f°$ for the following reaction:

$$H_2 + 1/2\ O_2 \rightarrow H_2O$$

To be more specific, the standard enthalpy of formation of water ΔH_f° is the enthalpy change during the reaction:

$$H_2(g) + 1/2O_2(g) \xrightarrow[1\text{ atm}]{25\ ^\circ C} H_2O(l)$$

where the reactants are in their natural physical state under standard temperature and pressure.

Note that according to these definitions, several of the reactions considered in the previous sections were in fact examples of reactions of formation. For instance, in CHM 8.3 discussing Hess's law, reaction (R1) is the reaction of formation of two moles of water, the reversed reaction (R3) would be the reaction of formation of two moles of CaO and the overall reaction (R) is the reaction of formation of 1 mole $Ca(OH)_2$. Also note that although one could use the reverse of reaction (R2) to form $Ca(OH)_2$, this reaction, even reversed, is not the reaction of formation of $Ca(OH)_2$. The reason is that the constitutive elements of this molecule are: calcium (Ca), hydrogen (H_2) and oxygen (O_2) and not CaO and H_2O. Enthalpies of formation are also referred to as heats of formation. As previously explained, if the reaction of formation is carried out at constant pressure, the change in the enthalpy represents the amount of heat released or absorbed during the reaction.

8.6 Bond Dissociation Energies and Heats of Formation

The bond dissociation energy, also known as the bond dissociation enthalpy, is a measure of bond strength within a particular molecule defined as a standard enthalpy change in the *homolytic* cleavage (= 2 free radicals formed; CHM 9.4) of any studied chemical bond. An example of bond dissociation energies would be the successive homolytic cleavage of each of the C-H bonds of methane (CH_4) to give, CH_3• + •H, CH_2• + •H, CH• + •H and finally C• + •H. The bond dissociation energies for each of the homolytic CH bond cleavage of methane are determined to be as follows: 435 KJ/mol, 444 KJ/mol, 444 KJ/mol and 339 KJ/mol, respectively. The average of these four individual bond dissociation energies is known as the bond energy of the CH bond and is 414 KJ/mol. Thus, with the exception of all diatomic molecules where only one chemical bond is involved so that bond energy and bond dissociation energy are in this case equivalent, the bond dissociation energy is not exactly the same as bond energy. Bond energy is more appropriately defined as the energy required to sever 1 mole of a chemical bond in a gas and not necessarily the measure of a chemical bond strength within a particular molecule. Bond energy is therefore a measure of bond strength. Moreover as just described, bond energy may be considered as an average energy calculated from the sum of bond dissociation energies of all bonds within a particular compound. Bond energies are always positive values as it always takes energy to break bonds apart.

The difficulty in defining bond dissociation energies in polyatomic molecules is that the amounts of energy required to break a given bond (say an O–H bond) in two different polyatomic molecules (H_2O and CH_3OH, for instance) are different. Bond dissociation energies in polyatomic molecules are approximated to an average value for molecules of the same nature. Within the framework of this commonly made approximation we can calculate the enthalpy change of any reaction using the *sum* of bond energies of the reactants and the products in the following way:

$$\Delta H^{\circ}_{(reaction)} = \Sigma BE_{(reactants)} - \Sigma BE_{(products)}$$

where BE stands for bond energies.

Standard enthalpy changes of chemical reactions can also be computed using enthalpies of formation in the following way:

$$\Delta H^{\circ}_{(reaction)} = \Sigma\Delta H_{(bonds\ broken)} + \Sigma\Delta H_{(bonds\ formed)}$$
$$= \Sigma BE_{(reactants)} - \Sigma BE_{(products)}$$

Note how this equation is similar but not identical to the one making use of bond energies. This comes from the fact that a bond energy is defined as the energy required to break (and not to form) a given bond. Also note that the standard enthalpy of formation of a mole of any **element** is zero.

Medium-level Importance

8.7 Calorimetry

Measurements of changes of temperature within a reaction mixture allow the experimental determination of heat absorbed or released during the corresponding chemical reaction. Indeed the amount of heat required to change the temperature of any substance X from T_1 to T_2 is proportional to $(T_2 - T_1)$ and the quantity of X:

$$Q = mC(T_2 - T_1)$$

or

$$Q = nc(T_2 - T_1)$$

where m is the mass of X, n the number of moles. The constant C or c is called the heat capacity. The standard units for C and c are, respectively, the $Jkg^{-1}K^{-1}$ and the $Jmol^{-1}K^{-1}$. C which is the heat capacity per unit mass is also referred to as the specific heat capacity. If you refer back to the definition of the calorie (*see* CHM 7.3) you will understand that the specific heat of water is necessarily: 1 cal g^{-1} °C^{-1}.

Note that heat can be absorbed or released without a change in temperature (CHM 4.3.3). In fact, this situation occurs whenever a phase change takes place for a pure compound. For instance, ice melts at a constant temperature of 0 °C in order to break the forces that keep the water molecules in a crystal of ice we need to supply an amount of heat of 6.01 kJ/mol. There is no direct way of calculating the heat corresponding to a phase change.

Heats of phase changes (heat of fusion, heat of vaporisation, heat of sublimation) are generally tabulated and indirectly determined in calorimetric experiments. For instance, if a block of ice is allowed to melt in a bucket of warm water, we can determine the heat of fusion of ice by measuring the temperature drop in the bucket of water and applying the law of conservation of energy. The relevant equation is:

$$Q = mL$$

where L is the latent heat which is a constant.

Calorimetry is the science of measuring the heat evolved or exchanged due to a chemical reaction. The thermal energy of a reaction (defined as the system) is measured as a function of its surroundings by observing a temperature change (ΔT) on the surroundings due to the system. The magnitude in temperature change is essentially a measure of a system's or sample's energy content which is measured either while keeping the volume constant (*bomb calorimetry*) or while keeping the pressure constant (*coffee-cup calorimetry*).

In a constant-volume calorimetry measurement, the bomb calorimeter is kept at a constant volume and there is essentially no heat exchange between the calorimeter and the surroundings and thus, the net heat exchange for the system is zero. The heat exchange for the reaction is then compensated for by the heat change for the water and bomb calorimeter material steel (or surroundings). Thus, $\Delta q_{system} = \Delta q_{reaction} + \Delta q_{water} + \Delta q_{steel} = 0$ in bomb calorimetry, and so $q_{cal} = -q_{reaction}$ in which the temperature change is related to the heat absorbed by the calorimeter (q_{cal}) and if no heat escapes the constant volume calorimeter, the amount of heat gained by the calorimeter then equals that released by the system and so, $q_{cal} = -q_{reaction}$ as stated previously. Note that since $Q = mc\Delta T$ as previously defined, and $q_{reaction} = -(q_{water} + q_{steel})$ therefore, $q_{reaction} = -(m_{water})(c_{water})\Delta T - (m_{steel})(c_{steel})\Delta T$.

For aqueous solutions, a coffee-cup calorimeter is usually used to measure the enthalpy change of the system. This is simply a polystyrene (Styrofoam) cup with a lid, a stirrer and a thermometer. The cup is partially filled with a known volume of water. When a chemical

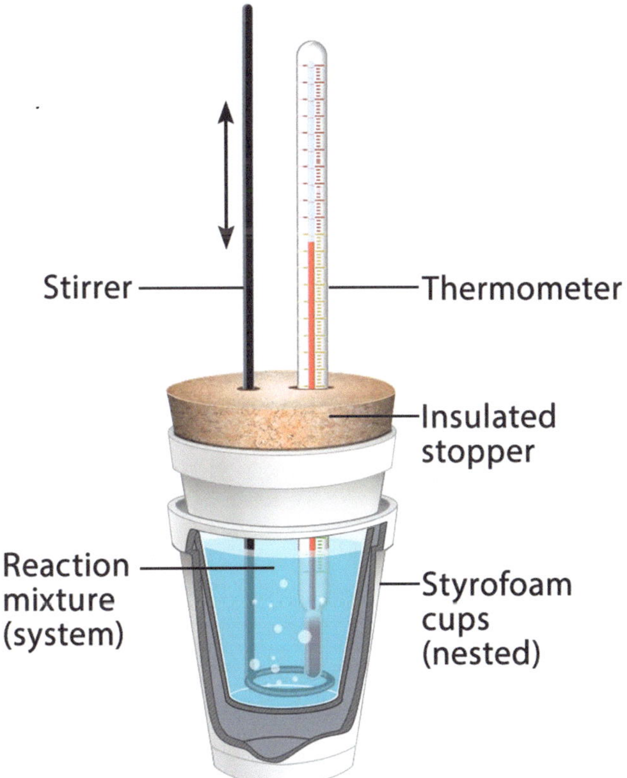

Figure III.A.8.3: Coffee-cup calorimeter.

Medium-level Importance

reaction occurs in the coffee-cup calorimeter, the heat of the reaction is absorbed by the water. The change in water temperature is used to calculate the amount of heat that has been absorbed (*used to make products, so water temperature decreases; endothermic*) or evolved (*lost to the water, so its temperature increases; exothermic*) in the reaction.

8.8 The Second Law of Thermodynamics

The first law of thermodynamics allows us to calculate energy transfers during a given transformation of the system. It does not allow us to predict whether a transformation can or cannot occur spontaneously. Yet our daily observations tell us that certain transformations always occur in a given direction. For instance, heat flows from a hot source to a cold source. We cannot spontaneously transfer heat in the other direction to make the hot source hotter and the cold source colder. The second law of thermodynamics states that entropy (S) of an isolated system will never decrease. In order for a reaction to proceed, the entropy of the system must increase. For any spontaneous process, the entropy of the universe increases which results in a greater dispersal or randomisation of the energy ($\Delta S > 0$). The second law of thermodynamics allows the determination of the preferred direction of a given transformation. Transformations which require the smallest amount of energy, and lead to the largest disorder of the system, are the most spontaneous.

Medium-level Importance

8.9 Entropy

Entropy is regarded as the main driving force behind all the chemical and physical changes known within the universe. All natural processes tend toward an increase in energy dispersal or, in other words, an entropy increase within our universe. Thus, a chemical system or reaction proceeds in a direction of universal entropy increase.

Entropy S is the state function which measures the degree of "disorder" in a system. For instance, the entropy of ice is lower than the entropy of liquid water since ice corresponds to an organised crystalline structure (*virtually no disorder*). In fact, generally speaking, the entropy increases as we go from a solid to a liquid to a gas. For similar reasons, the entropy decreases when an elastic band is stretched. Indeed, in the "unstretched" elastic band, the molecules of the rubber polymer are coiled up and form a disorganised structure. As the rubber is stretched these molecules will tend to line up with each other and adopt a more organised structure.

Entropy has the dimension of energy as a function of temperature as J/K or cal/K. Entropy can therefore be related to temperature and is thus a measure of energy dispersal (*joules*) per unit of temperature (*kelvin*).

The second law of thermodynamics can be expressed in the alternative form: a spontaneous transformation corresponds to an increase of the entropy of the system plus its surroundings. Hence, a chemical system is known to proceed in a direction that increases the entropy of the universe. As a result, ΔS must be incorporated in an expression that includes both the system and its surroundings so that, $\Delta S_{universe} = \Delta S_{surroundings} + \Delta S_{system} > 0$. When a system reaches a certain temperature equilibrium, it then also reaches its maximal entropy and so, $\Delta S_{universe} = \Delta S_{surroundings} + \Delta S_{system} = 0$. The entropy of the thermodynamic system is therefore a measure of how far the equalisation has progressed.

Entropy, like enthalpy, is a state function and is therefore path independent. Hence, a change in entropy depends only on the initial and final states ($\Delta S = S_{final} - S_{initial}$) and not on how the system arrived at that state. Under standard conditions, for any process or reaction, the entropy change for that reaction will be the difference between the entropies of products and reactants as follows:

$$\Delta S°_{reaction} = \Delta S°_{products} - \Delta S°_{reactants}$$

Considering the equation above, we can deduce the following: If the products have more entropy (*randomness*) than the reactants, the ΔS of the reaction is positive. If the products have less entropy (*randomness*) than the reactants, then the ΔS of the reaction is negative.

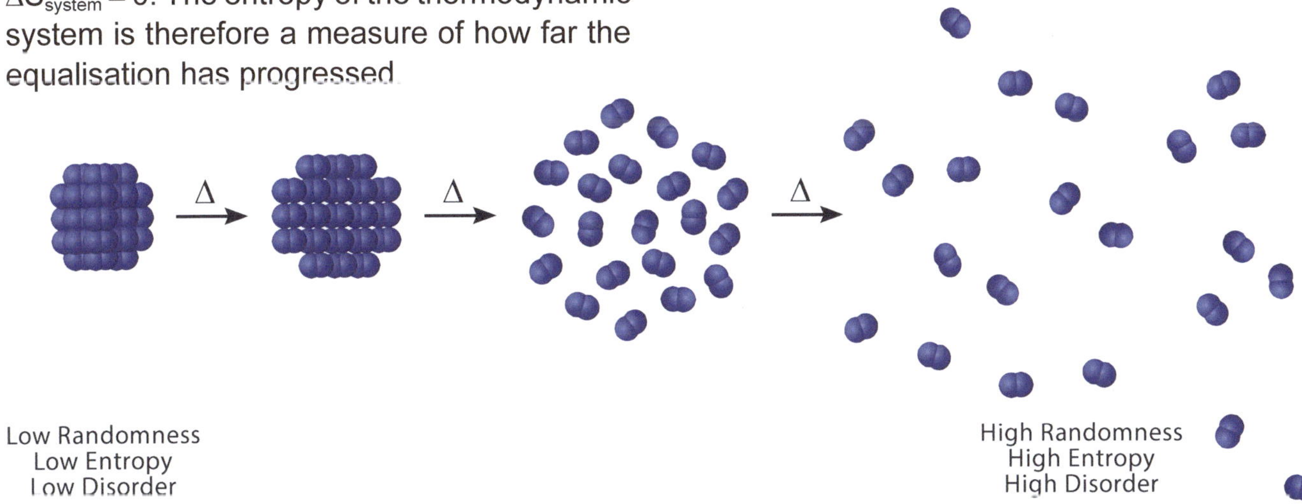

Figure III.A.8.4: Diatomic nitrogen, energy and entropy. Nitrogen (N_2) crystals have many different repeating forms including the cubic structure, which we saw for salt crystals (NaCl; CHM 3.1.1), a hexagonal close-packed structure, and several others. At 63 K and standard pressure, nitrogen crystals liquefy, and at 77 K, liquid nitrogen boils and becomes a gas. Increasing levels of disorder, and thus entropy: solid $\rightarrow$ liquid $\rightarrow$ gas. Note that if a reaction requires energy, a capital Greek letter delta (Δ) is associated with the chemical-reaction arrow to show that energy in the form of heat is added to the reaction; *hv* or hf is written if the energy is added in the form of light (energy E = hf; PHY 9.2.4).

Medium-level Importance

8.9.1 Identifying Entropy Changes from a Chemical Equation

From time to time, there will be an exam question asking students to identify the change in entropy based on an assessment of a chemical equation. Sometimes the question is based on a quantitative determination (i.e. based on a calculation using either the equation in CHM 8.9, or the Gibbs free energy equation in CHM 8.10); however, sometimes the question is based on a qualitative determination (i.e. simply by observing the phase changes, CHM 4.4.1, and/or changes in the number of moles or molecules as indicators of a change in entropy).

Consider the following reactions designed to produce and then isolate nitrogen gas. Before looking at the analysis, form an opinion as to which reactions have an increase in entropy and which reactions have a decrease in entropy.

Ammonium nitrate is first decomposed to give nitrogen gas.

$$2\ NH_4NO_3(s) \rightarrow 2\ N_2(g) + O_2(g) + 4\ H_2O(g)$$

Reaction I

Then water is removed by passing the gas over P_4O_{10}.

$$n\ P_4O_{10}(s) + 2n\ H_2O(g) \rightarrow 4\ (HPO_3)_n(s)$$

Reaction II

And finally, oxygen is removed by passing the gas over hot copper metal.

$$2\ Cu(s) + O_2(g) \rightarrow 2\ CuO(s)$$

Reaction III

After considering your opinion on the entropic changes in the preceding reactions, continue reading below.

Reaction I: There are 3 indicators to suggest a great increase in entropy (*more randomness*; $\Delta S > 0$; positive entropy). First, we are shown that $(s) \rightarrow (g) + (g) + (g)$, which means that a solid (*structured molecules, crystals*) has turned to gases (*unstructured molecules, random motion*). Second, 2 moles of a molecule (which means: $2 \times 6.02 \times 10^{23}$ molecules; CHM 1.3) has become more molecules ($2\ N_2 + O_2 + 4\ H_2O = 2 + 1 + 4 = 7$ moles, thus $7 \times 6.02 \times 10^{23}$ molecules). Third, one molecule (NH_4NO_3) has been fragmented into 3 molecules ($N_2 + O_2 + H_2O$). The latter two points are akin to having a nice drinking glass, dropping it on the floor, and watching it shatter into several pieces: a clear increase in randomness.

Reaction II: A solid compound and a gas combine to produce a solid compound is the strongest indicator of an increase in order (i.e. *decrease in randomness*; $\Delta S < 0$; negative entropy). Additionally, 2 molecules become 1 molecule which is a more ordered circumstance. Note that the issue of moles requires the value of n to be specified.

Reaction III: Again, a solid compound and a gas combine to produce a solid compound which is the strongest indicator of an increase in order (i.e. *decrease in randomness*; $\Delta S < 0$; negative entropy). Additionally, 2 molecules become 1 molecule which is a more ordered circumstance; and finally, 3 moles become 2 which also is more ordered.

8.10 Free Energy

The Gibbs free energy G is another state function which can be used as a criterion for spontaneity. This function is defined as:

$$G = H - T \cdot S$$

where:

- H is the enthalpy of the system in a given state (*in calories or SI unit: joules*);
- T is the absolute temperature (in kelvin, K) and thus must always have a positive value (CHM 7.4);
- S is the entropy of the system.

Consequently, Gibbs free energy (G) also determines the direction of a spontaneous change for a chemical system. The derivation for the formulation thus incorporates both the entropy and enthalpy parameters studied in the previous sections. Following various manipulations and derivations, one can then note that Gibbs free energy is an alternative form of both enthalpy and the entropy changes of a chemical process.

The standard Gibbs free energy of a reaction (ΔG°_{rxn}), is determined at 25 °C and a pressure of 1 atm. For a reaction carried out at constant temperature we can write that the change in the Gibbs free energy is:

$$\Delta G = \Delta H - T\Delta S$$

A reaction carried out at constant pressure is spontaneous if

$$\Delta G < 0, \textit{exergonic}$$

It is not spontaneous if:

$$\Delta G > 0, \textit{endergonic}$$

and it is in a state of equilibrium (reaction spontaneous in both directions) if:

$$\Delta G = 0.$$

	Spontaneous	Not spontaneous	Equilibrium
Gibbs free energy (ΔG)	Negative	Positive	0

As noted in the previous chapter, the study of thermodynamics generally describes the spontaneity or the direction and extent to which a reaction will proceed. It therefore enables one to predict if a reaction will occur spontaneously or not. Note that non-spontaneous processes may turn into spontaneous processes if coupled to another spontaneous process or more specifically by the addition of some external energy.

Thermochemistry then can be used to essentially calculate how much work a system can do or require. Thermodynamics basically then deals with the relative potentials of both the reactants and products of a chemical system. The next chapter will describe the

Medium-level Importance

actual rate (or *chemical kinetics* or *speed*) of a chemical reaction. In chemical kinetics, the chemical potential of intermediate states of a chemical reaction may also be described and thus enabling one to determine why a reaction may be slow or fast.

Consider the summary of Gibbs free energy below. Note that the table should not to be committed to memory; however, you should be able to deduce the results in the fourth column. The GAMSAT often has 1-2 questions covering Gibbs free energy.

$$\Delta G = \Delta H - T\Delta S$$

Enthalpy change	Entropy change	Gibbs free energy	Spontaneity
positive	positive	depends on T, may be + or –	yes, if the temperature is high enough
negative	positive	always negative	always spontaneous
negative	negative	depends on T, may be + or –	yes, if the temperature is low enough
positive	negative	always positive	never spontaneous

Medium-level Importance

CHAPTER 8: Enthalpy and Thermochemistry

GOLD STANDARD FOUNDATIONAL GAMSAT PRACTICE QUESTIONS

1) A student observes the melting of an ice cube. She correctly concludes that the overall observed process has led to:

A. the completion of real work.
B. an increase in the efficiency of the universe.
C. an increase in the entropy of the universe.
D. an increase in the total energy of the universe.

2) The heat capacity of a substance is 20 cal/(g)(°C). Suppose that 12 g of the substance is cooled at constant pressure. Which of the following describes the process?

A. Endothermic
B. Exothermic
C. Latent heat of fusion
D. Latent heat of vaporisation

3) Consider the following statement: A burn from steam at 100 °C is more severe than a burn from boiling water at 100 °C. Is the preceding statement valid?

A. No, because it is an isothermal process.
B. No, because there is no difference in the sum of kinetic and potential energy of the molecules.
C. Yes, because steam is hotter than the boiling water.
D. Yes, because the steam will give off a large amount of heat as it condenses.

4) If a chemical reaction is at equilibrium, which of the following is true?

A. The change in entropy is zero.
B. The number of reacting molecules is zero.
C. The change in enthalpy is zero.
D. The change in free energy is zero.

5) In the reaction $N_2(g) + 3H_2(g) \leftrightarrow 2NH_3(g)$, the entropy for the forward reaction:

A. increases.
B. remains the same.
C. decreases.
D. cannot be determined with the information given.

6) Which one of the following chemical reactions presents a change in entropy, ΔS, that is greater than zero?

A. $BaF_2(s) \rightarrow Ba^{2+}(aq) + 2F^-(aq)$
B. $2H_2(g) + O_2(g) \rightarrow 2H_2O(g)$
C. $CO_2(g) \rightarrow CO_2(s)$
D. $2NO_2(g) \rightarrow N_2O_4(g)$

7) Consider the following reaction:

$$H_2O + CH_2{=}CH_2 \rightarrow CH_3CH_2OH$$

Let ΔH be the change in enthalpy of the above reaction. If ΔH_1 is the heat of formation of H_2O, and ΔH_2 is the heat of formation of CH_3CH_2OH, what is the heat of formation of $CH_2{=}CH_2$?

A. $\Delta H_2 - \Delta H$
B. $\Delta H_2 - \Delta H_1$
C. $\Delta H_2 \bullet \Delta H_1 - \Delta H$
D. $\Delta H_2 - \Delta H_1 - \Delta H$

Medium-level Importance

Medium-level Importance

Questions 8–9

Consider the following relations:

$$Q = mc\Delta T$$

and

$$Q = mL$$

Note that:

- Q is the heat energy (calories or joules); m is the mass of the object or substance being heated; c is the specific heat of the object or substance being heated; T is the temperature; and L is the latent heat, which is the amount of energy released or absorbed at constant temperature due to a phase change. For example, the phase change from solid to liquid uses the latent heat of fusion, and from liquid to vapor (gas) is the latent heat of vaporisation.
- A calorie is the amount of thermal energy required to raise the temperature of liquid water by 1 degree Celcius. Thus, the specific heat c of liquid water is 1 cal g^{-1} $°C^{-1}$.

8) The heat capacity of a substance was determined to be 8 cal/(g)(°C). Suppose that 6 g of the substance is cooled from 40 °C to 10 °C at constant pressure. What is the enthalpy change for the substance?

A. –1.44 kcal
B. –1.92 kcal
C. –240 cal
D. –480 cal

9) At constant pressure, how much heat is needed to convert a 10-gram ice cube at 0 °C to steam at 100 °C?

Note that:

- Latent heat of fusion = 80 kcal/kg
- Latent heat of vaporisation = 540 kcal/kg

A. 620 cal
B. 1.0 kcal
C. 1.6 kcal
D. 7.2 kcal

10) Consider the following chemical reaction involving silver sulfide and aluminium:

$$3Ag_2S\ (s) + 2Al\ (s) \rightarrow Al_2S_3\ (s) + 6Ag\ (s)$$

Tarnish can be removed from silver by employing the reaction above. What is the change in enthalpy for this reaction, as calculated from the following data?

$$2Al\ (s) + 3H_2S\ (g) \rightarrow Al_2S_3\ (s) + 3H_2\ (g) \quad \Delta H_1 = -107.2 \text{ kcal}$$

$$2Ag\ (s) + H_2S\ (g) \rightarrow Ag_2S\ (s) + H_2\ (g) \quad \Delta H_2 = -2.8 \text{ kcal}$$

A. –98.8 kcal
B. –104.4 kcal
C. –110.0 kcal
D. –115.6 kcal

GOLD STANDARD GAMSAT-LEVEL PRACTICE QUESTIONS

Questions 11–13

As the temperature of a crystalline solid is raised, the vibrations of the structural units become more vigorous. Eventually, a temperature is reached at which the crystalline structure is destroyed by these vibrations. The conversion of a solid to a liquid is called *melting*, and the temperature at which a solid melts is its *melting point*. Conversely, the conversion of a liquid to a solid is called *freezing*, and the temperature at which a liquid freezes is called its *freezing point*.

The quantity of heat required to melt a given amount of solid is called the *enthalpy of fusion*, ΔH fusion. For example, the enthalpy of fusion of water is 6.01 kJ/mol.

Reaction 1:

$H_2O_{(s)} \rightarrow H_2O_{(l)}$ $\Delta H_{fusion} = +6.01$ kJ/mol

Reaction 2:

$H_2O_{(l)} \rightarrow H_2O_{(s)}$ $\Delta H_{fusion} = -6.01$ kJ/mol

Note that the melting of water is an endothermic process, and the freezing of water is an exothermic process.

It is possible that the temperature of a liquid could drop below the freezing point without any solid appearing; this is the called supercooling. It results from there being a lack of small particles in the liquid on which the crystals can form. When a supercooled liquid does begin to freeze its temperature rises to the normal freezing point temperature. The melting point and enthalpy of fusion of some common substances are listed in Table 1.

Substance	Melting Point	ΔH_{fusion} (kJ/mol)
Sodium, Na	97.8	2.64
Methyl alcohol, CH_3OH	–97.9	3.18
Propyl alcohol, $CH_3CH_2CH_2OH$	–131.1	6.96
Lead, Pb	327.4	4.77

Table 1

11) In order for Reaction 1 to occur which of the following is necessary?

A. Energy must be put into the system.

B. A catalyst must be present in the system.

C. Small particles must be present in the system.

D. Energy must be given off by the system.

12) If heat is added to a solid-liquid mixture at equilibrium, the solid gradually melts while the temperature remains constant. When all the solid has melted, the temperature rises again. Why?

A. The ΔH_{fusion} of a substance requires that its temperature remain constant.

B. The added heat goes into breaking up the crystalline structure as opposed to increasing the average velocity of the molecules.

C. The added heat goes into increasing the average velocity of the molecules thus increasing the entropy of the system.

D. The added heat is absorbed by the container in which the mixture is held.

13) Which of the following would be most consistent with the likely melting point of ethyl alcohol (CH_3CH_2OH)?

A. –81.3 °C

B. –99.8 °C

C. –114.5 °C

D. –126.3 °C

High-level Importance

14) The specific latent heat (L) of a material is a measure of the heat energy (Q) per mass (m) released or absorbed during a phase change, and is thus defined through the formula Q = mL.

The dimension of a physical quantity can be expressed as a product of the basic physical dimensions of mass (M), length (L) and time (T). For example, the dimension of the physical quantity speed or velocity (m/s) is length/time (= L/T).

Which of the following would be consistent with the dimensional formula for the specific latent heat?

A. MLT^{-2}
B. ML^2T^{-2}
C. ML^2T^{-1}
D. L^2T^{-2}

Questions 15–18

In 1873, Willard Gibbs published *A Method of Geometrical Representation of the Thermodynamic Properties of Substances by Means of Surfaces* in which he introduced the preliminary outline of the principles of his new equation able to predict or estimate the tendencies of various natural processes to occur when bodies or systems are brought into contact. By studying the interactions of homogeneous substances in contact, i.e. bodies, being in composition part solid, part liquid, and part vapor, and by using a 3-D volume-entropy-internal energy graph, Gibbs was able to determine three distinct states of equilibrium.

As a result of his research, chemical reactions can be viewed from a thermodynamic perspective. Changes in enthalpy (ΔH) and entropy (ΔS) are the two driving factors that determine whether a reaction is spontaneous or not. Gibbs free energy (ΔG) combines both of these two factors as such:

$$\Delta G = \Delta H - T\,\Delta S$$

where T is the temperature in kelvin (K).

Note that the standard enthalpy of formation (i.e. ΔH°_f, *the standard heat of formation*) of a compound is the change of enthalpy during the formation of 1 mole of the substance from its constituent elements, with all substances in their standard states.

	ΔH°_f (kJ/mol)
$N_2(g)$	0
$H_2(g)$	0
$NH_3(g)$	–46

Table 1: Changes in standard enthalpy of formation

	S° (J/mol-K)
$N_2(g)$	192
$H_2(g)$	131
$NH_3(g)$	192

Table 2: Standard entropy

The following relations may be of help. For enthalpy (H) and entropy (S):

$$\Delta H^\circ = \Sigma\Delta H^\circ_{f\,(products)} - \Sigma\Delta H^\circ_{f\,(reactants)}$$

$$\Delta S^\circ = \Sigma S^\circ_{products} - \Sigma S^\circ_{reactants}$$

15) What is ΔH° for the reaction: $N_2(g) + 3H_2(g) \rightarrow 2NH_3(g)$?

A. 0 J
B. 46 kJ
C. –46 kJ
D. –92 000 J

16) What is $\Delta S°$ for the reaction: $N_2(g) + 3H_2(g) \rightarrow 2NH_3(g)$?

A. −201 J/K
B. −192 J/K
C. −131 J/K
D. 201 J/K

17) At standard temperature, the reaction $N_2(g) + 3H_2(g) \rightarrow 2NH_3(g)$ is:

A. spontaneous.
B. not spontaneous.
C. rapid.
D. slow.

18) Consider Figure 1.

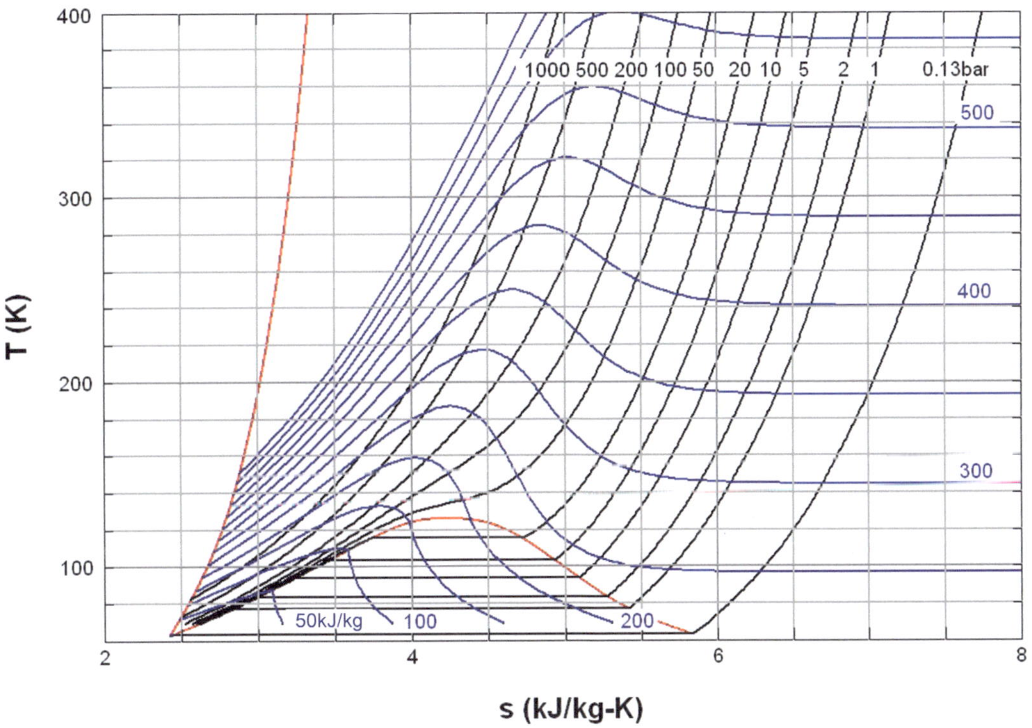

Figure 1: Temperature-entropy diagram of nitrogen (N_2). The red curve at the left is the melting curve. The red dome represents the two-phase region, with saturated liquid on the low-entropy side, and saturated gas on the high-entropy side. The black curves are isobars: each one provides constant pressure in "bar" units. The blue curves are isenthalps: each one provides constant enthalpy in kJ/kg. (Adwaele, Lumen Candela; Boundless, 2021)

Based on Figure 1, at a temperature of 273 K (0 °C, 32 °F) and an absolute pressure of 10^5 Pa (100 kPa, 1 bar), which of the following is the best estimate of the entropy of N_2?

A. 6.75 kJ/g-K
B. 6.75 J/g-K
C. 7.5 kJ/g-K
D. 7.5 J/g-K

High-level Importance

Questions 19–23

It is well known that there are two major forms of carbon, that is, carbon has two main allotropes: graphite and diamond. These differ greatly from each other with respect to their physical properties as shown in Table 1. The physical properties of silicon are also shown in Table 1 for comparison as carbon and silicon belong to the same group in the periodic table.

Physical properties	Graphite	Diamond	Silicon
Density (g cm^{-3})	2.26	3.51	2.33
Enthalpy of combustion to yield oxide (ΔHc) kJ mol^{-1}	–393.3	–395.1	–910
Melting point (°C)	2820	3730	1410
Boiling point (°C)		4830	2680
Conductivity (electrical)	Fairly good	Non-conductor	Good
Conductivity (thermal)	Fairly good	Non-conductivity	Good

Table 1

Graphite possesses what is commonly known as a layer structure: carbon atoms form three covalent bonds with each other to yield layers of carbon assemblies parallel with each other. These layers are held together via weak Van der Waals' forces which permit some movement of the layers relative to one another.

A phase diagram is a graph that shows the relation between the solid, liquid and gaseous states. Any point in the graph is where 2 phases exist at equilibrium except the triple point where all 3 exist at equilibrium. Solid CO_2 is called "dry ice" because it can go directly from solid to vapour (sublimation) at room pressure (i.e. 101.3 kPa). The triple point of CO_2 occurs at 217 K and 515 kPa. A reduction in CO_2 pressure directly correlates with changes in its sublimation, melting and boiling points.

19) The properties of the layer-like structure of solid graphite stated in the passage would lend it to which of the following industrial uses?

A. Insulator
B. Structural
C. Corrosive
D. Lubricant

20) Using the information in the table, calculate the enthalpy change for the following process:

$$C_{graphite} \rightarrow C_{diamond}$$

A. +1.8 kJ mol^{-1}
B. –1.8 kJ mol^{-1}
C. +1.0 kJ mol^{-1}
D. –1.0 kJ mol^{-1}

21) It is possible to convert graphite into diamond via various chemical processes. Based on the information in the passage, which of the following would facilitate increased amounts of diamond assuming that the system is in equilibrium?

A. Higher pressures
B. Lower temperatures
C. A catalyst
D. None of the above

Questions 22 and 23 refer to the following additional information:

At a given temperature T in kelvin, the relationship between the three thermodynamic quantities including the change in Gibbs free energy (ΔG), the change in enthalpy (ΔH) and the change in entropy (ΔS), can be expressed as follows:

$$\Delta G = \Delta H - T\Delta S$$

22) The sublimation of carbon dioxide occurs quickly at room temperature. At the same temperature, what might be predicted for the three thermodynamic quantities for the reverse reaction?

A. Only ΔS would be positive.
B. Only ΔS would be negative.
C. Only ΔH would be negative.
D. Only ΔG would be positive.

23) Which of the following statements is consistent with the triple point of carbon dioxide?

A. The absolute temperature dominates the effect on Gibbs free energy.
B. The reaction is spontaneous, Gibbs free energy is negative.
C. The enthalpy change is equal to the effect of the entropy change.
D. The entropy change is negative because there is more disorder overall.

24) Consider Figure 1 below which was created using data from an artificial lung model. The dark dots represent expiration (*deflation*) and the light dots represent inspiration (*inflation*).

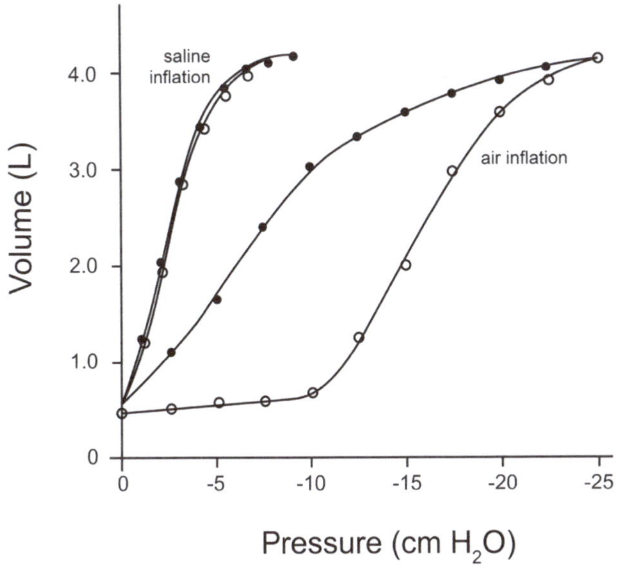

Figure 1

Based on Figure 1, which of the following represents a significant difference between the saline and air inflation of the lungs?

A. Maximum volume
B. Minimum volume
C. Work done
D. None of the above

High-level Importance

25) The total area of the Hubble telescope exposed to the sun is 70 000 m^2. The rate of solar energy incident on the telescope is 120 W m^{-2}.

If a channel covering the entire exposed surface contains water and the temperature of the water must rise by at least 10 °C in order to keep the telescope cool, at what approximate rate must the water be made to flow assuming that energy transfer is instantaneous?

Note that:

- Specific heat (*specific heat capacity*) of water = 4.2 J g^{-1} $°C^{-1}$
- Density of water = 1000 kg m^{-3}
- The following equation may be of help: $Q = mc\Delta T$, where Q is the heat energy (joules, J); m is the mass of the object; c is the specific heat; T is the temperature.

A. 200 L s^{-1}
B. 3150 L s^{-1}
C. 2.0×10^5 L s^{-1}
D. 3.1×10^6 L s^{-1}

SPOILER ALERT

Gold Standard has cross-referenced the content in this chapter to examples from ACER's official GAMSAT practice materials. It is for you to decide when you want to explore these questions since you may want to preserve some of ACER's materials for timed mock-exam practice.

Examples – Gibbs free energy, with enthalpy, entropy and a twist: 42-43 of 2; straightforward Gibbs free energy: Q102-103 of 3; Gibbs free energy and spontaneity: Q71 of 4; heat exchange but the equation and sign convention are given (no assumed knowledge; not counted as referring to this chapter): Q71 of 3. Note that "Q" is followed by the question number, and, for example, "of 1" refers to booklet number 1 which is referenced in the Spoiler Alert table at the end of Chapter 1. The 15 full-length GAMSAT practice tests by Gold Standard, HEAPS-1 through HEAPS-15, contain specific cross-references to this chapter within the worked solutions. Note that the unit with forms of carbon including a table of data and Gibbs free energy questions is from HEAPS-6, and the independent question asking about skin burns from water vs steam is from HEAPS-9.

Chapter Checklist

- ☐ Access your online account to view answers, worked solutions and discussion boards.
- ☐ Reassess your 'learning objectives' for this chapter: Go back to the first page of this chapter and re-evaluate the top 3 boxes and the Introduction.
    - ☐ Please be sure that you have completed the *Need for Speed* exercises at the beginning of this chapter.
- ☐ Complete a maximum of 1 page of notes using symbols/abbreviations to represent the entire chapter based on your learning objectives. These are your Gold Notes.
- ☐ Consider your multimedia options based on your optimal way of learning:
    - ☐ Download the free Gold Standard GAMSAT app for your Android device or iPhone.
    - ☐ Create your own, tangible study cards or try the free app: Anki.
    - ☐ Record your voice reading your Gold Notes onto your smartphone (audio files, e.g., *memo* or MP3s) and listen during exercise, transportation, etc.
    - ☐ Try out the Gold Standard GAMSAT online videos at gamsat-prep.com, or you can try other options on YouTube like Khan Academy or Crash Course Chemistry.
- ☐ Reassess your schedule for your full-length GAMSAT practice tests: ACER and/or HEAPS exams. Ensure that you have scheduled one full day to complete a practice test and 1-2 days for a thorough assessment of worked solutions while adding to your abbreviated Gold Notes.
- ☐ Reassess your progress in scheduling and/or evaluating stress reduction techniques such as regular exercise (sports), yoga, meditation and/or mindfulness exercises (*see* YouTube for suggestions).

High-level Importance

RATE PROCESSES IN CHEMICAL REACTIONS
Chapter 9

Memorise

* Reaction order
* Define: rate-determining step
* Generalised potential energy diagrams
* Define: activation energy, catalysis
* Define: saturation kinetics, substrate

Understand

* Reaction rates, rate law, determine exponents
* Rate constant equation; apply Le Chatelier's
* Law of mass action, equations for Gibbs free energy, saturation kinetics, Keq

Importance

High level: 26% of GAMSAT General Chemistry questions released by ACER are related to content in this chapter (in our estimation).

* Note that approximately 80% of the questions in GAMSAT General Chemistry are related to just 4 chapters: 4, 5, 6, and 9.

GAMSAT-Prep.com

Introduction

Rate processes involve the study of the velocity (*speed*) and mechanisms of chemical reactions. **Reaction rate** (= *velocity*) tells us how fast the concentrations of reactants change with time. **Reaction mechanisms** show the sequence of steps to get to the overall change. Experiments show that 4 important factors generally influence reaction rates: **(1)** the nature of the reactants, **(2)** their concentration, **(3)** temperature, and **(4)** catalysis.

The ideas presented in this chapter represent the most tested content in GAMSAT General Chemistry. Frankly, many of the equation manipulations and graph analyses within this chapter could apply to many other types of GAMSAT questions (though, of course, those were not counted as part of the percent importance of this chapter). Note: Most of the graphs that appear in the *Need for Speed* exercises can be found in ACER's materials (*see* Spoiler Alert).

Multimedia Resources at GAMSAT-Prep.com

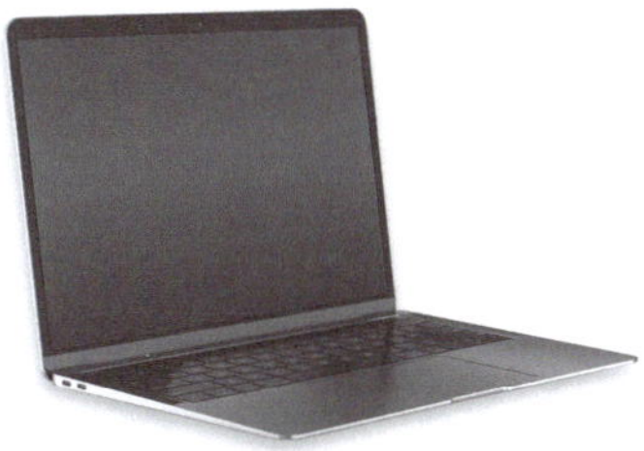

Open Discussion Boards
(*gamsat-prep.com/forum*)

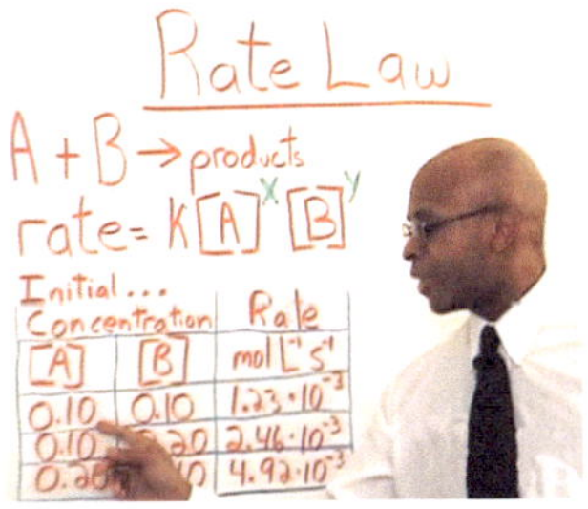

Science Preparation Videos

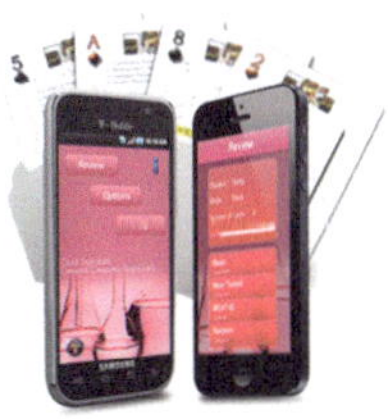

Flashcards

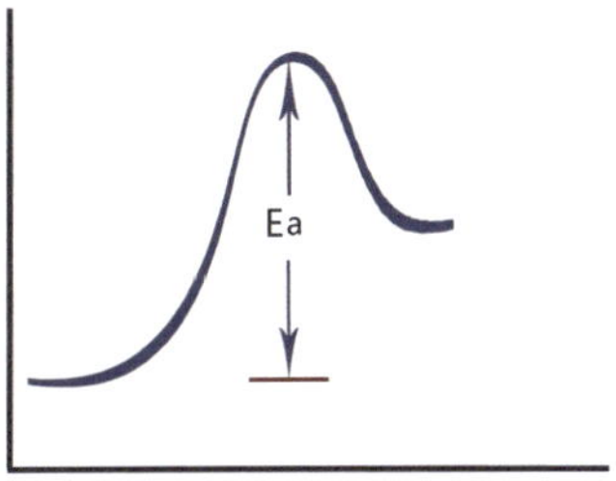

Special Guest

* The real GAMSAT may have advanced-level information presented (i.e. in a passage) but previous knowledge of said information is not required to answer the questions that would follow. Practice questions at the end of this chapter, as well as ACER and GS (HEAPS) practice GAMSATs can help you clarify this point.

9.0 GAMSAT has a *Need for Speed*!

High-level Importance

Section	GAMSAT General Chemistry *Need for Speed* Exercises
9.2	Consider the following rate law and complete the missing fields. rate = k $[A]^m [B]^n$ where [ ] is the concentration of the corresponding reactant in ________ (*units*) ________ is the order of the reaction with respect to A ________ is the order of the reaction with respect to B ________ is the overall reaction order ________ is the rate constant
	Complete the 2 missing fields with the appropriate reaction order.

Reactant Concentration versus Time

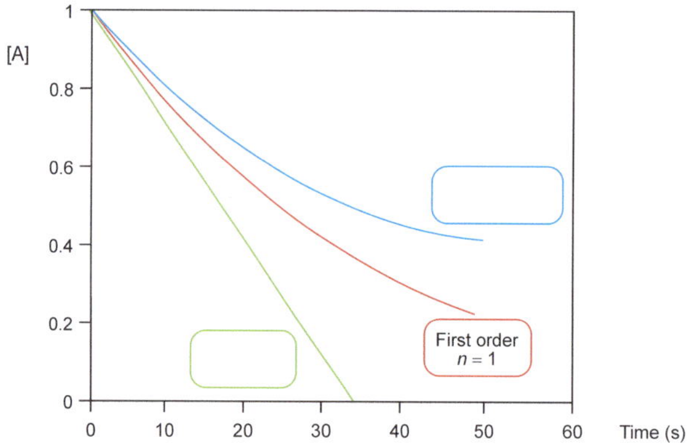

Section	
9.2.1	Based only on the integrated rate law, draw the general direction of the curve or line.

Integrated Rate Law	Graph
$[A]_t = -kt + [A]_0$	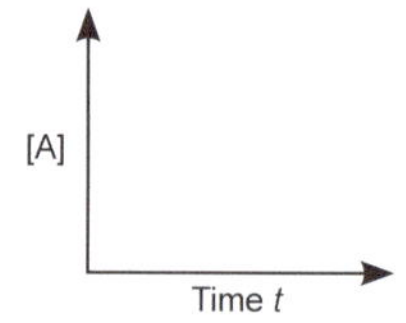
$\ln[A]_t = -kt + \ln[A]_0$ $\ln\frac{[A]_t}{[A]_0} = -kt$	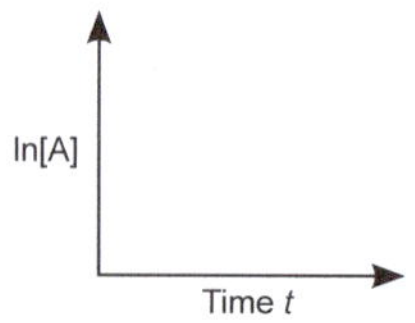
$\frac{1}{[A]_t} = kt + \frac{1}{[A]_0}$	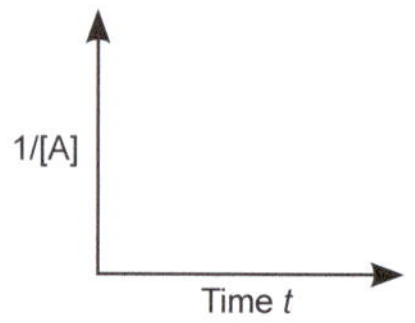

9.4

Circle either 'fastest' or 'slowest': The rate of the overall chemical reaction is naturally limited by the (fastest / slowest) step; therefore, the rate-determining step in the mechanism of a reaction is the (fastest / slowest) step. In other words, the overall rate law of a chemical reaction is basically equal to the rate law of the (fastest / slowest) step.

9.5

Apply the following (**labels**) to each of the two graphs: Reactants (**A + B**), Products (**C + D**), Activation energy (**E$_a$**), Activated complex (**AC**).

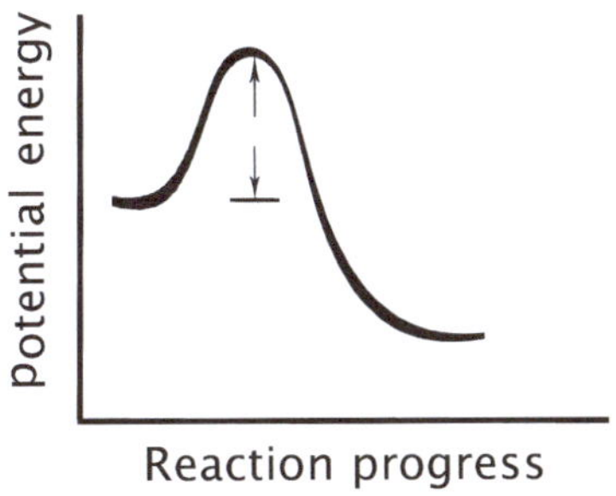

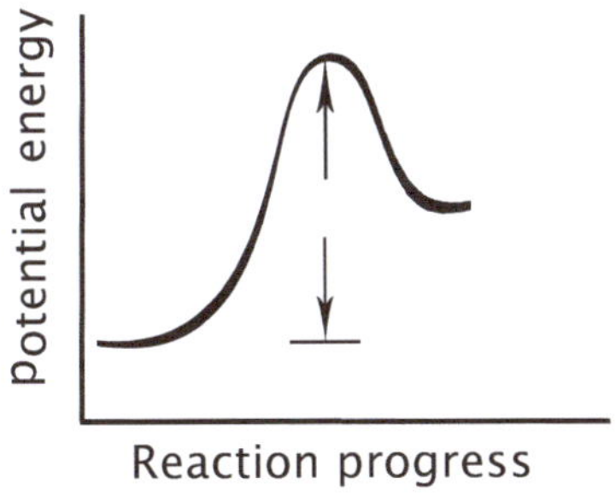

9.7

Consider the graph below.

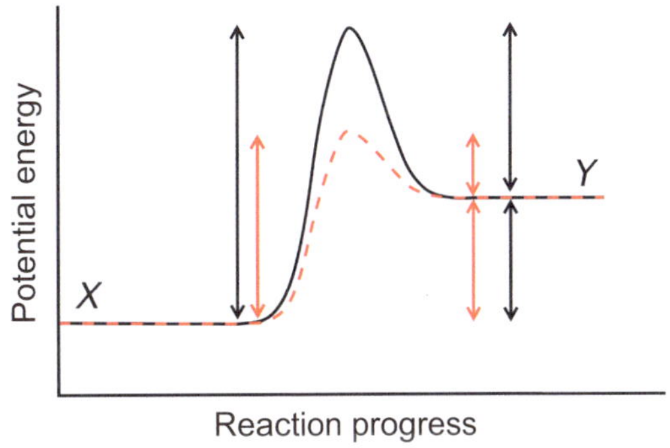

Is the forward reaction ($X \rightarrow Y$) exothermic or endothermic? (exothermic / endothermic)

Is the reverse reaction ($Y \rightarrow X$) exothermic or endothermic? (exothermic / endothermic)

Label the graph with a number: **1.** ΔH (*the change in enthalpy*); **2.** E_a ($X \rightarrow Y$) [*the activation energy for the forward reaction*]; **3.** E_a ($Y \rightarrow X$) [*the activation energy for the reverse reaction*].

Point to the curve which represents the reaction in the presence of a catalyst.

9.8

Consider the following balanced chemical reaction:

$$aA + bB \rightleftharpoons cC + dD$$

where a, b, c and d are the corresponding stoichiometric coefficients. Write the expression for the equilibrium constant.

$K_{eq} =$

Choose one of the following three options for the three conditions below in terms of which is favored: **(1)** forward reaction; **(2)** reverse reaction; **(3)** neither.

$K_{eq} > 1$ ____________________ $K_{eq} < 1$ ____________________ $K_{eq} = 1$ ____________________

9.1 Reaction Rate

Consider a general reaction:

$$2\,A + 3\,B \rightarrow C + D$$

The rate or the velocity (*speed*) at which this reaction proceeds can be expressed by one of the following:

(i) rate of disappearance of A: $-\Delta[A]/\Delta t$

(ii) rate of disappearance of B: $-\Delta[B]/\Delta t$

(iii) rate of appearance or formation of C: $\Delta[C]/\Delta t$

(iv) rate of appearance or formation of D: $\Delta[D]/\Delta t$

Where [ ] denotes the concentration of a reactant or a product in moles/litre (CHM 5.3.1). Thus, the reaction rate is usually expressed as a change in reactant or product concentration ($\Delta_{conc.}$) per unit change in time (Δt).

Since A and B are disappearing in this reaction, [*A*] and [*B*] are decreasing with time, i.e. $\Delta[A]/\Delta t$ and $\Delta[B]/\Delta t$ are negative quantities. On the other hand, the quantities $\Delta[C]/\Delta t$ and $\Delta[D]/\Delta t$ are positive since both C and D are being formed during the process of this reaction. By convention: rates of reactions are expressed as positive numbers; as a result, a negative sign is necessary in the first two expressions.

Suppose that A disappears at a rate of 6 (moles/litre)/s. In the same time interval (1s), in a total volume of 1L we have:

$(3 \text{ mol B}/2 \text{ mol A}) \times 6 \text{ mol A}$
$= 9$ moles of B disappearing
$(1 \text{ mol C}/2 \text{ mol A}) \times 6 \text{ mol A}$
$= 3$ moles of C being formed
$(1 \text{ mol D}/2 \text{ mol A}) \times 6 \text{ mol A}$
$= 3$ moles of D being formed

Therefore individual rates of formation or disappearance are not convenient ways to express the rate of a reaction. Indeed, depending on the reactant or product considered the rate will be given by a different numerical value unless the stoichiometric coefficients are equal (e.g. for C and D in our case).

A more convenient expression of the rate of a reaction is the overall rate. This rate is simply obtained by dividing the rate of formation or disappearance of a given reactant or product by the corresponding stoichiometric coefficient, i.e.:

$$\text{overall rate} = -(1/2)\,\Delta[A]/\Delta t, \text{ or } -(1/3)\,\Delta[B]/\Delta t,$$
$$\text{or } \Delta[C]/\Delta t, \text{ or } \Delta[D]/\Delta t.$$

A simple verification on our example will show you that these expressions all lead to the same numerical value for the overall rate: 3 (moles/L)/s. Therefore for a generic equation such as, $aA + bB \rightarrow cC + dD$, a generalisation of the overall reaction rate would be as follows:

$$\text{Rate} = \frac{-1}{a}\frac{\Delta[A]}{\Delta t} = \frac{-1}{b}\frac{\Delta[B]}{\Delta t} = \frac{+1}{c}\frac{\Delta[C]}{\Delta t} = \frac{+1}{d}\frac{\Delta[D]}{\Delta t}$$

It can be seen from the preceding overall rate relationship that the rate is the same whether we use one of the reactants or one of the products to calculate the rates. Generally, one can see that knowing the rate of change in the concentration of any one reactant or product at a certain time point allows one to invariably determine the rate of change in the concentration of any other reactant or product at the same time point using the stoichiometrically balanced equation.

Whenever the term "rate" is used (with no other specification) it refers to the "overall rate" unless individual and overall rates are equal.

9.2 Dependence of Reaction Rates on Concentration of Reactants

The rate of a reaction (given in moles per litre per second) can be expressed as a function of the concentration of the reactants. In the previous chemical reaction we would have:

$$\text{rate} = k\,[A]^m\,[B]^n$$

- [ ] is the concentration of the corresponding reactant in moles per litre
- k is referred to as the rate constant
- m is the order of the reaction with respect to A
- n is the order of the reaction with respect to B
- m + n is the overall reaction order.

The rate constant k is reaction specific. It is directly proportional to the rate of a reaction. It increases with increasing temperature since the proportion of molecules with energies greater than the activation energy E_a of a reaction increases with higher temperatures.

According to the rate law above, the reaction is said to be an (m + n)*th* order reaction, or, an m*th* order reaction with respect to A, or, an n*th* order reaction with respect to B.

The value of the m or n*th* rate orders of the reaction describes how the rate of the reaction depends on the concentration of the reactant(s).

For example, a zero rate order for reactant A (where m = 0), would indicate that the rate of the reaction is independent of the concentration of reactant A and therefore has a constant reaction rate (this is also applicable to reactant B). The rate equation can therefore be expressed as a rate constant k or the rate = k. The rate probably depends on temperature or other factors excluding concentration.

A first rate order for reactant A (where m = 1) would indicate that the rate of the reaction is directly proportional to the concentration of the reactant A (or B, where n = 1). Thus, the rate equation can be expressed as follows: rate = $k[A]^1$ or rate = $k[B]^1$.

A second rate order for reactant A (m = 2) would indicate that the rate is proportional to the square of the reactant concentration. The rate equation can thus be expressed as follows: rate = $k[A]^2$.

Hence, the rate orders or exponents in the rate law equation can be integers, fractions, or zeros and are not necessarily equal to the stoichiometric coefficients in the given reaction except when a reaction is the rate-determining step (*slowest step in a reaction sequence*, or, elementary step; CHM 9.4). Consequently, although there are other orders, including both higher and mixed orders or fractions that are possible as described, the three described orders (0, 1st and 2nd), are amongst the most common orders studied.

As shown by the graphical representation below, for the zero-order reactant, as the concentration of reactant A decreases over time, the slope of the line is constant and thus the rate is constant. Moreover, the rate does not change regardless of the decrease in reactant A concentration over time and thus the zero order rate order. For first order, the decrease in reactant A concentration is shown to affect the rate of reaction in direct proportion. Thus, as the concentration decreases, the rate decreases proportionally. Lastly, for second order, the rate of the reaction is shown to decrease proportionally to the square of the reactant A concentration. In fact, the curves for 1st and 2nd order reactions resemble exponential decay.

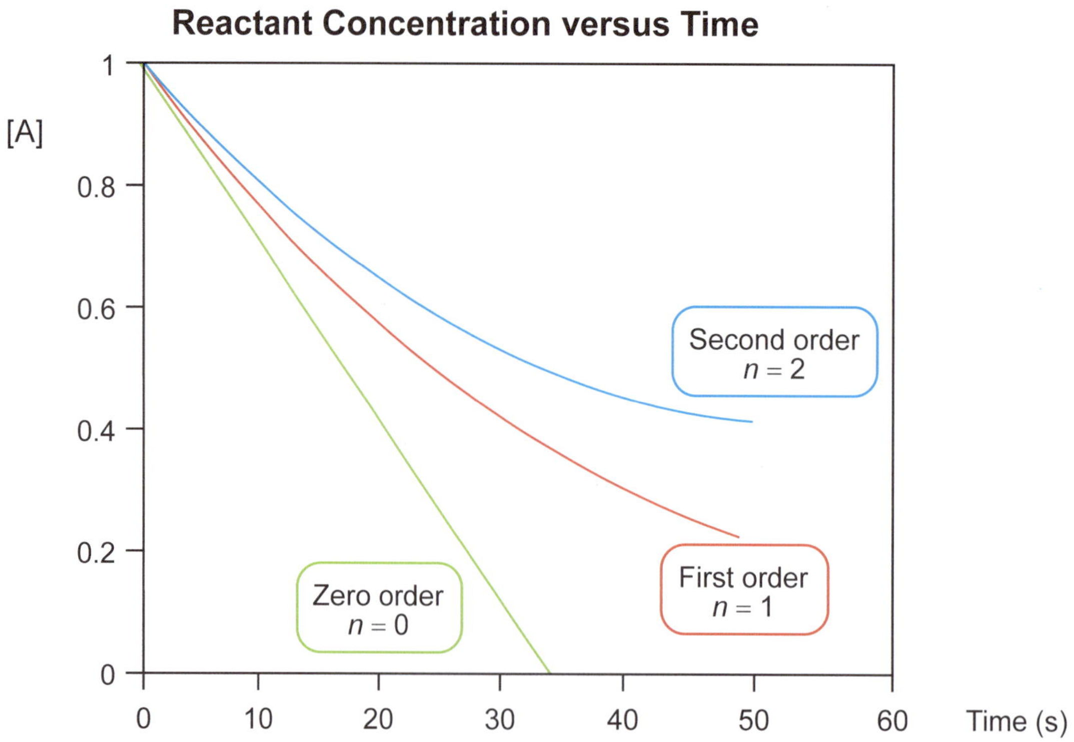

Figure III.A.9.0: Reactant concentration vs. time curves. Notice that first and second order reactions have exponential decay curves (PHY 10.5) but, of course, second order reactions decay faster. It is expected that you can recognise the graphs above and those in the next section (CHM 9.2.1).

9.2.1 Differential Rate Law vs. Integrated Rate Law

Rate laws may be expressed as differential equations or as integrated rate laws. As differential equations, the relationship is shown between the rate of a reaction and the concentration of a reactant. Alternatively, the integrated rate law expresses a rate as a function of concentration of a reactant or reactants and time.

For example, for a zero-order rate, Rate = $k[A]^0$ = k, and since Rate = $-\Delta[A]/\Delta t$, then $-\Delta[A]/\Delta t$ = k, and following the integration of the differential function, the following zero-order integrated rate law is obtained: $[A]_t = -kt + [A]_o$, where $[A]_t$ = is the concentration of A at a particular time point t, and $[A]_0$ is the initial concentration of A, and k is the rate constant.

The following table summarises the main rate laws of the 0th, 1st and 2nd rate orders and their respective relationships.

Table 9.2.1: The graphs below do not need to be memorised but you may be expected to match any Integrated Rate Law equation with its graph since they follow the simple standard of y = mx + b (GM 3.4.4, 3.5.1). The negative slopes (–k) go downhill, and the positive slope (k) goes uphill; no graph begins at the origin (0,0) since they all have a *y*-intercept based on the initial concentration of A.

Rate Law Summary					
Reaction Order	**Rate Law**	**Units of *k***	**Integrated Rate Law**	**Straight-Line Plot**	**Half-Life Equation**
0	Rate = $k[A]^0$	$M \cdot s^{-1}$	$[A]_t = -kt + [A]_0$	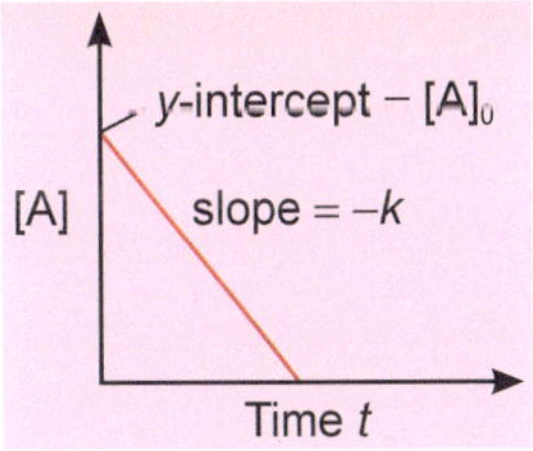	$t_{1/2} = \frac{[A]_0}{2k} = \frac{1}{k}\frac{[A]_0}{2}$
1	Rate = $k[A]^1$	s^{-1}	$\ln[A]_t = -kt + \ln[A]_0$ $\ln\frac{[A]_t}{[A]_0} = -kt$	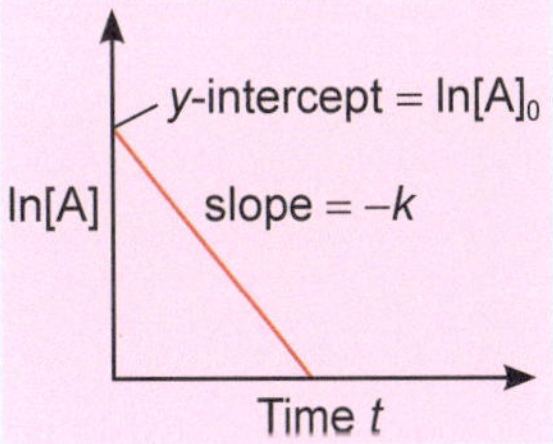	$t_{1/2} = \frac{0.693}{k} = \frac{1}{k}(0.693)$
2	Rate = $k[A]^2$	$M^{-1} \cdot s^{-1}$	$\frac{1}{[A]_t} = kt + \frac{1}{[A]_0}$	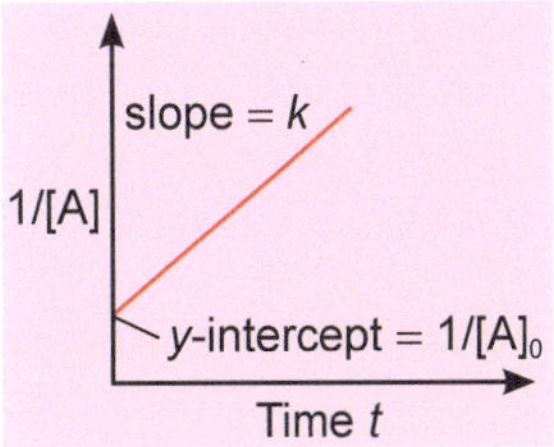	$t_{1/2} = \frac{1}{k[A]_0} = \frac{1}{k}\frac{1}{[A]_0}$

High-level Importance

As depicted by the table, the first and second order rate laws are also derived in a similar manner as the zero-order rate law.

Included within the table is also the half-lives of the three described rate laws. The half-life of a reaction is defined as the time needed to decrease the concentration of the reactant to one-half of the original starting concentration (PHY 12.4). Each rate order has its own respective half-life (*see* graphs below).

The rate order of a reactant may be determined experimentally by either the isolation or initial rates method as described in the following section or by plotting concentration, or some function of concentration such as ln[ ] or 1/[ ] of reactant as a function of time. A linear relationship between the dependent concentration variable of reactant and the independent time variable will then delineate the actual order of the reactant. Moreover, if a linear curve is obtained when plotting [reactant] versus time, the order would be zero whereas, if a linear relationship is noted when plotting ln [reactant] versus time, this would be first order, and second order would be for a linear relationship between 1/[reactant] versus time.

Therefore, the rate law of a reaction with a multi-step mechanism cannot be deduced from the stoichiometric coefficients of the overall reaction; it must be determined experimentally for a given reaction at a given temperature as will be described in the following section.

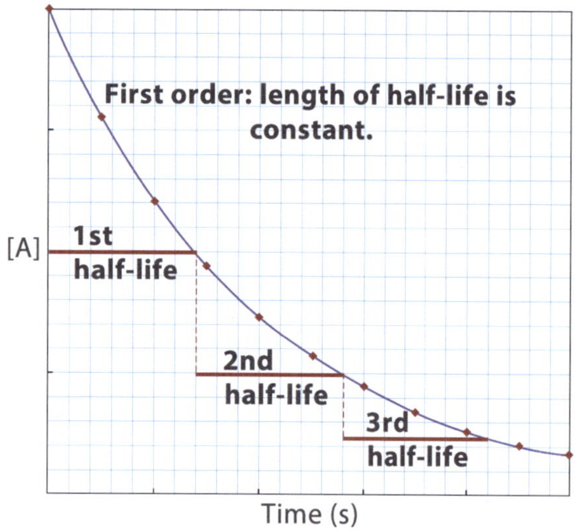

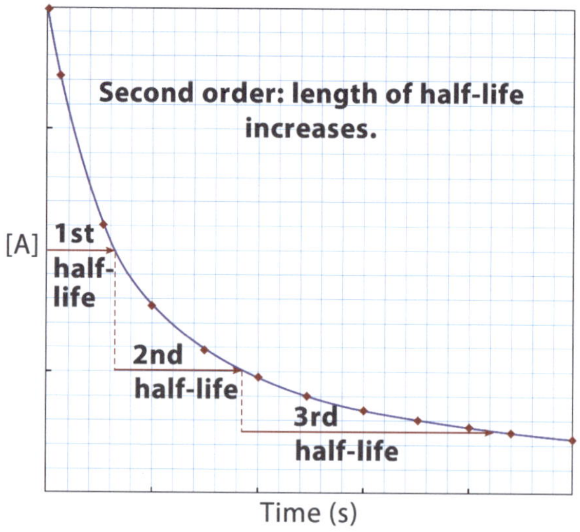

9.3 Determining Exponents of the Rate Law

The only way to determine the exponents with certainty is via experimentation. The rate law for any reaction must therefore always be determined by experimentation, often by a method known as the "initial rates method or the isolation method".

Exp. #	Initial Concentration		Initial Rate ($mol\ L^{-1}\ s^{-1}$)
	[A]	[B]	
1	0.10	0.10	0.20
2	0.20	0.10	0.40
3	0.30	0.10	0.60
4	0.30	0.20	2.40
5	0.30	0.30	5.40

In the initial rates method, if there are two or more reactants involved in the reaction, the reactant concentrations are usually varied independent of each other so that, for example, in a two reactant reaction, if one reactant concentration is altered the other reactant concentration would be kept constant and the effect on the initial rate of the reaction would be measured. Consider the following five experiments varying the concentrations of reactants A and B with resulting initial rates of reaction:

$$A + B \rightarrow \text{products}$$

In the first three experiments the concentration of A changes but B remains the same. Thus the resultant changes in rate only depend on the concentration of A. Note that when [A] doubles (Exp. 1, 2) the reaction rate doubles, and when [A] triples (Exp. 1, 3) the reaction rate triples. Because it is directly proportional, the exponent of [A] must be 1. Thus the rate of reaction is first order with respect to A.

In the final three sets of experiments, [B] changes while [A] remains the same. When [B] doubles (Exp. 3, 4) the rate increases by a factor of 4 (= 2^2). When [B] triples (Exp. 3, 5) the rate increases by a factor of 9 (= 3^2). Thus the relation is exponential where the exponent of [B] is 2. The rate of reaction is second order with respect to B.

$$\text{initial rate} = k[A]^1[B]^2$$

The overall rate of reaction (n+m) is third order. The value of the rate constant k can be easily calculated by substituting the results from any of the five experiments. For example, using experiment #1:

$$k = \frac{\text{initial rate}}{[A]^1\ [B]^2}$$

$$k = \frac{0.20\ \text{mol}\ L^{-1}\ s^{-1}}{(0.10\ \text{mol}\ L^{-1})\ (0.10\ \text{mol}\ L^{-1})^2}$$

$$= 2.0 \times 10^2\ L^2 mol^{-2} s^{-1}$$

k is the rate constant for the reaction which includes all five experiments.

Note: The units of the resultant rate constant "k" will differ depending on the overall rate order of a reaction.

9.4 Reaction Mechanism - Rate-determining Step

Chemical equations fail to describe the detailed process through which the reactants are transformed into the products. For instance, consider the reaction of formation of hydrogen chloride from hydrogen and chlorine:

$$Cl_2(g) + H_2(g) \rightarrow 2\ HCl(g)$$

The equation above fails to mention that in fact this reaction is the result of a chain of reactions proceeding in three steps:

Initiation step: formation of free chlorine radicals by photon irradiation or introduction of heat (= *radicals*, the mechanism will be discussed in organic chemistry):

$$1/2\ Cl_2 \rightleftharpoons Cl\cdot$$

The double arrow indicates that in fact some of the Cl free radicals recombine to form chlorine molecules; the whole process eventually reaches a state of equilibrium where the following ratio is constant:

$$K = [Cl\cdot]/[Cl_2]^{1/2}$$

The determination of such a constant will be dealt with in the sub-section on "equilibrium constants" (CHM 9.8.1).

Propagation step: formation of reactive hydrogen free radicals and reaction between hydrogen free radicals and chlorine molecules:

$$Cl\cdot + H_2 \rightarrow HCl + H\cdot$$

$$H\cdot + Cl_2 \rightarrow HCl + Cl\cdot$$

Termination step: Formation of hydrogen chloride by reaction between hydrogen free radicals and chlorine free radicals.

$$H\cdot + Cl\cdot \rightarrow HCl$$

The detailed chain reaction process above is called the mechanism of the reaction. Each individual step in a detailed mechanism is called an elementary step. Any reaction proceeds through some mechanism which is generally impossible to predict from its chemical equation. Such mechanisms are usually determined through an experimental procedure. Generally speaking, each step proceeds at its own rate.

The rate of the overall reaction is naturally limited by the slowest step; therefore, the rate-determining step in the mechanism of a reaction is the slowest step. In other words, the overall rate law of a reaction is basically equal to the rate law of the slowest step. The faster processes have an indirect influence on the rate: they regulate the concentrations of the reactants and products. The chemical equation of an elementary step reflects the exact molecular process that transforms its reactants into its products. For this reason its rate law can be predicted from its chemical equation: in an elementary process, the orders with respect to the reactants are equal to the corresponding stoichiometric coefficients.

In our example, experiments show that the rate-determining step is the reaction between chlorine radicals and hydrogen molecules, all the other steps are much faster. According to the principles stated, the rate law of the overall reaction is equal to the rate law of this rate-determining step. Therefore, the rate of the overall reaction is proportional to the concentration of hydrogen molecules and chlorine radicals but is not directly proportional to the concentration of chlorine molecules. However, since the ratio of concentrations of Cl and Cl_2 is regulated by the initiation step concentration, it can be shown that according to the mechanism provided the rate law is:

$$\text{rate} = k[H_2] \cdot [Cl_2]^{1/2}$$

It is important to note that the individual orders of a reaction are generally not equal to the stoichiometric coefficients.

9.5 Dependence of Reaction Rates upon Temperature

Rates of chemical reactions are generally very sensitive to temperature fluctuations. In particular, many reactions are known to slow down by decreasing the temperature or vice versa. How does one therefore explain the temperature dependence on reaction rates? The rate of a reaction is essentially equal to the reactant concentration raised to a reaction order (n) times the rate constant k or rate $= k[A]^x$. From the collision theory of chemical kinetics, it was established that the rate constant of a reaction can be expressed as follows:

$$k = A\, e^{-Ea/RT}$$

- A is a constant referred to as the "Arrhenius constant" or the frequency factor which includes two separate components known as, the orientation factor (p) and the collision frequency (z). More specifically, the collision frequency (z) is defined as the number of collisions that molecules acquire per unit time and the orientation factor (p) is defined as the proper orientation reactant molecules require for product formation. Thus, the Arrhenius constant, A, is related to both the frequency of collisions (z) and the proper orientation (p) of the molecular collisions required for final product formation, and so $A = pz$.
- e is the base of natural logarithms (GM 3.7);
- E_a is the activation energy, it is the energy required to get a reaction started. For reactants to transform into products, the reactants must go through a high energy state or "transition state" which is the minimum energy (activation energy) required for reactants to transform into products. If two molecules of reactants collide with proper orientation and sufficient energy

or force in such a way that the molecules acquire a total energy content surpassing the activation energy, E_a, the collisions will result in a complete chemical reaction and the formation of products. Note: only a fraction of colliding reactant molecules will have sufficient kinetic energy to exceed an activation energy barrier.

- R is the ideal gas constant (1.99 cal mol^{-1} K^{-1})
- *T* is the absolute temperature.

It can therefore be seen that the rate constant, k, contains the temperature component as an exponent and thus, temperature affects a reaction rate by affecting the actual rate constant k. Note: A rate constant remains constant only when temperature remains constant. The rate constant equation otherwise known as the "Arrhenius equation" thus describes the relationship between the rate constant (k) and temperature.

Either an increase in temperature or decrease in activation energy will result in an increase in the reaction constant k and thus an increase in the reaction rate. The species formed during an efficient collision, before the reactants transform into the final product(s), is called the activated complex or the transition state.

Within the framework of this theory, when a single-step reaction proceeds, the potential energy of the system varies according to Figure III.A.9.1.

The change in enthalpy (ΔH) during the reaction is the difference between the total energy of the products and the reactants.

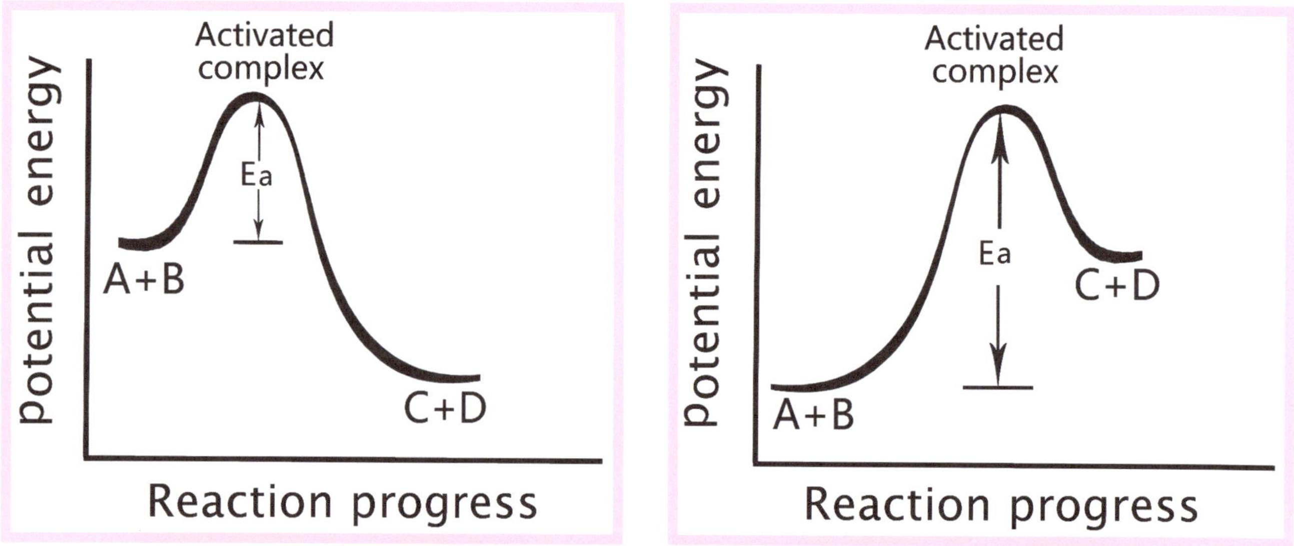

Figure III.A.9.1: Potential energy diagrams: exothermic vs. endothermic reactions.

The left curve of Figure III.A.9.1 shows that the total energy of the reactants is higher than the total energy of the products: this is obviously the case for an exothermic reaction. The right curve of Figure III.A.9.1, shows the profile of an endothermic reaction. A negative enthalpy change indicates an exothermic reaction and a positive enthalpy change depicts an endothermic reaction. The difference in potential energy between the reactant(s) and the activated complex is the activation energy of the forward reaction and the difference between the product(s) and the activated complex is the activation energy of the reverse reaction. Also note that the bigger the difference between the total energy of the reactants and the activated complex, i.e. the activation energy E_a, the slower the reaction.

If a reaction proceeds through several steps one can construct a diagram for each step and combine the single-step diagrams to obtain the energy profile of the overall reaction.

9.6 Kinetic Control vs. Thermodynamic Control

Consider the case where two molecules A and B can react to form either products C or D. Suppose that C has the lowest Gibbs free energy (i.e. the most thermodynamically stable product). Also suppose that product D requires the smallest activation energy and is therefore formed faster than C. If it is product C which is exclusively observed when the reaction is actually performed, the reaction is said to be thermodynamically controlled (i.e. out of a list of possible pathways the reactants choose the one leading to the most stable product). If on the other hand the reactants choose the pathway leading to the product which is produced more quickly, it is said to be kinetically controlled.

9.7 Catalysis

A catalyst increases the rate of a chemical reaction without being consumed by the reaction (*the initial number of moles of this compound in the reaction mixture is equal to the number of moles of this compound once the reaction is completed*). Catalysts work by providing an alternative mechanism for a reaction that involves a different transition state, one in which a lower activation energy occurs at the rate-determining step. Catalysts help lower the activation energy of a reaction and help the reaction to proceed. Enzymes are the

High-level Importance

typical biological catalysts. They are protein molecules with very large molar masses containing one or more active sites (BIO 4.1-4.4). Enzymes are very specialised catalysts. They are generally specific and operate only on certain biological reactants called substrates. They also generally increase the rate of reactions by large factors. The general mechanism of operation of enzymes is as follows:

$$\text{Enzyme (E)} + \text{Substrate (S)} \rightarrow \text{ES (complex)}$$

$$\text{ES} \rightarrow \text{Product (P)} + \text{Enzyme (E)}$$

If we were to compare the energy profile of a reaction performed in the absence of an enzyme to that of the same reaction performed with the addition of an enzyme we would obtain Figure III.A.9.2.

As you can see from Figure III.A.9.2, the reaction from the substrate to the product is facilitated by the presence of the enzyme because the reaction proceeds in two fast steps (low E_a's). Generally, catalysts (or enzymes) stabilise the transition state of a reaction by lowering the energy barrier between reactants and the transition state. Catalysts (or enzymes) do not change the energy difference between reactants and products. Therefore, catalysts do not alter the extent of a reaction or the chemical equilibrium itself. Generally, the rate of an enzyme-catalysed reaction is:

$$\text{rate} = k[\text{ES}]$$

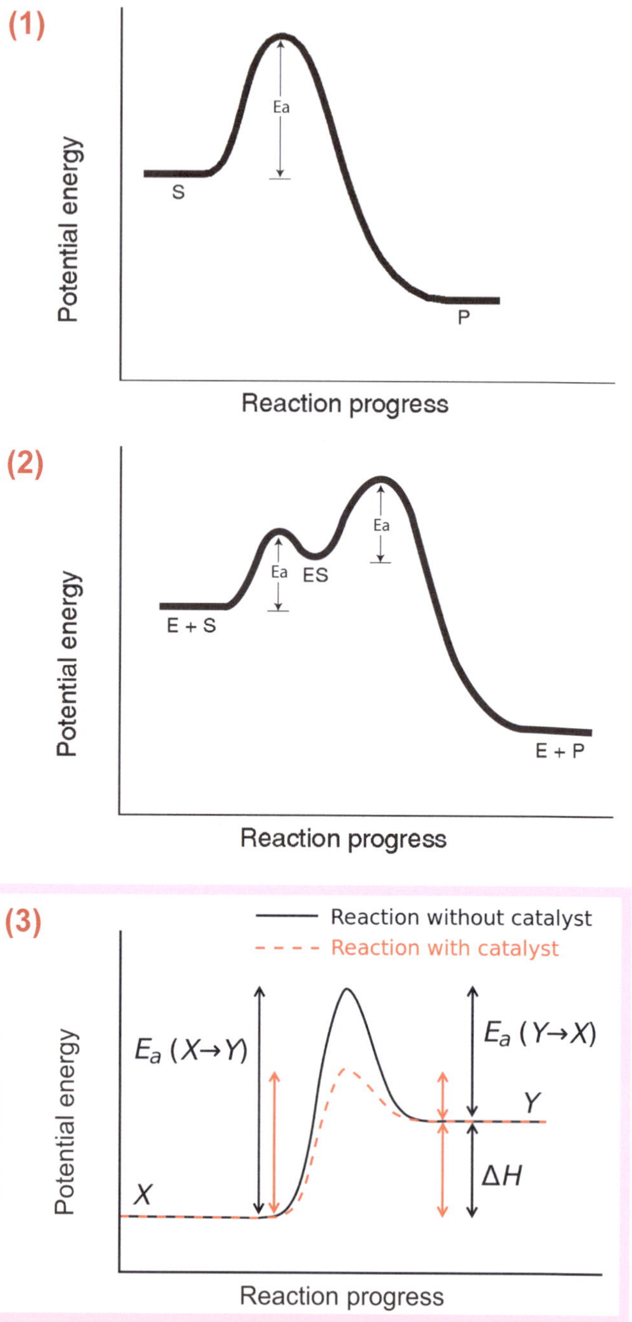

Figure III.A.9.2: Potential energy diagrams: (1) exothermic (CHM 9.5) without a catalyst; (2) exothermic with a catalyst; (3) showing both with and without a catalyst - the forward reaction being endothermic, thus the reverse reaction is exothermic.

The rate of formation of the product $\Delta[P]/\Delta t$ vs. the concentration of the substrate $[S]$ yields a plot as in Figure III.A.9.3.

When the concentration of the substrate is large enough for the substrate to occupy all the available active sites on the enzyme, any further increase would have no effect on the rate of the reaction. This is called *saturation kinetics* (BIO 1.1.2).

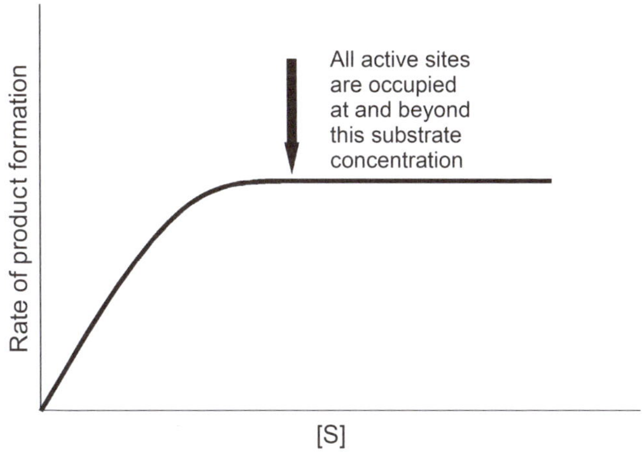

Figure III.A.9.3: Saturation kinetics.

9.8 Equilibrium in Reversible Chemical Reactions

In most chemical reactions once the product is formed, it reacts in such a way to yield back the initial reactants. Eventually, the system reaches a state where there are as many molecules of products being formed as there are molecules of reactants being generated through the reverse reaction. At equilibrium, the concentrations of reactants and products will not necessarily be equal, however, the concentrations remain the same. Hence, the relative concentrations of all components of the forward and reverse reactions become constant at equilibrium. This is called a state of "dynamic equilibrium". It is characterised by a constant K:

$$aA + bB \rightleftharpoons cC + dD$$

where a, b, c and d are the corresponding stoichiometric coefficients:

$$K_{eq} = \frac{[C]^c\,[D]^d}{[A]^a\,[B]^b}$$

The equilibrium constant K (sometimes symbolised as K_{eq}) has a given value at a given temperature. If the temperature changes the value of K changes. At a given temperature, if we change the concentration of A, B, C or D, the system evolves in such a way as to re-establish the value of K. This is called the law of mass action. {Note: catalysts speed up the rate of reaction *without* affecting K_{eq}}

The following is an example of how an equilibrium constant K is calculated based on a chemical reaction at equilibrium. Remember that the equilibrium constant K can be directly calculated only when the equilibrium concentrations of reactants and products are known or obtained.

As an example, suppose that initially, 5 moles of reactant X are mixed with 12 moles of Y and both are added into an empty 1 litre container. Following their reaction, the system eventually reaches equilibrium with 4 moles of Z formed according to the following reaction:

$$X\ (g) + 2Y\ (g) \rightleftharpoons Z\ (g)$$

For this gaseous, homogeneous mixture (CHM 1.1), what is the value of the equilibrium constant K?

At equilibrium, 4 moles of Z are formed and therefore, 4 moles of X and 8 moles of Y are consumed based on the mole:mole ratio of the balanced equation. Since 5 moles X and 12 moles Y were initially available prior to equilibrium, at equilibrium following the reaction, there remains 1 mol X and 4 moles Y. Since all of the reaction takes place in a 1 L volume, the equilibrium concentrations are therefore, 1 mol/L for X, 4 mol/L for Y and Z, respectively.

Thus, the equilibrium constant can then be calculated as follows:

$$K = [Z]/[X][Y]^2 = [4]/[1][4]^2 = 0.25.$$

The K value is an indication of where the equilibrium point of a reaction actually lies, either far to the right or far to the left or somewhere in between. The following is a summary of the significance of the magnitude of an equilibrium constant K and its meaning:

1. If $K_{eq} > 1$, this means that the forward reaction is favored and thus, the reaction favors product formation. If K is very large, the equilibrium mixture will then contain very little reactant compared to product.
2. If $K_{eq} < 1$, the reverse reaction is favored and so the reaction does not proceed very far towards product formation and thus very little product is formed.
3. If $K_{eq} = 1$, neither forward nor reverse directions are favored.

Note: Pure solids and pure liquids do not appear in the equilibrium constant. Thus in heterogeneous equilibria, since the liquid and solid phases are not sensitive to pressure, their "concentrations" remain constant throughout the reaction and so, mathematically, their values are denoted as 1.

Naturally, H_2O is one of the most common liquids dealt with in reactions. Remember to set its activity equal to 1 when it is a liquid but, if H_2O is written as a gas, then its concentration must be considered.

And finally, it is important to understand that we are not discussing *static* equilibrium. The latter would suggest that equilibrium concentrations are not changing because the chemical reaction has stopped. We introduced the idea of a *dynamic* equilibrium when discussing Raoult's law (CHM 5.1.1). The analogy was of a closed water bottle: Liquid constantly evaporating and vapor constantly condensing to liquid water; however, the level of the water in the water bottle does not rise nor fall. And so it is with chemical equilibria, there is a constant interplay between molecules (*dynamic equilibrium*) but, at a given temperature, the equilibrium constant K_{eq} remains constant (i.e. there is no *net* change in concentrations).

9.8.1 The Reaction Quotient Q to Predict Reaction Direction

The reaction quotient Q is the same ratio as the equilibrium constant K (cf. CHM 5.3.4). Q defines all reaction progresses including the K value. In other words, the equilibrium constant K is a special case of the reaction quotient Q.

Thus, the Q ratio has many values dependent on where the reaction lies prior to or subsequent to the concentrations at equilibrium. One may therefore determine if a reaction is going towards an equilibrium by making more products or, alternatively, if a reaction is moving towards equilibrium by making more reactants. The following is a summary of what Q means in relation to K.

Consider the following reaction:

$$aA + bB \rightleftharpoons cC + dD,$$

$$Q = [C]^c[D]^d/[A]^a[B]^b$$

The reaction quotient Q relative to the equilibrium constant K is essentially a measure

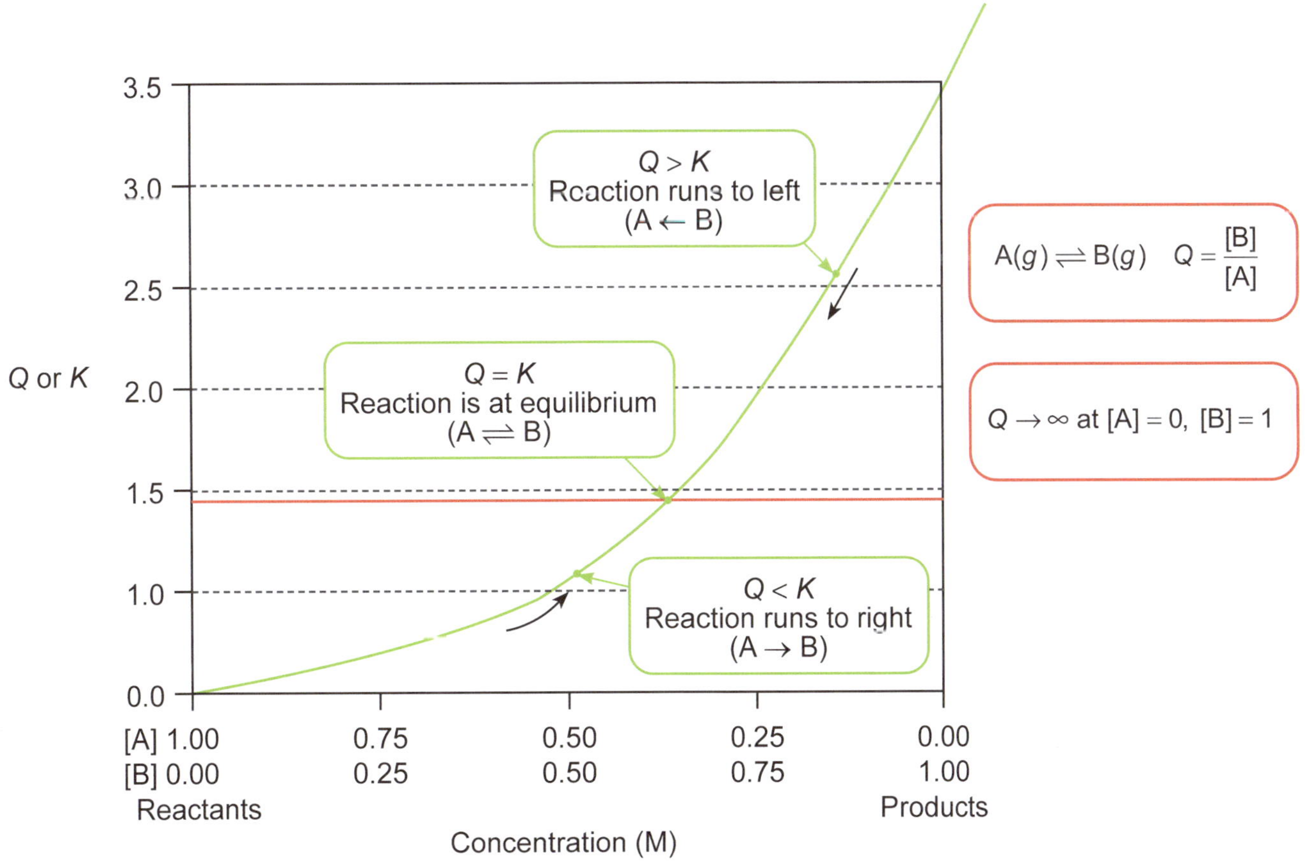

of the progress of a reaction toward equilibrium. The reaction quotient Q has many different values and changes continuously as a reaction progresses and depends on the current state of a reaction mixture. However, once all equilibrium concentrations have been reached, Q = K.

If Q = K, the reaction is at equilibrium and all concentrations are at equilibrium. If Q > K, there are more products initially than there are reactants so the reaction proceeds in reverse direction towards a decrease in product concentrations and a simultaneous increase in reactant concentrations until equilibrium is reached. If Q < K, there are more reactants then products and so the reaction proceeds forward towards product formation until equilibrium is reached.

9.9 Le Chatelier's Principle

Le Chatelier's principle states that whenever a perturbation is applied to a system at equilibrium, the system evolves in such a way as to compensate for the applied perturbation. For instance, consider the following equilibrium:

$$N_2(g) + 3H_2(g) \rightleftharpoons 2NH_3(g)$$

If we introduce more hydrogen (H_2) into the reaction mixture at equilibrium, i.e. if we increase the concentration of hydrogen gas, the system will evolve in the direction that will decrease the concentration of hydrogen (*from left to right*). The consequence of this *shift to the right* is that nitrogen gas (N_2) will go down in concentration (*because it is being used up for the shift to the right*) and, naturally, the concentration of ammonia (NH_3) will rise. In the end, equilibrium is reestablished. A different perspective: Adding hydrogen is a stress to the equilibrium, to relieve the stress, the reaction shifts to the right which produces more ammonia to return to balance.

Let us consider an alternative scenario: If more ammonia is introduced into the reaction mixture, the equilibrium would shift from the right-hand side to the left-hand side (*a shift to the left*) producing more nitrogen and hydrogen; of course, the removal of ammonia from the reaction vessel would do the opposite (i.e. shifting the equilibrium from the left-hand side to the right-hand side: *a shift to the right*) which would produce more ammonia and reestablish equilibrium.

In a similar fashion, an increase in total pressure (*decrease in volume*) favors the direction which decreases the total number of compressible (i.e. *gases*) moles (from the left-hand side where there are 4 moles to the right-hand side where there are 2 moles).

It can also be said that when there are different forms of a gaseous substance, an increase in total pressure (*decrease in volume*) favors the form with the greatest density, and a decrease in total pressure (*increase in volume*) favors the form with the lowest density.

Finally, if the temperature of a reaction mixture at equilibrium is increased, the equilibrium evolves in the direction of the endothermic (heat-absorbing) reaction. For instance, the forward reaction of the equilibrium:

$$N_2O_4(g) \rightleftharpoons 2NO_2(g)$$

is endothermic; therefore, an increase in temperature favors the forward reaction over the backward reaction. In other words, the dissociation of N_2O_4 increases with temperature.

An easy way to remember how to handle exothermic or endothermic reactions, in context with Le Chatelier's principle without memorisation, is to simply add "heat" as a reactant (endothermic), or product (exothermic). For example, since we were told that the forward reaction was endothermic, we could illustrate that fact by adding the word "heat" to the reactant:

$$\text{heat} + N_2O_4(g) \rightleftharpoons 2NO_2(g)$$

Now it is easier to visualise that if the temperature is increased, heat becomes the stress, thus the reaction shifts to the right. Conversely, if the temperature decreases, the reaction must do the opposite by shifting to the left to increase the heat and return to equilibrium.

9.10 Relationship between the Equilibrium Constant and the Change in the Gibbs Free Energy

In the "thermodynamics" section we defined the Gibbs free energy (CHM 8.10). The *standard* Gibbs free energy ($G°$) is determined at 25 °C (298 K) and 1 atm. The change in the standard Gibbs free energy for a given reaction can be calculated from the change in the standard enthalpy and entropy of the reaction using:

$$\Delta G° = \Delta H - T\,\Delta S°$$

where T is the absolute temperature at which the reaction is carried out. If this reaction happens to be the forward reaction of an equilibrium, the equilibrium constant associated with this equilibrium is simply given by:

$$\Delta G° = -R\;T\;ln\;K_{eq}$$

where R is the ideal gas constant (1.99 cal mol^{-1} K^{-1}) and ln is the natural logarithm (i.e. log to the base *e*; *see* GM 3.7).

It is important to remember the sign for Gibbs free energy when the reaction is not spontaneous, spontaneous and at equilibrium (CHM 8.10).

High-level Importance

CHAPTER 9: Rate Processes in Chemical Reactions

GOLD STANDARD FOUNDATIONAL GAMSAT PRACTICE QUESTIONS

1) Choose the second order reaction from the following rate laws:

A. Rate = k [RX]
B. Rate = k [RX] [$^-$OH]
C. Rate = k $[RX]^2$ [$^-$OH]
D. Rate = k $[RX]^2$ $[^-OH]^2$

2) A reaction was found to be zero order with respect to X. Increasing the concentration of X by a factor of 3 would cause the reaction rate to:

A. increase by a factor of 3.
B. decrease by a factor of 9.
C. increase by a factor of 27.
D. remain constant.

3) The mechanism for the formation of product T is as follows:

$$P + Q \rightarrow R + S \quad (\textit{slow})$$
$$Q + S \rightarrow T \quad (\textit{fast})$$

Which of the following is an intermediate in the reaction?

A. P
B. Q
C. R
D. S

4) The overall reactions and rate laws are given below. Which one of the following represents an elementary step?

A. $2A \rightarrow P$ rate = k[A]
B. $A + B + C \rightarrow P$ rate = k[A][C]
C. $A + B \rightarrow P$ rate = k[A][B]
D. $A + 2B \rightarrow P$ rate = $k[A]^2$

5) Consider the following gas phase chemical reaction:

$$2\ NH_3(g) \rightleftharpoons N_2(g) + 3\ H_2(g)$$

The equilibrium constant K_{eq} is 230 at 300 °C. At the given temperature, which one of the following statements is true at equilibrium?

A. Only products are present.
B. Only the reactant is present.
C. The products predominate.
D. The reactant predominates.

6) The decomposition of hydrogen peroxide in the presence of the iodide anion is believed to occur via the following mechanism.

$$H_2O_2(aq) + I^-(aq) \rightarrow H_2O(l) + IO^-(aq)$$
$$H_2O_2(aq) + IO^-(aq) \rightarrow H_2O(l) + O_2(g) + I^-(aq)$$

In this mechanism, what must $I^-(aq)$ represent?

A. A catalyst
B. An intermediate
C. The activated complex
D. A product of the overall reaction

7) Consider the following rate law for a chemical reaction: rate = $k[X][Y]^2$. Which one of the following statements is **not** correct?

A. If [X] is doubled and [Y] is held constant, the reaction rate will be doubled.
B. If [Y] is doubled and [X] is held constant, the reaction rate will increase by a factor of 4.
C. The reaction is first order with respect to X.
D. The reaction is second order overall.

High-level Importance

8) The rate law of the overall chemical reaction $A + B \rightarrow C$ is experimentally determined to be rate = $k[A]^2$. Which one of the following is certain not to increase the rate of the reaction?

A. Increasing the concentration of reactant A
B. Increasing the concentration of reactant B
C. Adding a catalyst for the reaction
D. Increasing the temperature of the reaction

9) Consider the following reaction at equilibrium.

$$2\,CO_2(g) \rightleftharpoons 2\,CO(g) + O_2(g) \qquad \Delta H° = 514 \text{ kJ/mol}$$

Le Chatelier's principle predicts that adding $O_2(g)$ to the reaction container will:

A. decrease the value of the equilibrium constant.
B. increase the value of the equilibrium constant.
C. increase the partial pressure of $CO_2(g)$ at equilibrium.
D. increase the partial pressure of CO(g) at equilibrium.

10) Consider the following gas phase reaction at equilibrium.

$$H_2 + I_2 \rightleftharpoons 2HI \qquad \Delta H = -12.40 \text{ kcal}$$

Raising the temperature for the chemical reaction above would result in which of the following?

A. An increase in the concentration of H_2 and I_2
B. A decrease in entropy
C. No change in the equilibrium concentrations of reactants and products
D. Neither **A**, nor **B**, nor **C** is true.

11) Consider the following chemical reaction.

$$N_2 + 3H_2 \rightleftharpoons 2NH_3$$

Suppose that the concentrations of reactants and products at equilibrium for the gas phase reaction above are $[N_2] = 0.19$ M, $[H_2] = 0.10$ M, and $[NH_3] = 0.01$ M.

What is the approximate magnitude of the equilibrium constant for the reaction?

A. 0.05
B. 0.2
C. 0.5
D. 2.0

12) Consider the following chemical reaction.

$$2NO(g) + O_2(g) \rightarrow 2NO_2(g) \qquad \Delta H° = -116.2 \text{ kJ}$$

Which of the following represents the general shape of the potential energy diagram for the preceding reaction?

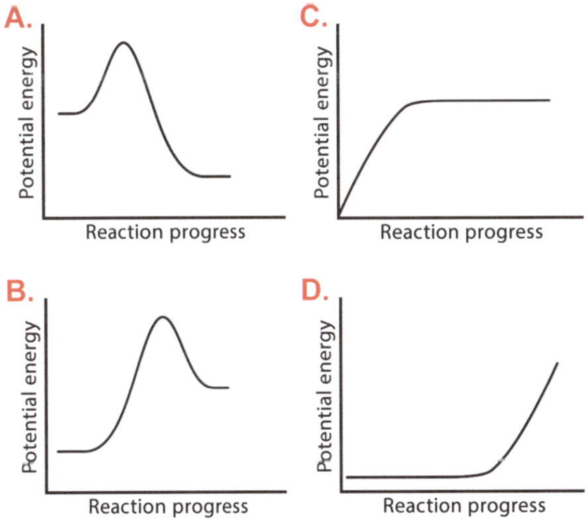

High-level Importance

GOLD STANDARD GAMSAT-LEVEL PRACTICE QUESTIONS

Questions 13–15

Consider the data in Table 1, which pertain to the following overall chemical reaction:

$$A + B \rightarrow C$$

Experiment no.	[A]	[B]	Initial rate of formation of C (M/s)
1	0.10	0.10	4.0×10^{-5}
2	0.10	0.20	4.0×10^{-5}
3	0.20	0.10	1.6×10^{-4}

Table 1

The rate of a reaction (given in moles per litre per second) can be expressed as a function of the concentration of the reactants. In the previous chemical reaction, we would have:

$$\text{rate} = k\,[A]^m\,[B]^n$$

where [ ] is the concentration of the corresponding reactant in moles per litre (M); k is the rate constant; m is the order of the reaction with respect to A; n is the order of the reaction with respect to B; m + n is the overall reaction order.

Note that the *molecularity* of a reaction is the number of molecules reacting in an elementary step. A *unimolecular* reaction is one in which only one reacting molecule participates in the reaction. Two reactant molecules collide with one another in a *bimolecular* reaction. A *termolecular* reaction involves three reacting molecules in one elementary step.

13) Based on Table 1, the rate law for the reaction is:

A. Rate = $k[A][B]$.
B. Rate = $k[A]^2[B]$.
C. Rate = $k[A]^2$.
D. Rate = $k[A][B]^2$.

14) Based on the information provided, the rate constant, k, is:

A. $4.0 \times 10^{-3}\ M^{-1}s^{-1}$
B. $4.0 \times 10^{-3}\ Ms^{-1}$
C. $4.0 \times 10^{-5}\ M^{-1}s^{-1}$
D. $4.0 \times 10^{-5}\ Ms^{-1}$

15) The mechanism of the reaction described in Table 1 most likely involves:

A. a termolecular rate-determining step.
B. a bimolecular rate-determining step involving two molecules of A, followed by a fast step involving a molecule of B.
C. a fast step involving a molecule of A and a molecule of B, followed by a bimolecular rate-determining step involving another molecule of A.
D. a bimolecular rate-determining step involving a molecule of A and a molecule of B, followed by a fast step involving another molecule of A.

Questions 16–18

Kidney stones (renal lithiasis) are small, hard mineral deposits that form inside kidneys. Kidney stones can affect any part of the urinary tract — from kidneys to bladder. Often, stones form when the urine becomes concentrated, allowing minerals to crystallise.

Passing (i.e. eliminating through the natural path) kidney stones can be quite painful, usually only requiring pain medication and increased water intake, but sometimes other medications or shock waves are needed. On rare occasion, stones become lodged in the urinary tract requiring surgical intervention.

Calcium oxalate, a derivative of the diprotic oxalic acid, is the most common component in kidney stones. The following is the structure of oxalic acid.

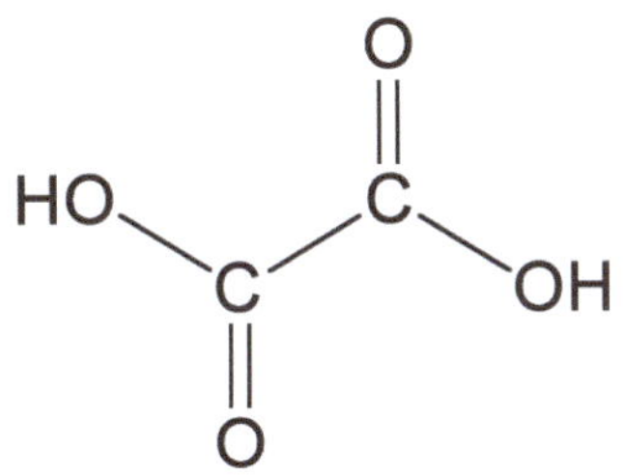

The first pKa value for oxalic acid is 1.27 and the second pKa value is 4.28. The Ksp for calcium oxalate is 2.7×10^{-9}. Consider the following sequence of reactions:

(1) $HOOCCOOH \rightleftharpoons HOOCCOO^{-} + H^{+}$

(2) $HOOCCOO^{-} \rightleftharpoons {}^{-}OOCCOO^{-} + H^{+}$

(3) $Ca^{++} + {}^{-}OOCCOO^{-}(aq) \rightleftharpoons Ca(OOCCOO)(s)$

Healthy kidneys can concentrate urine. This is accomplished in different ways including the countercurrent multiplier function of the loop of Henle, and the secretory function of the nephron.

	Plasma Concentration (millimol/L)	Typical concentration in urine
urea	5.1	60×
ammonia	0.062	500×
sodium ions	140	6×
calcium ions	2.0	1.5×
creatinine	0.85	100×

Table 1: Relative concentrations of solutes in urine as compared to approximate values in plasma

16. Based on the information provided, determine the minimum oxalate ion concentration in urine that would be required to form kidney stones.

A. 9.0×10^{-7} M
B. 9.0×10^{-4} M
C. 6.0×10^{-7} M
D. 6.0×10^{-4} M

17. When the body's intake of calcium is low, in order to maintain homeostasis, there is an increased renal absorption of calcium. Based on the information provided, which of the following changes in urine is most consistent with a decrease in calcium intake in a person with kidney stones?

A. Decreased oxalate ions
B. Increased solubility product
C. Decreased pH
D. Increased pH

18. Potassium citrate is a medication that can be used to treat gout. A side effect of potassium citrate is the alkalisation of urine. Would calcium oxalate kidney stones be more or less likely to be produced in a person taking potassium citrate?

A. Less likely, because the increased hydroxide concentration will bind the protons producing water.
B. Less likely, because the reaction is buffered by monohydrogen oxalate.
C. More likely, because the increased pH will lead to increased oxalate ion concentration.
D. More likely, because the conjugate base of oxalic acid is the oxalate ion.

High-level Importance

Questions 19–22

The essential stages in the manufacture of H_2SO_4 and H_2SO_3 involve the burning of sulfur or roasting of sulfide ores in air to produce SO_2. This is then mixed with air, purified and passed over a vanadium catalyst (either VO_3^- or V_2O_5) at 450 degrees Celsius. Thus the following reaction occurs.

$$2SO_2(g) + O_2(g) \rightleftharpoons 2SO_3(g) \qquad \Delta H = -197 \text{ kJ mol}^{-1}$$

Reaction I

If the SO_2 is very carefully dissolved in water, sulfurous acid (H_2SO_3) is obtained. The first proton of this acid ionises as if from a strong acid while the second ionises as if from a weak acid.

$$H_2SO_3 + H_2O \rightarrow H_3O^+ + HSO_3^-$$

Reaction II

$$HSO_3^- + H_2O \rightleftharpoons H_3O^+ + SO_3^{2-} \qquad K_a = 5.0 \times 10^{-6}$$

Reaction III

The concentration of H_2SO_3 in cleaning fluid was determined by titration with 0.10 M NaOH (strong base) as shown in Fig.1. Two equivalence points were determined using 30 ml and 60 ml of NaOH, respectively:

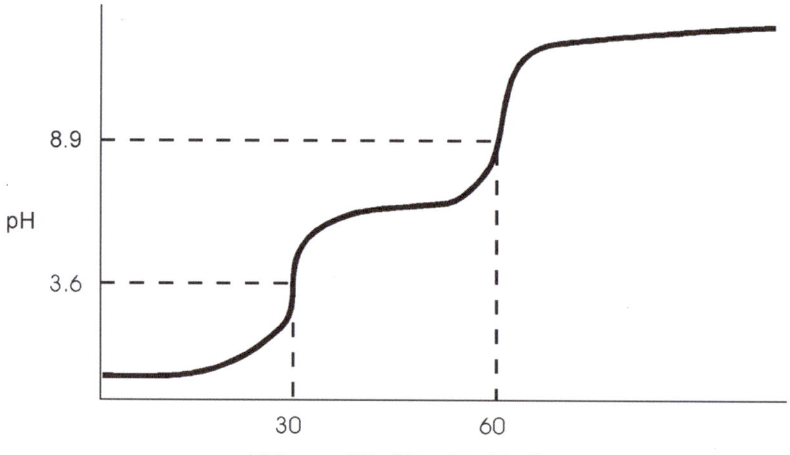

Figure 1

Note: You may find some of the following information helpful. Relative atomic masses: H = 1.0, N = 14.0, O = 16.0, S = 32, Cl = 35.5

19) What is the percent by mass of oxygen in sulfurous acid?

A. 31.9%
B. 19.7%
C. 39.0%
D. 58.5%

20) If no catalyst was used in Reaction I, which of the following would experience a change in its partial pressure when the same system reaches equilibrium?

A. There will be no change in the partial pressure of any of the reactants
B. $SO_3(g)$
C. $SO_2(g)$
D. $O_2(g)$

21) If the temperature was decreased in Reaction I, which of the following would experience an increase in its partial pressure when the same system reaches equilibrium?

A. There will be no change in the partial pressure of any of the reactants

B. $SO_3(g)$

C. $SO_2(g)$

D. $O_2(g)$ and $SO_2(g)$

22) Which of the following acid-base indicators is most suitable for the determination of the first end point of the titration shown in Figure 1?

A. Cresol red (colour change between pH = 0.2 and pH = 1.8)

B. p-Xylenol blue (colour change between pH = 1.2 and pH = 2.8)

C. Bromophenol blue (colour change between pH = 3.0 and pH = 4.6)

D. Bromocresol green (colour change between pH = 3.8 and pH = 5.4)

23) According to the Arrhenius equation the rate constant k is equal to $Ae^{-Ea/RT}$, where A is the Arrhenius constant, e is the base of natural logarithms, Ea is the activation energy, R is the ideal gas constant, and T is the temperature in kelvin. Which of the following options represents a graph of ln k vs 1/T?

A.

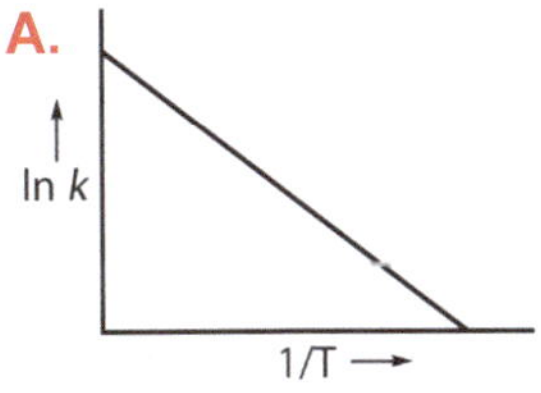

C.

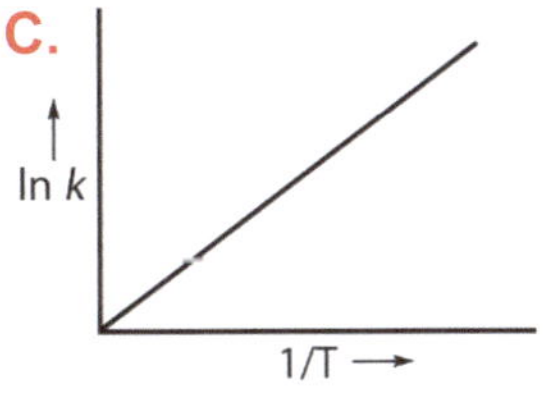

B.

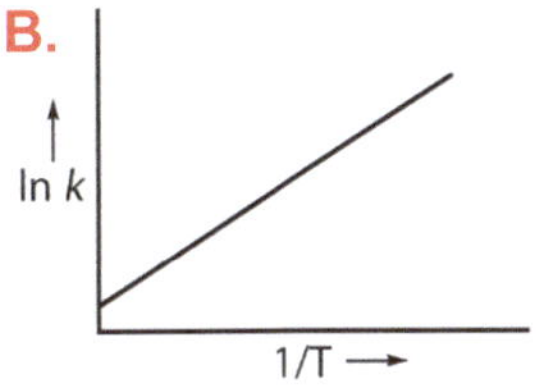

D.

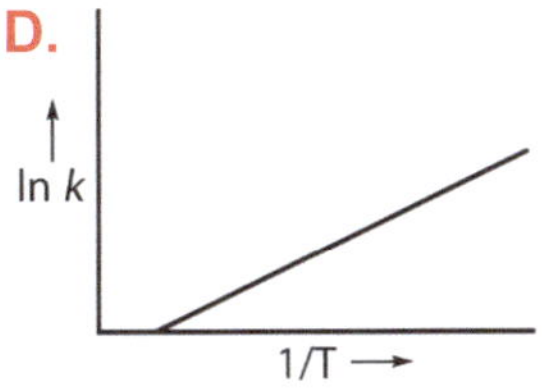

24) Ammonia is used as a key component to the production of food, fertilisers and household cleaning fluids. The balanced equation below represents the reaction that takes place in a sealed container.

$$N_2(g) + 3H_2(g) \rightleftharpoons 2NH_3(g) \qquad \Delta H < 0$$

To meet an increased demand for fertiliser, many companies try various techniques to increase the yield of ammonia. In a trial run on a small scale at a particular laboratory, the chemical engineer made adjustments to the temperature, pressure and concentration of the equilibrium mixture of the production of ammonia from nitrogen and hydrogen. The results are shown in Figure 1.

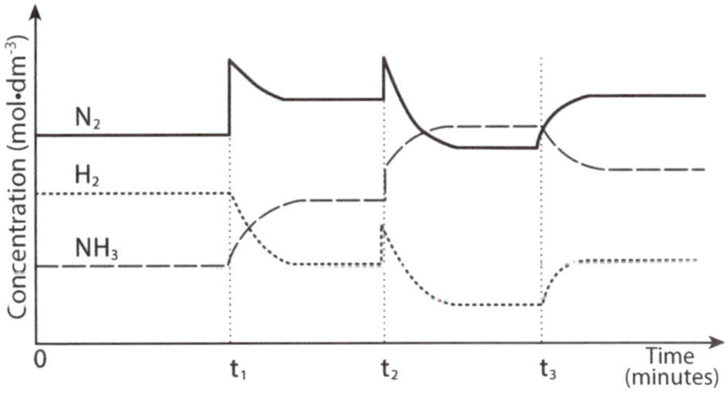

Figure 1

During the experiment, changes were made to the equilibrium mixture at the specific times identified in Figure 1 as t_1, t_2 and t_3. At each time, only one change was made. Identify the most likely change that occurred.

A. Additional NH_3 was added to the mixture at t_1.

B. The pressure on the system was decreased at t_2.

C. The temperature of the system was decreased at t_3.

D. Neither **A** nor **B** nor **C**.

High-level Importance

Questions 25–28

Silver is still one of the most versatile metals known to man, being used in almost everything from electrical wires to jewellery. It is also quite unreactive, and is resistant to attack by common agents such as acid and oxygen. Needless to say, the mining of this precious metal is the mainstay of the economy of many countries. Unfortunately, silver does not occur in its elemental state in nature. It is mined as argentite (Ag_2S containing ore) and horn silver (AgCl containing ore).

The main method used in industry for separating silver from its ores involves complexation and the cyanide ligand (CN^-). The cyanide ligand is used to produce the soluble silver cyanide complex according to Reaction I and Reaction II.

Reaction I

$$Ag_2S + 4CN^- \rightarrow 2[Ag(CN)_2]^- + S^{2-}$$

Reaction II

$$AgCl + 2CN^- \rightarrow [Ag(CN)_2]^- + Cl^-$$

The silver metal in its elemental form is then precipitated by adding zinc dust to the solution as shown in Reaction III.

Reaction III

$$2[Ag(CN)_2]^- + Zn \rightarrow [Zn(CN)_4]^{2-} + 2Ag(s)$$

Silver complexes provide one of the most fascinating demonstrations of the relative strengths of different ligands for a particular cation. This is a common occurrence with most complexes of this nature but what makes silver unique is that many of its complexes differ in colour. Table 1 is a list of a few of the silver complexes and their colours.

Complex	Colour
$[Ag(CN)_2]^-$	Clear solution
AgI	Yellow precipitate
$[Ag(EDTA)]^-$	Clear solution
Ag_2S	Black precipitate

Table 1

One will notice that precipitates are listed in the table. These can be regarded as neutral complexes and, as is often the case with neutral complexes, they are quite insoluble and hence precipitate out of solution.

25) Silverware tarnishes (*darkens on the surface*) because of a reaction between silver and tiny amounts of a gas in air. Based on information in the passage, that gas must be which of the following gases?

A. O_2
B. N_2
C. H_2O
D. H_2S

26) Given that $K_{a1}(H_2S) = 9.1 \times 10^{-8}$ and $K_{a2}(H_2S) = 1.2 \times 10^{-15}$, what would be the effect on Reaction I if protons were added to the reaction mixture at equilibrium? (note: the effect of protons on CN^- is relatively negligible)

A. The equilibrium would shift to the left.
B. The equilibrium would shift to the right.
C. There would be no change in the equilibrium position of the reaction.
D. The change in the equilibrium position cannot be determined from the information given.

27) One of the complexes formed by silver is silver bromide, AgBr. Why would you expect it to be insoluble?

A. Because it is a neutral complex.
B. Because Br^- is a large anion.
C. Because the relative molecular mass of AgBr is large.
D. Because most bromides are insoluble.

28) Given the data below, which of the following ligands would you add to a clear silver complex in solution to determine which of the clear complexes in Table 1 was present?

In order of decreasing affinity for silver ions:

$$\text{EDTA} > S^{2-} > CN^- > I^-$$

A. EDTA
B. S^{2-}
C. CN^-
D. I^-

29) Consider the Arrhenius equation arranged as:

$$2.303 \log_{10}\left(\frac{k_2}{k_1}\right) = \frac{E_a}{R}\left(\frac{T_2 - T_1}{T_1 T_2}\right)$$

Note that:

- the rate constants k_1 and k_2 are at two different temperatures T_1 and T_2
- the activation energy for a reaction is given by E_a
- R is the gas constant, 8.31 J mol^{-1} K^{-1}

If the rate of reaction is one hundred times faster at 34 °C than it is at 24 °C, which of the following would be the best approximation of the activation energy as determined from the Arrhenius equation?

A. 35 J
B. 3500 J
C. 350 kJ
D. 3.5×10^4 kJ

30) Consider the following potential energy (PE) diagram:

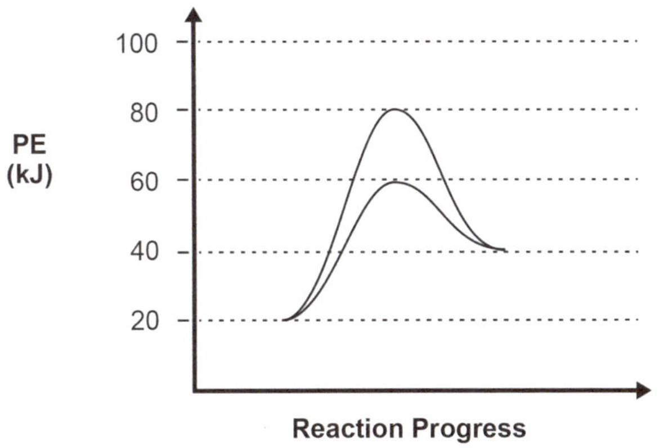

Which of the following best describes this chemical reaction?

	ΔH (kJ)	Activation Energy (kJ)	Reaction
A.	−20	40	catalysed
B.	−20	60	catalysed
C.	+20	40	uncatalysed
D.	+20	60	uncatalysed

31) The data in Table 1 were collected for Reaction I:

$$2X + Y \rightarrow Z \qquad \text{Reaction I}$$

Exp.	[X] in M	[Y] in M	Initial rate of reaction
1	0.050	0.100	8.5×10^{-6}
2	0.050	0.200	3.4×10^{-5}
3	0.200	0.100	3.4×10^{-5}

Table 1

What is the rate law for the reaction?

A. Rate = $k[X]^2[Y]$
B. Rate = $k[X]^2[Y]^2$
C. Rate = $k[X][Y]^2$
D. Rate = $k[X][Y]$

32) Consider the following reaction:

$$2A \rightarrow B$$

The integrated rate law for the preceding reaction is given below, where the rate constant is k_1, the concentration of A at any time t is $[A]$, and at time 0 is $[A]_0$:

$$k_1 t = \ln \frac{[A]_0}{[A]}$$

The following graph illustrates the relationship between the change in concentration and time for the preceding reaction.

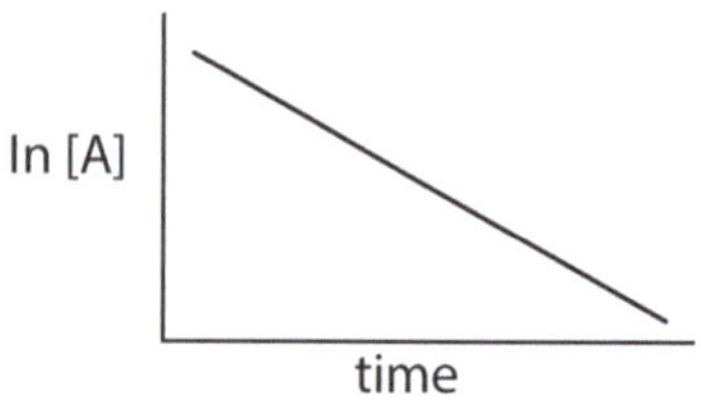

The slope of the line is equal to which of the following?

A. $-1/k_1$
B. $-k_1$
C. $-\ln[A]$
D. k_1

Questions 33–35

Sparsomycin is an antibiotic that inhibits peptidyl transferase activity. Figure 1 shows the kinetics of inhibition of rabbit red blood cell peptidyltransferase by Sparsomycin. The time plots shown were done using Sparsomycin concentrations of (✱) 0.1×10^{-6} M, (▲) 0.2×10^{-6} M, and (●) 0.4×10^{-6} M. The percentage (x′) of the remaining active peptidyltransferase is shown, as well as the percentage at equilibrium (x'_{eq}) for each curve which is indicated by the dashed --- lines.

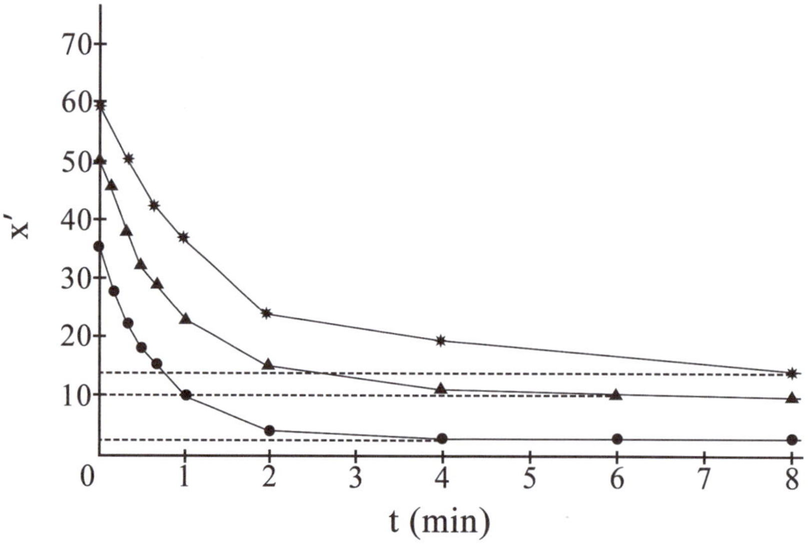

Figure 1

Adapted from D. Synetos, Molecular Pharmacology June 1, 1998 vol. 53 no. 6 1089-1096.

33) Which of the following graphs is consistent with the data in Figure 1?

The following estimates may be of assistance: log 6 = 0.8, log 4 = 0.6.

A.

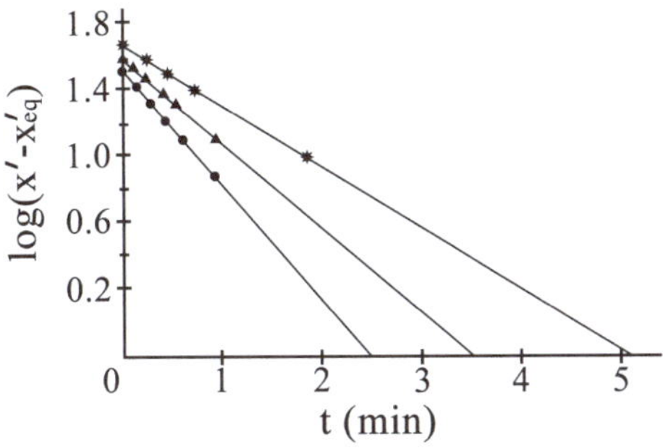

B.

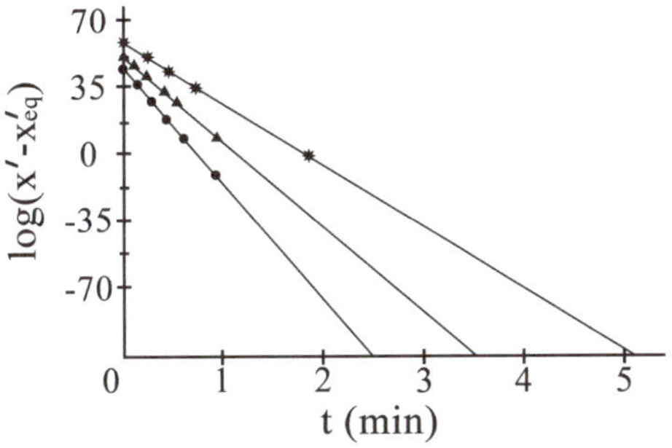

C.

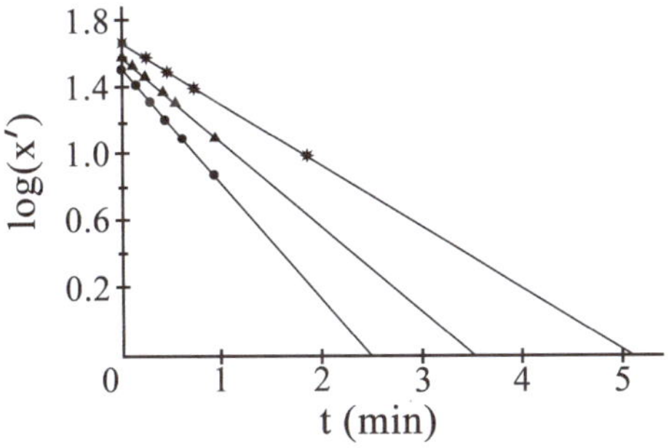

D.

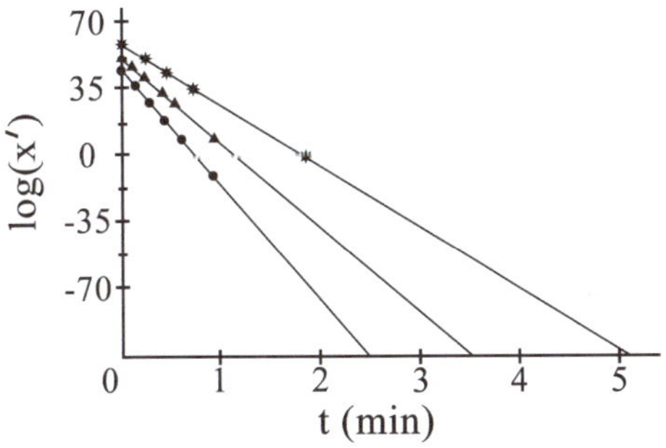

34) According to Figure 1, if 0.2×10^{-6} M of Sparsomycin is applied to 70 picograms of peptidyltransferase from rabbit red blood cells, estimate the rate of inhibition at t = 2 minutes.

A. 30 picograms/minute
B. 25 picograms/minute
C. 15 picograms/minute
D. 3.5 picograms/minute

35) Which of the following is NOT true concerning the curves in Figure 1?

A. The equilibrium point of the curve using 0.4×10^{-6} M Sparsomycin is obtained at a point where more than 95% of the peptidyltransferase is not active.
B. The fact that the 3 plots are curved, does not in itself indicate if the reaction is first order or second order.
C. The curve where 0.2×10^{-6} M Sparsomycin is used is most consistent with a first-order reaction because the active concentration of peptidyltransferase decreases by approximately 50% at just under 1 minute, and then by another 50% (approximately) at just under 1 minute later.
D. If the curves were linear, they would be most consistent with zero-order and first-order reactions.

High-level Importance

SPOILER ALERT

Gold Standard has cross-referenced the content in this chapter to examples from ACER's official GAMSAT practice materials. It is for you to decide when you want to explore these questions since you may want to preserve some of ACER's materials for timed mock-exam practice.

Examples – Reaction rates including a table of data and recognising the correct rate law graph (a little acid/base and log rules): Q28-30 of 2; Gibbs free energy, with enthalpy, entropy and a twist: Q42-43 of 2 (not counted, because it was counted for Chapter 8); Arrhenius equation, potential energy graph (can you label it?): Q49-51 of 3 (note that ACER did not give the conversion factor between kelvin and Celsius, + 273, which is necessary to correctly answer Q50-51; that is why we did not give the conversion factor for Q29, Chapter 9); rate law with table of data and one calculation: Q77-78 of 3; Le Chatelier (with a bit of acid/base): Q92 of 3; rate law with graph and reaction order: Q6-9 of 4; Le Chatelier (again, with a bit of acid/base): Q47-48 of 4; rate law classic unit: Q55-58 of 4; equilibrium constant Keq: Q69 of 4; basic rate law (maths): Q70 of 4; Gibbs free energy Q71 of 4 (not counted, because it was counted for Chapter 8); Note that "Q" is followed by the question number, and, for example, "of 1" refers to booklet number 1 which is referenced in the Spoiler Alert table at the end of Chapter 1. The 15 full-length GAMSAT practice tests by Gold Standard, HEAPS-1 through HEAPS-15, contain specific cross-references to this chapter within the worked solutions. Note that the kidney-stones unit at equilibrium with Le Chatelier is a rare visitor from HEAPS-1; HEAPS-5 and HEAPS-6 have a few independent questions including several using the rate law with a table of data, and one Le Chatelier unit with acids and bases.

Chapter Checklist

- ☐ Access your online account to view answers, worked solutions and discussion boards.
- ☐ Reassess your 'learning objectives' for this chapter: Go back to the first page of this chapter and re-evaluate the top 3 boxes and the Introduction.
  - ☐ Please be sure that you have completed the *Need for Speed* exercises at the beginning of this chapter.
- ☐ Complete a maximum of 1 page of notes using symbols/abbreviations to represent the entire chapter based on your learning objectives. These are your Gold Notes.
- ☐ Consider your multimedia options based on your optimal way of learning:
  - ☐ Download the free Gold Standard GAMSAT app for your Android device or iPhone.
  - ☐ Create your own, tangible study cards or try the free app: Anki.
  - ☐ Record your voice reading your Gold Notes onto your smartphone (audio files, e.g., *memo* or MP3s) and listen during exercise, transportation, etc.
  - ☐ Try out the Gold Standard GAMSAT online videos at gamsat-prep.com, or you can try other options on YouTube like Khan Academy or Crash Course Chemistry.
- ☐ Reassess your schedule for your full-length GAMSAT practice tests: ACER and/or HEAPS exams. Ensure that you have scheduled one full day to complete a practice test and 1-2 days for a thorough assessment of worked solutions while adding to your abbreviated Gold Notes.
- ☐ Reassess your progress in scheduling and/or evaluating stress reduction techniques such as regular exercise (sports), yoga, meditation and/or mindfulness exercises (*see* YouTube for suggestions).

High-level Importance

ELECTROCHEMISTRY

Chapter 10

Memorise

- Rules for oxidation numbers (*optional*)
- Define: anode, cathode, anion, cation
- Define: standard half-cell potentials
- Define: strong/weak, oxidising/reducing agents

Understand

- Calculations involving oxidation numbers
- Basics: Electrochemical cells
- Calculation involving Faraday's law
- Half reaction, reduction potentials
- Direction of electron flow

Importance

Medium level: 7% of GAMSAT General Chemistry

questions released by ACER are related to content in this chapter (in our estimation).

* Note that approximately 80% of the questions in GAMSAT General Chemistry are related to just 4 chapters: 4, 5, 6, and 9.

Introduction

Electrochemistry links chemistry with electricity (*the movement of electrons through a conductor*). If a chemical reaction produces electricity (i.e. a battery or galvanic/voltaic cell) then it is an **electrochemical cell**. If electricity is applied externally to drive the chemical reaction then it is **electrolysis**. In general, oxidation/reduction reactions occur and are separated in space or time, connected by an external circuit. If you need to balance redox reactions using the "half-reaction method of balancing" (CHM 10.1) during the GAMSAT, you will be reminded of the rules (i.e. do not memorise them).

Multimedia Resources at GAMSAT-Prep.com

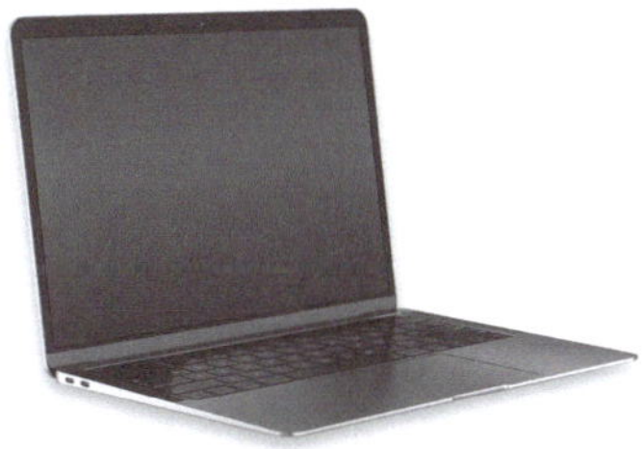

Open Discussion Boards
(*gamsat-prep.com/forum*)

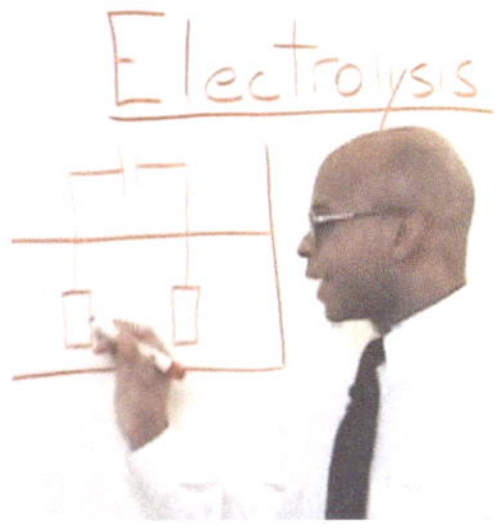

Science Preparation Videos

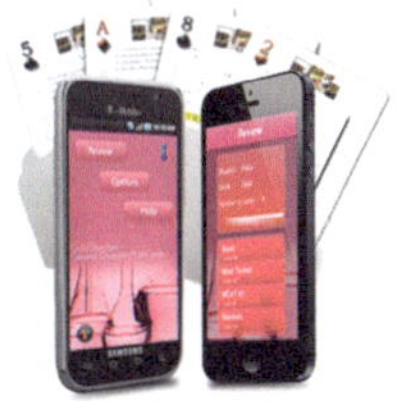

Flashcards

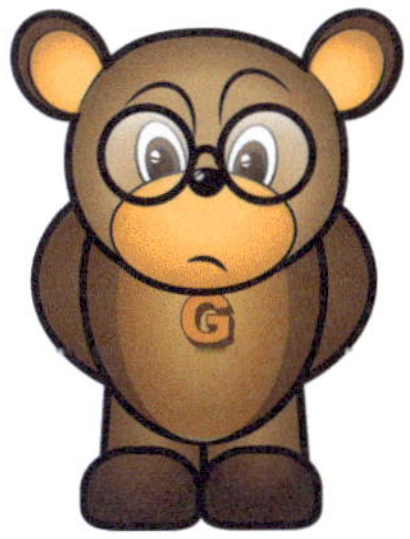

Special Guest

* The real GAMSAT may have advanced-level information presented (i.e. in a passage) but previous knowledge of said information is not required to answer the questions that would follow. Practice questions at the end of this chapter, as well as ACER and GS (HEAPS) practice GAMSATs can help you clarify this point.

10.0 GAMSAT has a *Need for Speed*!

Section	GAMSAT General Chemistry *Need for Speed* Exercises
10.0.1	For the statements below, circle either increase or decrease, and gain or loss. Oxidation is defined as either an (increase / decrease) in oxidation number, or a (gain / loss) of one or more electrons. Reduction is defined as either an (increase / decrease) in oxidation number, or a (gain / loss) of one or more electrons.
	What is the oxidation number of the atoms below? O in O_2: ______________ Fe in Fe^{3+}: ______________ For H in most compounds: ______________ For O in most compounds: ______________ For alkali metals (first column in the periodic table): ______________ For alkaline earth metals (second column in the periodic table): ______________
	$Zn(s) + CuSO_4(aq) \longrightarrow ZnSO_4(aq) + Cu(s)$ Oxid.#: 0, +2, +2, 0 Circle either oxidising or reducing. During the redox reaction above, Cu is reduced while Zn is oxidised. Zn can be referred to as the (oxidising / reducing) agent. Cu is the (oxidising / reducing) agent.
10.1	In the statements below, circle either oxidised or reduced, and circle either oxidising or reducing. The more positive the reduction potential (E°), the more likely the species is to be (oxidised / reduced). Thus, the species would be regarded as a strong (oxidising / reducing) agent.

	Circle the correct statement for the empty field below. (be at equilibrium / occur spontaneously / not occur spontaneously) The more positive the E° value, the more likely the reaction will ____________ as written.
	In the statement below, circle either oxidised or reduced. The oxidising agent is (oxidised / reduced); the reducing agent is (oxidised / reduced).
10.2	In the diagram of an electrochemical (*galvanic*) cell below, the voltmeter is connected to a wire on its left, and a wire on its right. Draw an arrow along the wire on the left, and the wire on the right, to indicate the direction of electron flow. 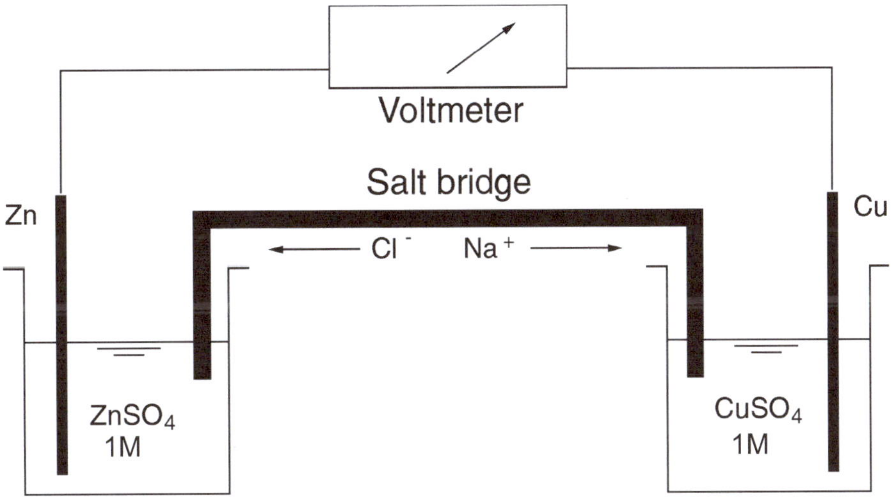 There are 2 beakers in the image above: Identify which one is the cathode compartment, and which one is the anode compartment.
10.4	In the statement below, circle either cations or anions. A cathode is defined as the electrode to which (cations / anions) flow, and an anode is defined as the electrode to which (cations / anions) flow.

10.0.1 Oxidation Numbers, Redox Reactions, Oxidising vs. Reducing Agents

The special class of reactions known as *redox* reactions are better balanced using the concept of oxidation state. In a redox reaction, oxidation and reduction must occur simultaneously. Oxidation is defined as either an increase in oxidation number or a loss of one or more electrons. Reduction is defined as a decrease in oxidation number or a gain of one or more electrons.

To begin with, it is very important to understand the difference between the ionic charge and the oxidation state of an element. Let us consider the two compounds sodium chloride (NaCl) and water (H_2O). NaCl is made up of the charged species or ions: Na^+ and Cl^-. During the formation of this ionic compound, one electron is transferred from the Na atom to the Cl atom. It is possible to verify this fact experimentally and determine that the charge of sodium in NaCl is indeed +1 and that the one for chlorine is −1.

The elements in the periodic table tend to lose (*oxidation*) or gain (*reduction*) electrons to different extents. Therefore, even in non-ionic compounds electrons are always transferred, to different degrees, from one atom to another during the formation of a molecule of the compound. The actual partial charges that result from these partial transfers of electrons can also be determined experimentally. The oxidation state is not equal to such partial charges. It is rather an artificial concept that is used to perform some kind of "electron bookkeeping."

In a molecule like H_2O, since oxygen tends to attract electrons more than hydrogen, one can predict that the electrons that allow bonding to occur between hydrogen and oxygen will be displaced towards the oxygen atom. For the sake of "electron bookkeeping", we assign these electrons to the oxygen atom. The charge that the oxygen atom would have in this artificial process would be −2: this defines the oxidation state of oxygen in the H_2O molecule. In the same line of reasoning, one defines the oxidation state of hydrogen in the water molecule as +1. The actual partial charges of hydrogen and oxygen are in fact smaller; but, as we will see later, the concept of oxidation state is very useful in stoichiometry.

Here are the general rules one needs to follow to assign oxidation numbers (= *oxidation states*) to different elements in different compounds:

1. In elementary substances, the oxidation number of an uncombined element, regardless of whether it is monatomic (1 atom), diatomic (2 atoms) or polyatomic (multiple atoms), is **zero**. This is, for instance, the case for N in N_2 or Na in sodium element, O in O_2, or S in S_8.
2. In monatomic ions, the oxidation number of the element that make up this ion is equal to the charge of the ion. This is the case for Na in Na^+ (+1), or Cl in Cl^- (−1), or Fe in Fe^{3+} (+**3**). Clearly, monatomic ions are the only species for which atomic charges and oxidation numbers coincide.
3. In a neutral molecule, the sum of the oxidation numbers of all the elements that make up the molecule is zero. In a polyatomic ion (e.g. SO_4^{2-}) the sum of the oxidation numbers of the elements that make up this ion is equal to the charge of the ion.

Medium-level Importance

4. Some useful oxidation numbers to memorise:

For H: +**1** in most compounds; except in metal hydrides (general formula: XH where X is from the first two columns of the periodic table; CHM 2.4.1) where it is equal to –1.

For O: –**2** in most compounds. In peroxides (e.g. in H_2O_2) the oxidation number for O is –1, it is +2 in OF_2 and –1/2 in superoxides (e.g. potassium superoxide: KO_2 which contains the O_2^- ion as opposed to the O^{2-} ion).

For alkali metals (first column in the periodic table): +**1**.

For alkaline earth metals (second column): +**2**.

Aluminium usually has an oxidation number of +3 (e.g. chlorides $AlCl_3$, nitrites $Al(NO_2)_3$) and rarely lower (e.g. +2 in AlO, +1 in AlBr).

The oxidation number of each Group VIIA element is –1; however, when it is combined with an element of higher electronegativity, the oxidation number is +1. For example, the oxidation number of Cl is –1 in HCl, and the oxidation number of Cl is +1 in HClO.

An element is said to have been *reduced* during a reaction if its oxidation number decreased during this reaction. It is said to have been oxidised if its *oxidation* number increased. A simple example is:

	Zn(s)	+	$CuSO_4$(aq)	⟶
Oxid.#:	0		+2	
	$ZnSO_4$(aq)	+	Cu(s)	
Oxid.#:	+2		0	

During this reaction Cu(s) is reduced (oxidation number decreases from +2 to 0) while Zn(s) is oxidised (oxidation number increases from 0 to +2). Since, in a sense, Cu is reduced by Zn, Zn can be referred to as the reducing agent. Similarly, Cu is the oxidising agent.

In the next section, we will use oxidation numbers in chemical reactions related to electricity: *electrochemistry* (CHM 10.1). Many of the reduction-oxidation (*redox*) agents in the table below will be explored in GAMSAT Organic Chemistry.

Medium-level Importance

Common Redox Agents

Reducing Agents	Oxidising Agents
* Lithium aluminium hydride ($LiAlH_4$) * Sodium borohydride ($NaBH_4$) * Metals * Ferrous ion (Fe^{2+})	* Iodine (I_2) and other halogens * Permanganate (MnO_4) salts * Peroxide compounds (i.e. H_2O_2) * Ozone (O_3); osmium tetroxide (OsO_4) * Nitric acid (HNO_3); nitrous oxide (N_2O)

10.1 Redox Reactions and Half-cell Potentials

Medium-level Importance

Electrochemistry is based on oxidation-reduction (*redox*) reactions in which one or more electrons are transferred from one ionic species to another. Recall that oxidation is defined as the loss of one or more electrons and reduction is defined as the gain in electron(s). In a redox reaction, reduction and oxidation must occur simultaneously. Before you read this section you should revise the rules that allow the determination of the oxidation state of an element in a polyatomic molecule or ion, and the definition of oxidation and reduction processes. We had previously applied the rules for the determination of oxidation numbers in the case of the following overall reaction (*see* CHM 10.0.1):

$$CuSO_4(aq) + Zn(s) \rightleftharpoons$$
Oxid.#: +2 0
$$Cu(s) + ZnSO_4(aq)$$
Oxid.#: 0 +2

The reduction and oxidation half reactions of the forward process are:

reduction half reaction:
$Cu^{2+}(aq) + 2e^- \rightarrow Cu(s)$

oxidation half reaction:
$Zn(s) \rightarrow Zn^{2+}(aq) + 2e^-$

A half reaction does not occur on its own merit. Any reduction half reaction must be accompanied by an associated oxidation half reaction, or vice versa, as electrons need to be transferred accordingly from one reactant to another. To determine the number and the side on which to put the electrons one follows the simple rules:

(i) The electrons are always on the left-hand side of a reduction half-reaction.

(ii) The electrons are always on the right-hand side of an oxidation half-reaction.

(iii) For a reduction half-reaction:

# of electrons required = initial oxidation # – final oxidation #

(iv) For an oxidation half-reaction:

# of electrons required = final oxidation # – initial oxidation #

The next step is to balance each half-reaction, i.e. the charges and the number of atoms of all the elements involved have to be equal on both sides. The preceding example is very simple since the number of electrons required in the two half-reactions is the same. Consider the following more complicated example:

reduction: $Sn^{2+}(aq) + 2e^- \rightarrow Sn(s)$
oxidation: $Al(s) \rightarrow Al^{3+}(aq) + 3e^-$

To balance the overall reaction (*$6e^-$ on both sides*), you need to multiply the first half reaction by a factor of 3 and the second by a factor of 2 (*thus the electrons can cancel*).

Balancing redox reactions in aqueous solutions may not always be as straightforward as balancing other types of chemical reactions. For redox reactions, both the mass and the charge must be balanced. In addition, when looking at redox reactions occurring in aqueous solutions one must also consider at times if the solution is acidic or basic. The procedure used to balance redox reactions in acidic versus basic solutions is slightly different. Generally, the recommended steps used in balancing redox reactions is as follows and the method used is called the "*half-reaction method of balancing*":

1) Identify all the oxidation states of all elements within the redox reaction.

2) Identify the elements being oxidised and those being reduced.

3) Separate the overall redox reaction into its corresponding oxidation and reduction half reactions.

4) Balance all elements for each half reaction excluding hydrogen and oxygen.

5) Balance oxygen by the addition of water to the side missing the oxygen and balance the oxygen atoms by adding the appropriate coefficients in front of water.

6) Balance hydrogen by the addition of H^+ ion to the side missing the hydrogen atoms until hydrogen is balanced with the appropriate coefficients added. Note that the difference in balancing redox reactions in acidic versus basic aqueous solutions is at this step. In basic solutions, an additional step is required to neutralise the H^+ ions with the addition of OH^- ions so that both may then combine to form water.

7) Balance the half reactions with respect to charge by the addition of electrons on the appropriate side.

8) Balance the number of electrons for each half reaction by multiplying each of the half reactions (*if required*) with the appropriate coefficient.

9) Add the two half reactions making sure that all electrons are cancelled.

10) Finally, as a check: you should always verify that all elements and charges are balanced on both sides of the overall reaction and that the final overall reaction *never contains any free electrons.*

Example: In acidic solution, balance the following redox reaction:

$Fe^{2+}(aq) + MnO_4^-(aq) \rightarrow Fe^{3+}(aq) + Mn^{2+}(aq)$

Step 1: +2   +7 −2   +3   +2

Step 2: Fe is oxidised (+2 to +3)
Mn in MnO_4^- is reduced to Mn^{2+}
(+7 to +2, oxygen will be balanced with water)

Step 3: Oxidation: $Fe^{2+}(aq) \rightarrow Fe^{3+}(aq)$
Reduction: $MnO_4^-(aq) \rightarrow Mn^{2+}(aq)$

Step 4, 5 and 6: Oxidation: $Fe^{2+}(aq) \rightarrow Fe^{3+}(aq)$
Reduction: $8H^+(aq) + MnO_4^-(aq) \rightarrow Mn^{2+}(aq) + 4H_2O(l)$

Step 7: Oxidation: $Fe^{2+}(aq) \rightarrow Fe^{3+}(aq) + 1e^-$
Reduction: $5e^- + 8H^+(aq) + MnO_4^-(aq) \rightarrow Mn^{2+}(aq) + 4H_2O(l)$

Step 8: Oxidation: $5[Fe^{2+}(aq) \rightarrow Fe^{3+}(aq) + 1e^-]$
$5Fe^{2+}(aq) \rightarrow 5Fe^{3+}(aq) + 5e^-$
Reduction: $5e^- + 8H^+(aq) + MnO_4^-(aq) \rightarrow Mn^{2+}(aq) + 4H_2O(l)$

Step 9: Overall: $5Fe^{2+}(aq) + 8H^+(aq) + MnO_4^-(aq) \rightarrow 5Fe^{3+}(aq) + Mn^{2+}(aq) + 4H_2O(l)$

Step 10: Check if all is balanced.

The oxidation/reduction capabilities of substances are measured by their standard reduction half-reaction potentials E°(V). The reduction potential E°(V) is a measure of the tendency of a chemical species to acquire electrons and thereby be reduced. The more positive the reduction potential, the more likely the species is to be reduced. Thus, the species would be regarded as a strong oxidising agent. These potentials are relative. The reference half-cell electrode chosen to measure the relative potential of all other half cells is known as the **s**tandard **h**ydrogen **e**lectrode, or SHE, and it corresponds to the following half reaction:

$$2H^+(1\text{ molar}) + 2e^- \rightarrow H_2(1\text{ atm}) \quad E^\circ = 0.00\ (V).$$

As the reference SHE cell potential is defined as 0.00 V, any half-cell system that accepts electrons from a SHE cell is reduced and therefore defined by a positive redox potential. Alternatively, any half-cell that donates electrons to a SHE cell is defined by a negative redox potential. Thus, the larger the reduction potential value of a half-cell, the greater the tendency for that half-cell to gain electrons and become reduced.

Standard half-cell potentials for other half-reactions have been tabulated and you will see examples to follow, and more in the practice questions at the end of this chapter. They are defined for standard conditions, i.e., concentration of all ionic species equal to 1 molar and pressure of all gases involved, if any, equal to 1 atm. The standard temperature is taken as 25 °C. In the case of the Cu^{2+}/Zn reaction the relevant data is tabulated as reduction potentials as follows:

$$Zn^{2+}(aq) + 2e^- \rightarrow Zn(s) \quad E^\circ = -0.76\text{ volts}$$
$$Cu^{2+}(aq) + 2e^- \rightarrow Cu(s) \quad E^\circ = +0.34\text{ volts}$$

As shown, it can be seen that the Cu/Cu^{2+} electrode is positive relative to the SHE and that the Zn/Zn^{2+} is negative relative to the SHE. The more positive the E° value, the more likely the reaction will occur spontaneously as written. The strongest reducing agents have large negative E° values. The strongest oxidising agents have large positive E° values. Therefore, in our example Cu^{2+} is a stronger oxidising agent than Zn^{2+}. This conclusion can be expressed in the following practical terms:

(i) If you put Zn in contact with a solution containing Cu^{2+} ions a spontaneous redox reaction will occur.

$$Zn(s) \rightarrow Zn^{2+}(aq) + 2e^-; \quad E^\circ(V) = +0.76$$
$$Cu^{2+}(aq) + 2e^- \rightarrow Cu(s); \quad E^\circ(V) = +0.34$$
$$E^\circ_{cell} = E^\circ_{red} + E^\circ_{ox} = +0.34 + 0.76 = +\ 1.10\text{ V.}$$

(ii) If you put Cu directly in contact with a solution containing Zn^{2+} ions, no reaction takes place spontaneously.

$$Cu(s) \rightarrow Cu^{2+}(aq) + 2e^-; \quad E^\circ(V) = -0.34$$
$$Zn^{2+}(aq) + 2e^- \rightarrow Zn(s); \ E^\circ(V) = -0.76$$
$$E^\circ_{cell} = E^\circ_{red} + E^\circ_{ox} = -0.76 + (-0.34) = -\ 1.10\text{ V.}$$

Thus for the spontaneous reaction:

(1) $E^\circ = E^\circ_{red} - E^\circ_{ox}$
$= +0.34 - (-0.76) = 1.10$ V

(2) $E^\circ_{cell} = E^\circ_{red} + E^\circ_{ox}$
$= +0.34 + 0.76 = 1.10$ V.

The positive value confirms the spontaneous nature of the reaction. {The theme of many exam questions: the oxidising agent is *reduced*; the reducing agent is *oxidised*}

For a cell potential (E°) calculation, if one is to calculate it using the formula (1), then use the tabulated reduction potentials for both half-cell reduction reactions. Alternatively, if one were to calculate the cell potential using the second formula (2), the half-cell potential that has the lower potential value, or the oxidised half cell (*more negative value*), needs to be reversed to have it in an oxidised format, and therefore the electromotive (E°) potential sign itself is also inverted accordingly, and the sum of the two half cells is then calculated. Also, note that the stoichiometric factors are not used if one is simply calculating the E° of the cell (*because the concentrations are, of course, standard at 1 M*).

10.2 Galvanic Cells

As a result of a redox reaction, one may harvest a substantial amount of energy, and the energy generated is usually carried out in what is known as an *electrochemical cell*. There are two types of electrochemical cells: a galvanic (or *voltaic*) cell, and an electrolytic cell. A galvanic cell produces electrical energy from a spontaneous chemical reaction that takes place within an electrochemical cell. On the other hand, an electrolytic cell induces a nonspontaneous chemical reaction within an electrochemical cell by the consumption of electrical energy.

Batteries are self-contained galvanic cells (e.g. the batteries that power flashlights, or help cars to start). A galvanic cell uses a spontaneous redox reaction to produce electricity. For instance, one can design a galvanic cell based on the spontaneous reaction:

$$Zn(s) + CuSO_4(aq) \rightarrow Cu(s) + ZnSO_4(aq)$$

An actual view of a galvanic cell is depicted in Figure III.A.10.1a. In addition, Figure III.A.10.1b shows a sketch of a line diagram of the same galvanic cell outlining all the different parts. Note that in Figure III.A.10.1b, Zn is not in direct contact with the Cu^{2+} solution; otherwise, electrons will be directly transferred from Zn to Cu^{2+} and no electricity will be produced to an external circuit.

The half reaction occurring in the left-hand (*anode*) compartment is the oxidation:

$$Zn(s) \rightarrow Zn^{2+}(aq) + 2e^-$$

The half reaction occurring in the right-hand (*cathode*) compartment is the reduction:

$$Cu^{2+}(aq) + 2e^- \rightarrow Cu(s)$$

Therefore, electrons flow out of the compartment where the oxidation occurs to the compartment where the reduction takes place.

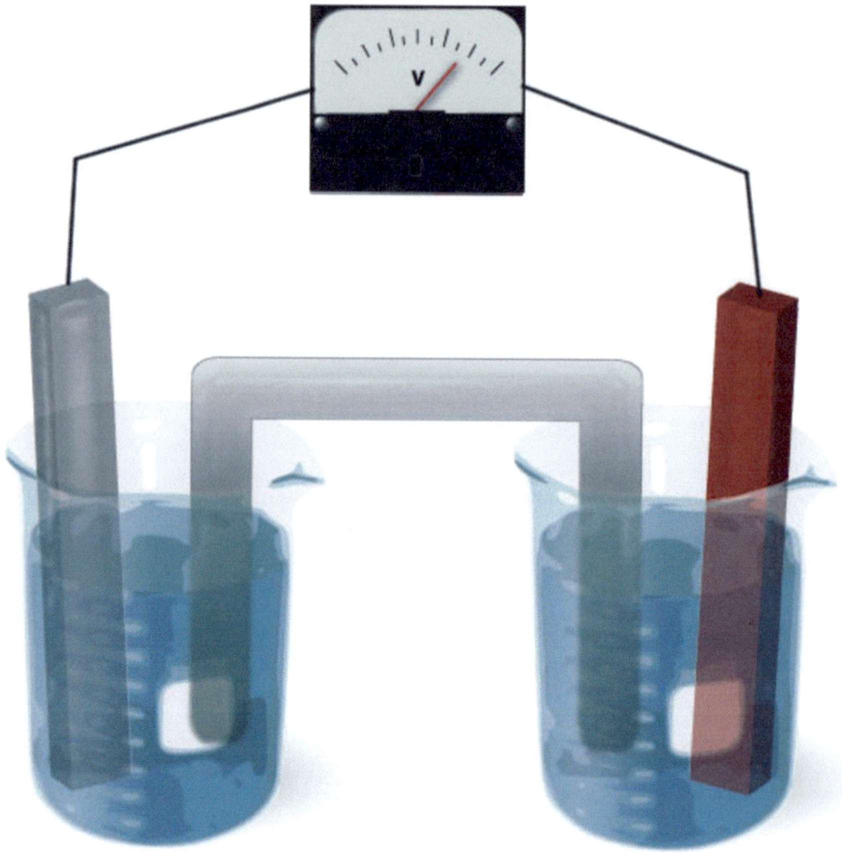

Figure III.A.10.1a: A galvanic (electrochemical) cell. As shown by the displacement in voltage via the voltmeter, the energy of a spontaneous redox reaction is essentially captured within the galvanic cell. A galvanic cell consists mainly of the following parts: **1)** Two separate half cells; **2)** Two solid element electrodes with differing redox potentials; **3)** Two opposing aqueous solutions each in contact with opposing solid electrodes; **4)** One salt bridge with an embedded salt solution; **5)** One ammeter or voltmeter and; **6)** An electrical solid element or wire to allow conductivity of electrons from anode to cathode. Note: The glass containers (*beakers*) are common in labs.

The metallic parts (Cu(*s*) and Zn(*s*) in our example) of the galvanic cell which allow its connection to an external circuit are called electrodes. The electrode out of which electrons flow is the anode; the electrode receiving these electrons is the cathode. In a galvanic cell the oxidation occurs in the anodic compartment and the reduction in the cathodic compartment. The voltage difference between the two electrodes is called the electromotive force (*emf*) of the cell. The voltage is measured by the voltmeter.

All of the participants belonging to each of the half cells are included within their respective half cell. Consequently, one half of the electrochemical cell consists of an appropriate metal (Zn) immersed within a solution containing the ionic form of the same metal ($ZnSO_4$). The other half then contains the

Medium-level Importance

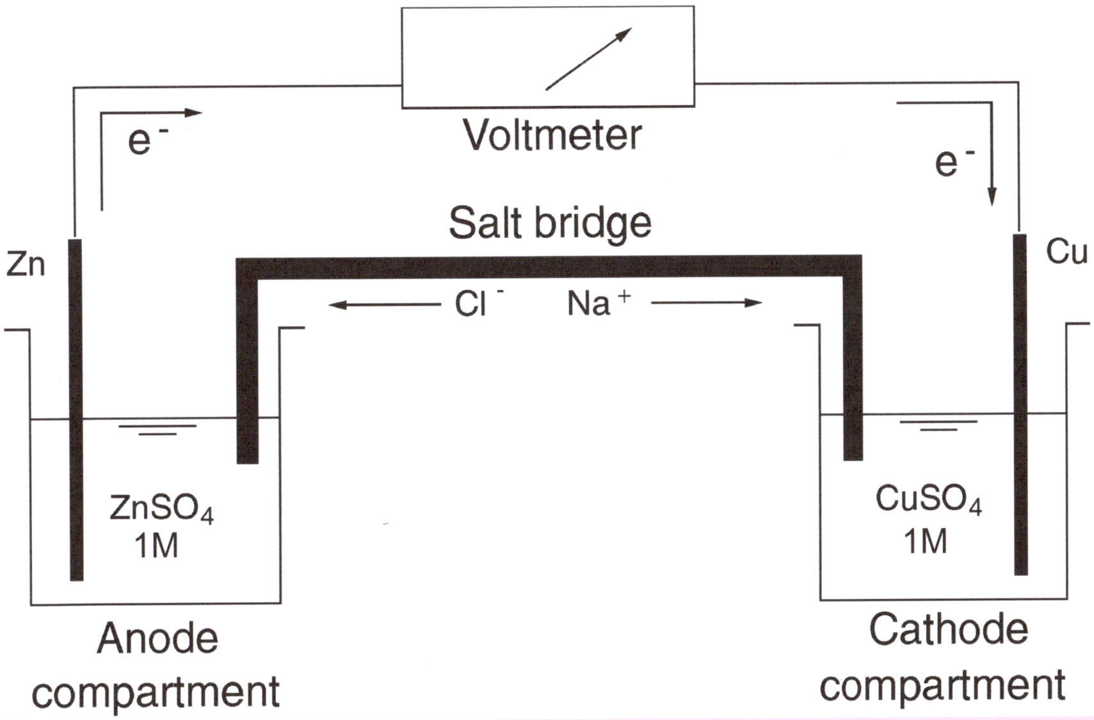

Figure III.A.10.1b: Line diagram of a galvanic (electrochemical) cell. Notice that the direction of movement of the ions from NaCl in the salt bridge indicates the nature of the two compartments, as well as the direction of electron flow. Cations (Na^+) are attracted to the cathode; anions (Cl^-) to the anode. The anions are part of a circuit (PHY 10.1-10.3): Electrons move negative charge through the wire and Cl^- carries the negative charge through the salt bridge completing the circuit (*circular route of negative charges*).

complementary metal (Cu) immersed into an aqueous solution consisting of its metal ion ($CuSO_4$) (Figure III.A.10.1b).

In certain cells, however, the participants involved in the reduction half reaction may all be part of the aqueous solution; in such a case, an inert electrode would replace the respective metal electrode. The inert electrode such as graphite or platinum would act as a conductive surface for electron transfer. An example of such a half-cell would be one where the reduction of manganese (Mn^{7+}) as MnO_4^- occurs in a solution which also contains manganese as ions (Mn^{2+}). To complete the electrochemical circuit, the two half-cells are then connected with a conducting wire which provides a means for electron flow. Electrons always flow from the anode (*oxidation half-cell*) to the cathode (*reduction half-cell*). The electrical energy from the flow of electrons may then be harvested and transformed into some alternative form of energy or mechanical work (*as required*). In order to prevent an excessive charge build up within each of the half-cell solutions as a result of oxidation and reduction reactions at the anode and cathode, a salt bridge is constructed and used to connect both half-cell solutions.

Mnemonic: LEO is A GERC
- Lose Electrons Oxidation is Anode
- Gain Electrons Reduction at Cathode

{A little less informative, but still helpful: LEO, the lion, says GER: Lose Electrons: Oxidation; Gain Electrons: Reduction.}

Electrochemical cells are usually represented as a cell diagram or a compact notation denoting all the parts of the cell. For example, the cell diagram of the cell that was previously discussed in which Zn is oxidised and Cu reduced would be represented as follows:

$$Zn(s) \mid Zn^{2+}(aq) \parallel Cu^{2+}(aq) \mid Cu(s).$$

The oxidation half reaction is on the left and the reduction half reaction is on the right side of the cell diagram. The single vertical lines represent the substances of each half-cell in different phases (solid and aqueous), and the double vertical line represents the salt bridge.

Medium-level Importance

10.2.1 The Salt Bridge

A salt bridge is a U-shaped tube (*see* Figure III.A.10.1b) with a strong electrolyte (CHM 5.3.2) suspended in a gel allowing the flow of the ions into the half-cell solutions. The salt bridge connects the two compartments chemically (for example, with Na^+ and Cl^-). It has two important functions:

1) Maintenance of Neutrality: As Zn(*s*) becomes Zn^{2+}(*aq*), the net charge in the anode compartment becomes positive. To maintain neutrality, Cl^- ions migrate to the anode compartment. The reverse occurs in the cathode compartment: positive ions are lost (Cu^{2+}), therefore positive ions must be gained (Na^+).

2) Completing the Circuit: Imagine the galvanic cell as a circuit (GAMSAT Physics Chapter 10). Negative charge leaves the anode compartment via *electrons* in a wire and then returns via *chemicals* (i.e. Cl^-) in the salt bridge. Thus the galvanic cell is an *electrochemical* cell.

As an alternative to a salt bridge, the solutions (i.e. $ZnSO_4$ and $CuSO_4$) can be placed in one container separated by a *porous* material which allows certain ions to cross (i.e. SO_4^{2-}, Zn^{2+}). Thus it would serve the same functions as the salt bridge.

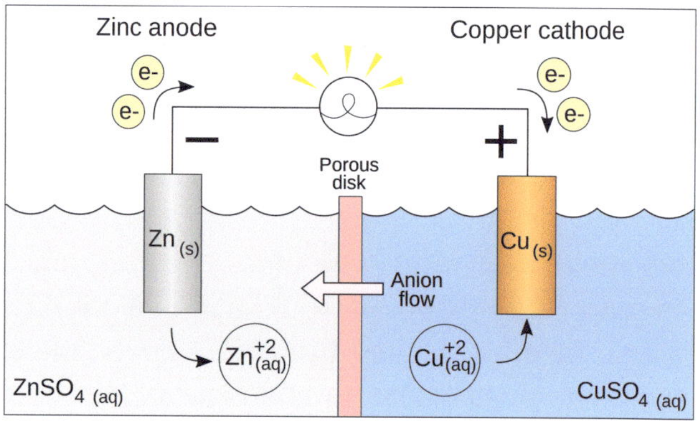

Figure III.A.10.2: Galvanic cell with porous material. (ref: α)

10.3 Concentration Cell

If the concentration of the ions in one of the compartments of a galvanic cell is not 1 molar, the half-cell potential E is either higher or lower than E°. Therefore, in principle, one could use the same substance in both compartments but with different concentrations to produce electricity.

Thus, one may construct a galvanic cell in which both half-cell reactions are the same, however, the difference in concentration is the driving force for the flow of current. The emf is equal in this case to the difference between the two potentials E. Such a cell is called a concentration cell.

To determine the direction of electron flow, the same rules as previously described are used. The cathodic compartment, in which the reduction takes place is the one corresponding to the largest positive (*smallest negative*) E.

The electromotive force varies with the differences in concentration of solutions in the half cells. When the concentration of solution is not equal to 1M, the emf (or E_{cell}) can be determined by the use of the Nernst equation as follows:

$$E_{cell} = E^{\circ}_{cell} - (RT/nF)(\ln Q)$$

or

$$E_{cell} = E^{\circ}_{cell} - 0.0592V/n\ (\log Q)$$

where; E°_{cell} is the standard electromotive force, R is the gas constant 8.314 J/Kmol, T is the absolute temperature in K, F is the Faraday's constant (CHM 10.5), n is the number of moles of electrons exchanged or transferred in the redox reaction, and Q is the reaction quotient (CHM 9.8.1).

Under standard conditions, Q = 1.00 as all concentrations are at 1.00 M and since log 1 = 0, $E_{cell} = E^{\circ}_{cell}$. {*GAMSAT Biology, and in this chapter's GAMSAT-level practice questions (General Chemistry Chapter 10), you will get to practice using the Nernst equation.*}

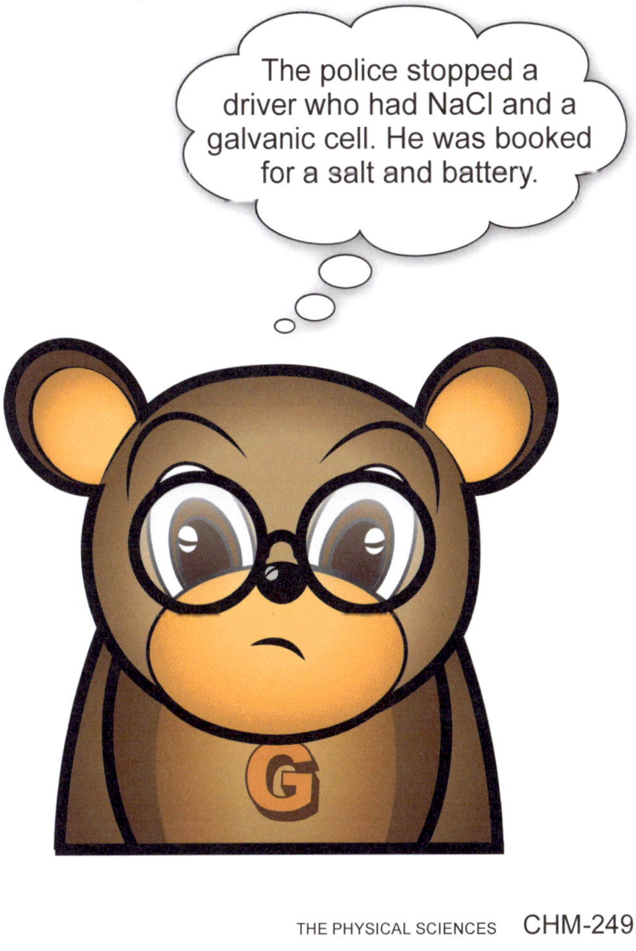

Medium-level Importance

10.4 Electrolytic Cell

There is a fundamental difference between a galvanic cell, or a concentration cell, and an electrolytic cell: in the first type of electrochemical cell, a spontaneous redox reaction is used to produce a current, in the second type, a current is actually imposed on the system to drive a non-spontaneous redox reaction. A cathode is defined as the electrode to which cations flow to, and an anode is defined as the electrode to which anions flow. Thus, a similarity between the two cells is that the cathode attracts cations, whereas the anode attracts anions. In both the galvanic cell and the electrolytic cell, reduction occurs always at the cathode and oxidation always occurs at the anode.

Remember the following key concepts:

(i) generally a battery is used to produce a current which is imposed on the electrolytic cell.

(ii) the battery acts as an electron pump: electrons flow into the electrolytic cell at the cathode and flow out of it at the anode.

(iii) the half reaction occurring at the cathode is a reduction since it requires electrons.

(iv) the half reaction occurring at the anode is an oxidation since it produces electrons.

In galvanic cells, a spontaneous oxidation reaction takes place at the cell's anode creating a source of electrons. For this reason, the anode is considered the negative electrode. However, in electrolytic cells, a non-spontaneous reduction reaction takes place at the cell's cathode using an external electrical energy as the source of electrons such as a battery. For this reason, the cathode is considered the negative electrode.

An electrolytic cell is composed of three parts: an electrolyte solution and two electrodes made from an inert material (i.e. platinum). The oxidation and reduction half reactions are usually placed in one container.

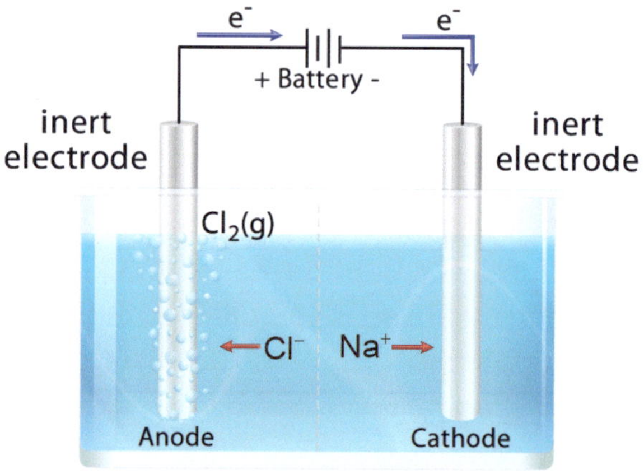

Figure III.A.10.3: Electrolytic cell.

The diagram is a depiction of the electrolysis of molten NaCl. As such, the Na^+ and Cl^- ions are the only species that are present in the electrolytic cell. Thus, the chloride anion (Cl^-) cannot be reduced any further and so it is oxidised at the anode, and the sodium cation (Na^+) is therefore reduced. The final products are sodium solid formation at the cathode, and chlorine (Cl_2) gas formation at the anode.

Note: the flow of electrons is still from anode to cathode as it is for galvanic cells.

Examples – The most common electrolytic cells are found in rechargeable batteries (*mobile phones, MP3's, etc.*), or electroplating (*adding gold or silver to a base metal to make jewelry*). When a rechargeable battery is being used in your mobile phone, it works like a galvanic cell since it uses redox energy to produce electricity. However, when the battery is charging, it works like an electrolytic cell since it uses outside electricity to reverse the completed redox reaction.

10.5 Faraday's Law

Faraday's law relates the amount of elements deposited or gas liberated at an electrode due to current (PHY 9.1, 10.1).

We have seen that in a galvanic cell, $Cu^{2+}(aq)$ can accept electrons to become Cu(*s*) which will actually plate onto the electrode. Faraday's law allows us to calculate the amount of Cu(*s*). In fact, the law states that the weight of product formed at an electrode is proportional to the amount of electricity transferred at the electrode and to the equivalent weight of the material.

Thus, we can conclude that 1 mole of $Cu^{2+}(aq)$ + 2 moles of electrons will leave 1 mole of Cu(*s*) at the electrode. One mole (= Avogadro's number; CHM 1.3) of electrons is called a *faraday* ($\mathfrak{F}$). A faraday is equivalent to 96 500 coulombs. A coulomb (GM 2.1.3; PHY 9.1, 10.1) is the amount of electricity that is transferred when a current of one ampere flows for one second (1C = 1A · s).

Medium-level Importance

10.5.1 Electrolysis Problem

How many grams of copper would be deposited on the cathode of an electrolytic cell if, for a period of 20 minutes, a current of 2.0 amperes is run through a solution of $CuSO_4$? {The molecular weight of copper is 63.5.}

Calculate the number of coulombs:

$$Q = It = 2.0\ A \times 20\ min \times 60\ sec/min = 2400\ C$$

Thus

$$\text{Faradays} = 2400\ C \times 1\mathfrak{F}/96\ 500\ C = 0.025\mathfrak{F}$$

Faradays can be related to moles of copper since

$$Cu^{2+} + 2e^- \rightarrow Cu$$

Since 1 mol Cu: 2 mol e^- we can write

$$0.025\mathfrak{F} \times (1\ mol\ Cu/2\mathfrak{F}) \times (63.5\ g\ Cu/mol\ Cu) = 0.79\ g\ Cu$$

Electrolysis would deposit 0.79 g of copper at the cathode.

To do the previous problem, you must know the definition of current and charge (CHM 10.5) but the value of the constant (a Faraday) would be given on the exam. You should be able to perform the preceding calculation efficiently as it involves dimensional analysis (GM 2.2); another awaits you in the GAMSAT-level practice questions.

10.6 Redox Titrations

Redox titrations are based on a redox reaction or reduction-oxidation reaction between an analyte (or sample) and a titrant. More specifically, redox titrations involve the reaction between an oxidising agent, which accepts one or more electrons, and a reducing agent, which reduces the other substance by donating one or more electrons.

The most useful oxidising agent for titrations is potassium permanganate - $KMnO_4$. Solutions of this salt are colourful since they contain the purple MnO_4^- ion. On the other hand, the more reduced form, Mn^{++}, is nearly colourless. So here is how this redox titration works: $KMnO_4$ is added to a reaction mixture with a reducing agent (i.e. Fe^{++}). MnO_4^- is quickly reduced to Mn^{++} so the colour fades immediately. This will continue until there is no more reducing agent in the mixture. When the last bit of reducing agent has been oxidised (i.e. all the Fe^{++} is converted to Fe^{+3}), the next drop of $KMnO_4$ will make the solution colourful since the MnO_4^- will have nothing with which to react. Thus if the amount of reducing agent was unknown, it can be calculated using stoichiometry guided by the amount of potassium permanganate used in the reaction.

CHAPTER 10: Electrochemistry

GOLD STANDARD FOUNDATIONAL GAMSAT PRACTICE QUESTIONS

Note: Often, but not always, ACER will provide the rules for assigning oxidation numbers, when needed. You can choose to look at the very basic rules below while completing practice questions, or you can cover the rules with Post-it notes!

Some of the rules for assigning oxidation numbers:

1. The oxidation number of an element in its free (uncombined) state is zero — for example, Cr(s) or Ag(s).
2. The oxidation number of a monatomic (1-atom) ion is the same as the charge on the ion.
3. The sum of all oxidation numbers in a neutral compound is zero. The sum of all oxidation numbers in a polyatomic (many-atom) ion is equal to the charge on the ion.
4. The oxidation number of oxygen in a compound can be taken as –2.
5. The oxidation state of hydrogen in a compound can be taken as +1.
6. The oxidation number of a Group IA element in a compound is +1 — for example, Na or K.
7. The oxidation number of a Group IIA element in a compound is +2 — for example, Mg or Ca.

Medium-level Importance

1) What is the oxidation number (*state*) of carbon in $NaHCO_3$?

A. 0
B. –4
C. +4
D. +6

2) What is the oxidation state of chromium in $Cr_2O_7^{2-}$?

A. 6
B. 7
C. 8
D. 12

3) What is the oxidation state of the halogen (Hal) in the halate ($HalO_3^-$) molecule?

A. –1
B. –5
C. 1
D. 5

4) What is the oxidation state of nitrogen in each of the two products in the following reaction, respectively?

$$H_2O + 3NO_2(g) \rightarrow 2HNO_3(aq) + NO(g)$$

A. +5, +2
B. –5, +2
C. –2, +2
D. +2, +2

5) What type of reaction is the following?

$$2MnO_4^- + 16H^+ + 10Cl^- \rightarrow 2Mn^{2+} + 5Cl_2(g) + 8H_2O$$

A. Combustion
B. Double replacement
C. Oxidation-reduction
D. Precipitation

High-level Importance

GOLD STANDARD GAMSAT-LEVEL PRACTICE QUESTIONS

Questions 6–9

In chemistry, a Pourbaix diagram, also known as a potential/pH diagram, maps out possible stable (equilibrium) phases of an aqueous electrochemical system. Predominant ion boundaries are represented by lines. The lines in the Pourbaix diagram show the equilibrium conditions, that is, where the activities are equal, for the species on each side of that line. On either side of the line, one form of the species will instead be said to be predominant.

Consider Figure 1.

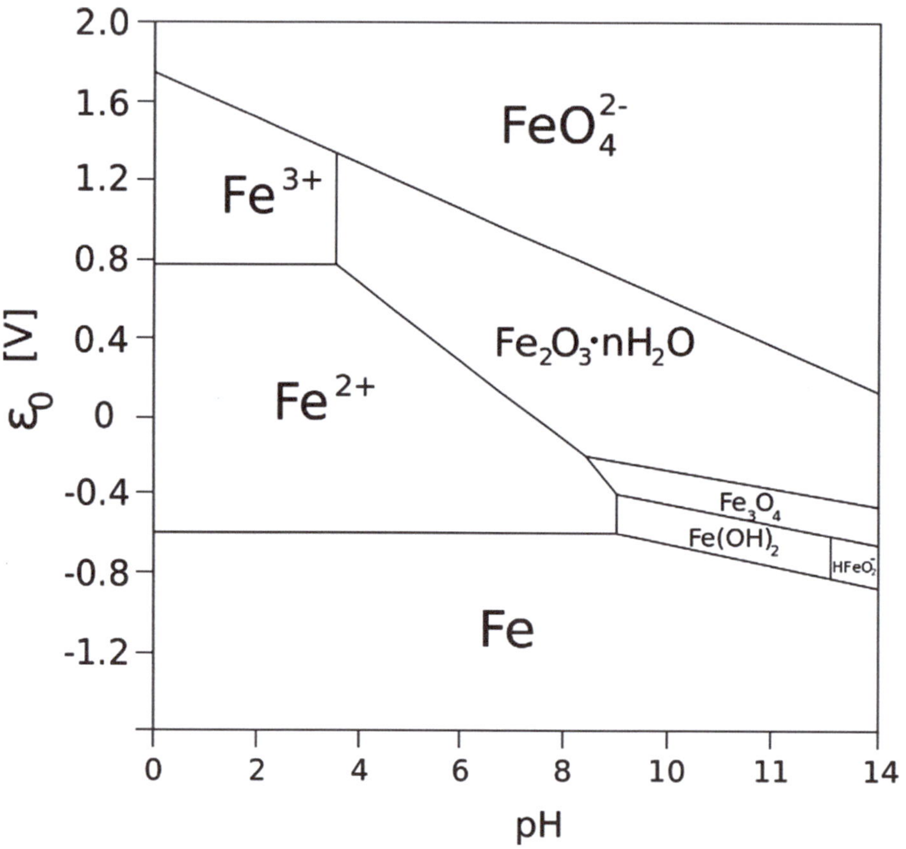

Figure 1: Pourbaix diagram for iron.
Modified from Andel Früh, University of Bath & Western Oregon University

Note that:

- All ionic forms of iron can be considered to be soluble and the non-ionic Fe is solid.
- A reducing agent is a substance that tends to bring about reduction by being oxidised and losing electrons, an oxidising agent is the opposite.

Rules for assigning oxidation numbers for this unit:

1. The oxidation number of an element in its free (uncombined) state is zero — for example, Al(s) or Zn(s).
2. The oxidation number of a monatomic (1-atom) ion is the same as the charge on the ion.
3. The sum of all oxidation numbers in a neutral compound is zero. The sum of all oxidation numbers in a polyatomic (many-atom) ion is equal to the charge on the ion.
4. The oxidation number of oxygen in a compound can be taken as –2.
5. The oxidation state of hydrogen in a compound can be taken as +1.

6) Which of the following statements is consistent with Figure 1?

A. The presence of solid iron increases across electric potential as the hydrogen ion concentration becomes lower.

B. At a potential of –0.4 V, as pH increases Fe^{2+} is reduced and may precipitate out as Fe_2O_3.

C. At pH of 1, as the potential changes from 0 to +1.0 V, Fe^{3+} is reduced to Fe^{2+}.

D. At a potential of –0.6 V, the equilibrium between solid iron and Fe^{2+} is independent of solution pH below a pH of 9.

7) Which of the following is the most oxidised form of iron?

A. Fe^{3+}

B. FeO_4^{-2}

C. Fe_3O_4

D. $Fe(OH)_2$

8) Which of the following would be the strongest oxidising agent?

A. Fe

B. Fe^{2+}

C. Fe^{3+}

D. $HFeO_2^-$

9) In electrochemistry, the Nernst Equation relates the reduction potential of an electrochemical reaction (half-cell or full-cell reaction) to the standard electrode potential, temperature, and activities (often approximated by concentrations) of the chemical species undergoing reduction and oxidation. It is the most important equation in the field of electrochemistry. At 25 °C, the Nernst equation can be simplified to the following equation:

$$(\varepsilon_0) = (0.06/z)\log_{10}K_{eq}$$

where z represents the number of electrons transferred in the reaction. What is K_{eq} for the following equilibrium at pH = 2?

$$Fe^{2+} + 2e^- \rightleftharpoons Fe$$

A. 10^{-20}

B. 10^{-10}

C. –20

D. –10

High-level Importance

Questions 10–12

An Ellingham diagram is a plot of the standard change in Gibbs free energy (ΔG^{o}) versus temperature. Reduction-oxidation (*redox*) reactions can be viewed from a thermodynamic perspective. Changes in enthalpy (ΔH) and entropy (ΔS) are the two driving factors that determine whether a reaction is spontaneous or not. Gibbs free energy (ΔG) combines both of these two factors as follows:

$$\Delta G = \Delta H - T\Delta S$$

where T is the temperature in kelvin (K).

Since ΔH and ΔS are essentially constant with temperature, unless a phase change occurs, the free energy versus temperature plot can be drawn as a series of straight lines. The slope of the line changes when any of the materials involved melt or vaporise.

The Ellingham diagram shown in Figure 1 is for metals reacting to form oxides. The oxygen partial pressure is taken as 1 atmosphere, and all of the reactions are normalised to consume one mole of O_2.

The position of the line for a given reaction in Figure 1 shows the stability of the oxide as a function of temperature. Reactions closer to the top of the diagram are the most "noble" metals (for example, gold and platinum), and their oxides are unstable and easily reduced. As we move down toward the bottom of the diagram, the metals become progressively more reactive and their oxides become harder to reduce.

A given metal can reduce the oxides of all other metals whose lines lie above theirs on the diagram. For example, the $2Mg + O_2 = 2MgO$ line lies below the $Ti + O_2 = TiO_2$ line, and so magnesium can reduce titanium oxide to metallic titanium; in other words, magnesium leads to the decomposition of titanium oxide.

When not coupled with another reaction that can drive the decomposition of an oxide, the decomposition temperature is the temperature at which the standard free energy of formation of the oxide just becomes positive.

Consider Figure 1.

10) The melting point for zinc (Zn) is approximately 400 °C, which can be identified in Figure 1 related to the following equation:

$$2Zn + O_2 = 2ZnO$$

Based on Figure 1, approximate the decomposition temperature for ZnO?

A. 400 °C
B. 900 °C
C. 1600 °C
D. 2000 °C

11) Which of the following statements is **not** consistent with the data presented in Figure 1?

A. The slope of each line with a positive slope is given by the absolute value of ΔS.
B. The melting points of metals are greater than that of their oxides.
C. Nickel(II) oxide (NiO) can be reduced by hydrogen at 1500 °C.
D. Carbon cannot reduce chromium(III) oxide (Cr_2O_3) at 1000 °C.

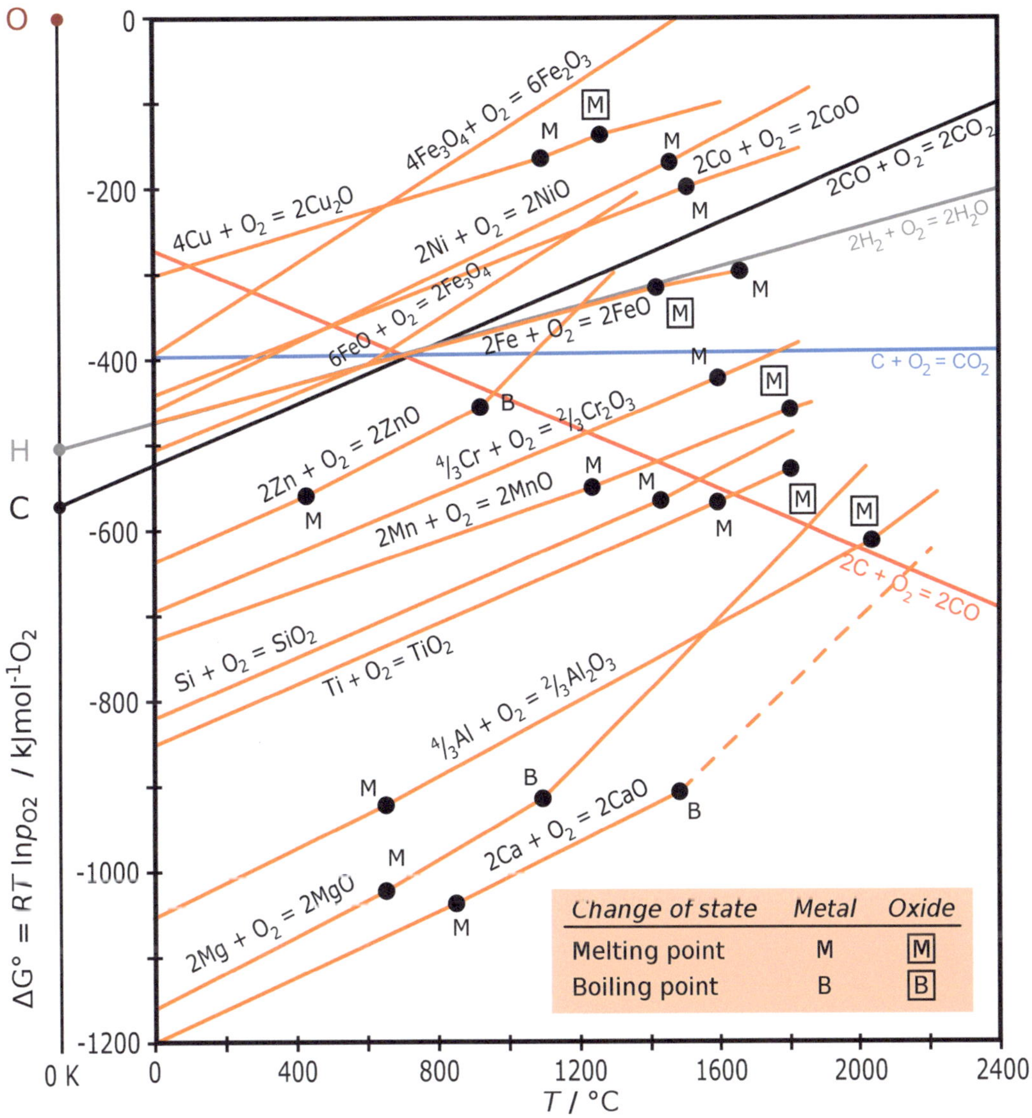

Figure 1: Ellingham diagram for several metals revealing the free energy of formation of metal oxides. (ref: β)

12) The black line for the oxidation of CO to produce CO_2 has a point of intersection C with a vertical line on the left of Figure 1. Based on the information provided, which of the following most accurately indicates that which would be predicted from the magnitude at point C in kJ/mol?

A. The equilibrium constant for the oxidation reaction

B. The approximate value of the standard entropy change

C. The approximate value of the standard enthalpy change

D. Neither **A**, nor **B**, nor **C** is correct

High-level Importance

Questions 13–17

Reduction potentials (also referred to as *redox potentials*) reveal the tendency of a chemical species to acquire electrons and thus be reduced. Each species has its own intrinsic redox potential; the more positive the potential, the greater the species' affinity for electrons and tendency to be reduced.

A reduction potential is measured in volts (V). Because the true or absolute potentials are difficult to accurately measure, reduction potentials are defined relative to the standard hydrogen electrode (SHE) which is arbitrarily given a potential of 0.00 volts. Standard reduction potential is measured under standard conditions: 25 °C, a 1M concentration for each ion participating in the reaction, a partial pressure of 1 atm for each gas that is part of the reaction, and metals in their pure state.

Half-reactions	Standard reduction potential (E°)
F_2 (g) + $2e^- \rightleftharpoons 2F^-$	2.87 V
Cl_2 (g) + $2e^- \rightleftharpoons 2Cl^-$	1.36 V
Br_2 (aq) + $2e^- \rightleftharpoons 2Br^-$	1.09 V
$Ag^+ + e^- \rightleftharpoons$ Ag (s)	0.80 V
$Fe^{3+} + e^- \rightleftharpoons Fe^{2+}$	0.77 V
$Cu^{2+} + 2e^- \rightleftharpoons$ Cu (s)	0.34 V
$2H^+ + 2e^- \rightleftharpoons H_2$(g)	0.00 V
$Pb^{2+} + 2e^- \rightleftharpoons$ Pb (s)	–0.13 V
$Ni^{2+} + 2e^- \rightleftharpoons$ Ni (s)	–0.41 V
$Zn^{2+} + 2e^- \rightleftharpoons$ Zn (s)	–0.76 V
$Na^+ + e^- \rightleftharpoons$ Na (s)	–2.71 V

Table 1: Standard State Reduction Potentials. Ions are in aqueous form.

13) What should happen when a piece of copper is placed in 1M HCl?

A. The copper is completely dissolved by the acid.
B. The copper is dissolved by the acid with the release of hydrogen gas.
C. The copper bursts into greenish flames.
D. Nothing happens.

14) What should happen when a piece of lead is placed in 1M HCl?

A. The lead is completely dissolved by the acid.
B. The lead begins to dissolve with the release of hydrogen gas.
C. The lead bursts into flames.
D. Nothing happens.

15) If standard state oxidation potentials are used instead of standard state reduction potentials and the half reactions are listed in descending order according to their standard state oxidation potentials, which one of the following would be true?

A. The lead reaction would be above the silver reaction.
B. The fluorine reaction would be above the chlorine reaction.
C. The iron reaction would be above the nickel reaction.
D. The hydrogen reaction would be below the copper reaction.

16) According to Table 1, which of the following species is the strongest reducing agent?

A. Fe^{3+}
B. Fe^{2+}
C. Zn^{2+}
D. Zn (s)

17) Only considering the standard half-cell reactions of the species listed in Table 1, how many different voltaic cells with a voltage greater than 2V can be made?

A. Fewer than 7
B. 7
C. 15
D. More than 15

---

18) Assume that the standard reduction potential for the reaction

$$A^{2+} + e^- \rightarrow A^+$$

is E^o_A, and the standard reduction potential for the reaction

$$B^+ + e^- \rightarrow B(s)$$

is E^o_B.

A solution initially containing 1.0 M A^{2+}, 1.0 M A^+ and 1.0 M B^+ is agitated with excess solid B metal. After equilibrium is reached, the solution contains 0.8 M of A^{2+}, 1.2 M of A^+ and 1.2 M of B^+. Which of the following is most consistent with the data as presented?

A. $E^o_A + E^o_B = 0$
B. $E^o_A < E^o_B$
C. $E^o_A > E^o_B$
D. $E^o_A = E^o_B$

19) A sample of solid iron was placed in a beaker of water and exposed to the atmosphere for one hour. After this, the solid iron that remained was removed from the beaker and a current of 0.2 A passed through the beaker which contained only Fe^{2+} in solution. After one hour and twenty minutes, all the iron present had been deposited on the cathode. Given that the Faraday constant F = 96000 C, what was the rate of rusting in grams per hour?

Note that:

1) the amu for Fe is approximately 56;

2) 1 Faraday is equivalent to 1 mole of electrons.

A. 0.218
B. 0.279
C. 0.340
D. 0.460

---

20) For an oxidation-reduction reaction, which of the following is a consistent set of relations?

A. $\Delta G^o > 0, \Delta E^o < 0, K_{eq} < 1$
B. $\Delta G^o < 0, \Delta E^o < 0, K_{eq} > 1$
C. $\Delta G^o < 0, \Delta E^o < 0, K_{eq} < 1$
D. $\Delta G^o < 0, \Delta E^o > 0, K_{eq} < 1$

High-level Importance

Questions 21–23

When one thinks of structural abnormalities in metals, invariably the first thing to come to mind is rusting. The rusting of iron in particular is a remarkable phenomenon, especially from the electrochemical point of view. Consider the following diagram.

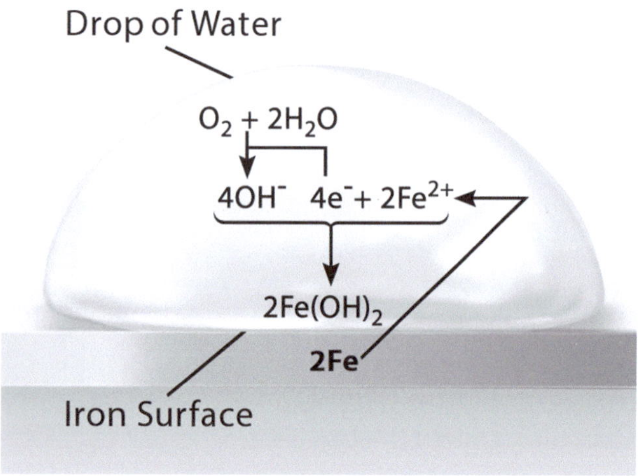

Figure 1

Metals have a tendency to "throw off" ions into solution (referred to as the *solution pressure*). Therefore, one would expect the metal to exert its full solution pressure at the centre of the drop. There is then an excess of electrons at the centre of the drop and a flow of electrons occurs from the inside to the outside of the drop. Here, since the outside of the drop is exposed to the atmosphere, oxygen reacts with the electrons to yield hydroxide ions.

Equation I

$$2Fe \leftrightarrow 2Fe^{2+} + 4e^- \qquad E^\circ = +0.440\ V$$

Equation II

$$O_2 + 2H_2O + 4e^- \leftrightarrow 4OH^- \qquad E^\circ = +0.401\ V$$

The Fe^{2+} and OH^- then react to produce iron (II) hydroxide. Further oxidation and subsequent dehydration eventually give rise to the hydrated iron (III) oxide (Fe_2O_3-xH_2O) which is not closely adhering and tends to "flake off."

Many processes can be used to reduce rusting. One involves coating the iron with "galvanising" zinc. When the surface is scratched and water enters, zinc hydroxide forms and this is a closely adhering salt which protects the iron underneath from further attack. Another method is the addition of bicarbonate (HCO_3^-) to remove the hydroxide ions produced before they can react with the iron.

Equation III

$$HCO_3^- + OH^- \rightarrow CO_3^{2-} + H_2O$$

Equations I to III are oxidation-reduction (*redox*) reactions. The voltage associated with a redox reaction at standard conditions can be summarised as $E^\circ(X/X^{+n})$ which describes the oxidation reaction, and $E^\circ(X^{+n}/X)$ which describes the reduction reaction.

21) For galvanising to be effective, which of the following must be true?

A. $K_{sp}\ Zn(OH)_2 < K_{sp}\ Fe(OH)_2$
B. $K_{sp}\ Zn(OH)_2 > K_{sp}\ Fe(OH)_2$
C. $E^\circ(Zn^{2+}/Zn) > E^\circ(Fe^{2+}/Fe)$
D. $E^\circ(Zn^{2+}/Zn) < E^\circ(Fe^{2+}/Fe)$

22) From the information in the passage, determine the E° for the overall reaction:

$$2Fe\ (s) + O_2\ (g) + 2H_2O\ (l) \rightarrow 2Fe^{2+}\ (aq) + 4OH^-\ (aq)$$

A. +0.382 V
B. +0.841 V
C. –0.058 V
D. –1.702 V

23) Why do you suppose that adding an electrolyte to the iron would increase its rate of rusting?

A. It causes the Fe_2O_3-xH_2O to flake off more rapidly.
B. It increases the charge-carrying capacity of the water.
C. It increases the solution pressure of the iron.
D. It inhibits the reactions involved.

---

24) Which of the species in Table 1 is best suited to oxidise NO given that:

$$HNO_2 + H^+ + e^- \leftrightarrow NO + H_2O$$

$$E^\circ = +1.00 \text{ V}$$

Electrochemical reaction	E° value (V)
$Ce^{4+} + e^- \leftrightarrow Ce^{3+}$	+1.695
$H_2O_2 + 2e^- \leftrightarrow 2OH^-$	+0.880
$MnO_4^- + e^- \leftrightarrow MnO_4^{2-}$	+0.564
$Cd^{2+} + 2e^- \leftrightarrow Cd$	−0.403

Table 1

A. Ce^{4+}
B. Ce^{3+}
C. Cd^{2+}
D. Cd

25) Which of the following is the strongest reducing agent?

Electrochemical reaction	E° value (V)
$MnO_2 + 4H^+ + 2e^- \leftrightarrow Mn^{2+} + 2H_2O$	+1.23
$Fe^{3+} + e^- \leftrightarrow Fe^{2+}$	+0.771
$N_2 + 5H^+ + 4e^- \leftrightarrow N_2H_5^+$	−0.230
$Cr^{3+} + e^- \leftrightarrow Cr^{2+}$	−0.410

A. Cr^{3+}
B. Cr^{2+}
C. Mn^{2+}
D. MnO_2

Bonus Question!

{Please be familiar with your log rules and exponents: CHM Primer 1.5.5, 3.7; GM 3.7.}

26) The attenuation coefficient (μ) is a constant representing the fraction of the reduction of intensity (*attenuation*) of, for example, incident electrons in a specific beam per unit thickness of a material. The SI unit for μ is m^{-1}.

The attenuation of an electron beam passing through a slab can be determined by a form of the Beer–Lambert law:

$$I = I_0 \cdot e^{-\mu x}$$

where I is the intensity at depth x metres, I_0 is the original intensity, μ is the attenuation coefficient, and e is approximately 2.718.

Note that: 1) ln 2 = 0.693 and ln 10 = 2.303; 2) if $y = e^x$ then $\ln y = x$.

Identify the best approximation of the attenuation coefficient of a slab of material which could stop half of the electrons from passing through a thickness of 7 cm.

A. 2.3 m^{-1}
B. 6.9 m^{-1}
C. 7.5 m^{-1}
D. 10 m^{-1}

High-level Importance

SPOILER ALERT

Gold Standard has cross-referenced the content in this chapter to examples from ACER's official GAMSAT practice materials. It is for you to decide when you want to explore these questions since you may want to preserve some of ACER's materials for timed mock-exam practice.

Examples – Standard reduction potential table, determine the reducing agent, modified Nernst equation question, absolute value of E° (absolute value: GM 1.1.3 and chapter-ending practice questions): Q29-33 of 1; oxidation numbers, although they give some rules, one of the questions is definitely easier if you know the rules already: Q14-15 of 3. Note that "Q" is followed by the question number, and, for example, "of 1" refers to booklet number 1 which is referenced in the Spoiler Alert table at the end of Chapter 1. The 15 full-length GAMSAT practice tests by Gold Standard, HEAPS-1 through HEAPS-15, contain specific cross-references to this chapter within the worked solutions. Note that the Pourbaix-diagram unit with the Nernst equation is a rare visitor from our Virtual Reality mock exam VR-1; the unit with the reduction potential table is from HEAPS-6; the chemistry that is occurring in a drop of water sitting quietly on iron is from HEAPS-7.

References

α: Figure III.A.10.2
OhiostandardVector, AntiComposite; Wikimedia Commons, 2021

β: Figure 1
Modified from DerSilberspiegel; Wikimedia Commons, 2021

Chapter Checklist

- ☐ Access your online account to view answers, worked solutions and discussion boards.
- ☐ Reassess your 'learning objectives' for this chapter: Go back to the first page of this chapter and re-evaluate the top 3 boxes and the Introduction.
    - ☐ Please be sure that you have completed the *Need for Speed* exercises at the beginning of this chapter.
- ☐ Complete a maximum of 1 page of notes using symbols/abbreviations to represent the entire chapter based on your learning objectives. These are your Gold Notes.
- ☐ Consider your multimedia options based on your optimal way of learning:
    - ☐ Download the free Gold Standard GAMSAT app for your Android device or iPhone.
    - ☐ Create your own, tangible study cards or try the free app: Anki.
    - ☐ Record your voice reading your Gold Notes onto your smartphone (audio files, e.g., *memo* or MP3s) and listen during exercise, transportation, etc.
    - ☐ Try out the Gold Standard GAMSAT online videos at gamsat-prep.com, or you can try other options on YouTube like Khan Academy or Crash Course Chemistry.
- ☐ Reassess your schedule for your full-length GAMSAT practice tests: ACER and/or HEAPS exams. Ensure that you have scheduled one full day to complete a practice test and 1-2 days for a thorough assessment of worked solutions while adding to your abbreviated Gold Notes.
- ☐ Reassess your progress in scheduling and/or evaluating stress reduction techniques such as regular exercise (sports), yoga, meditation and/or mindfulness exercises (*see* YouTube for suggestions).

"A diamond is merely a lump of coal that did well under pressure." Another big step in your GAMSAT prep is behind you! Revise your Gold Notes and practice, practice, practice! Good luck!

High-level Importance

GAMSAT GENERAL CHEMISTRY KEY POINTS

01
Atoms: Shapes, Classifications, Bonds to Make Molecules, and Balance

Chapter 1: Stoichiometry
Chapter 2: Electronic Structure and the Periodic Table
Chapter 3: Bonding

02
Solids, Liquids and Gases

Chapter 4: Phases and Phase Equilibria
Chapter 5: Solution Chemistry

03
Special Case: Protons in Water

Chapter 6: Acids and Bases

04
Chemical Reactions: Heat, Spontaneity, and Speed

Chapter 7: Thermodynamics
Chapter 8: Enthalpy and Thermochemistry
Chapter 9: Rate Processes in Chemical Reactions

05
Electricity from Chemicals: Redox Reactions

Chapter 10: Electrochemistry

GAMSAT-prep.com

Note: These final pages provide a summary of important facts, concepts and graphs for GAMSAT General Chemistry. The issue of what to memorise or understand, is dealt with clearly on the first page of each chapter.

CHAPTER 1: Stoichiometry

1.1 Atoms, Stuff, and Things that Matter

- That which occupies space and possesses mass...

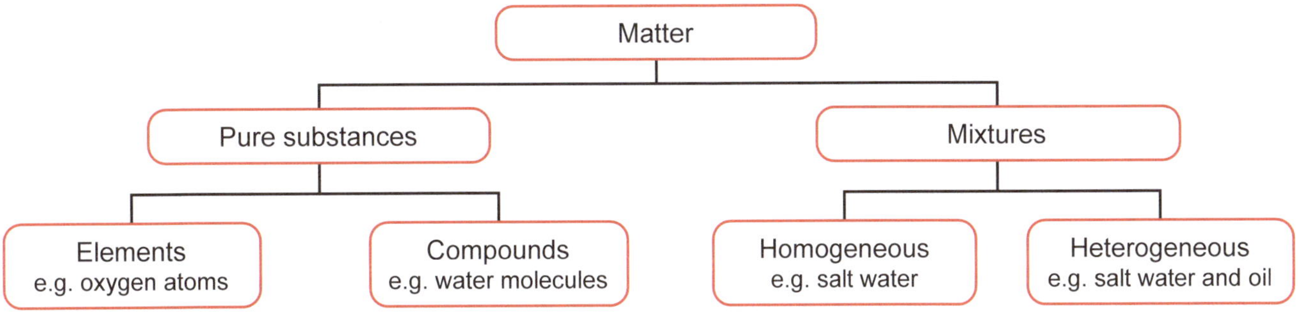

1.3 Mole - Atomic and Molecular Weights

For element:

$$\text{moles} = \frac{\text{weight of sample in grams}}{\text{GAW}}$$

1 mol = 6.02×10^{23} atoms

For compound:

$$\text{moles} = \frac{\text{weight of sample in grams}}{\text{GMW}}$$

1 mol = 6.02×10^{23} molecules

1.5.1 Categories of Chemical Reactions

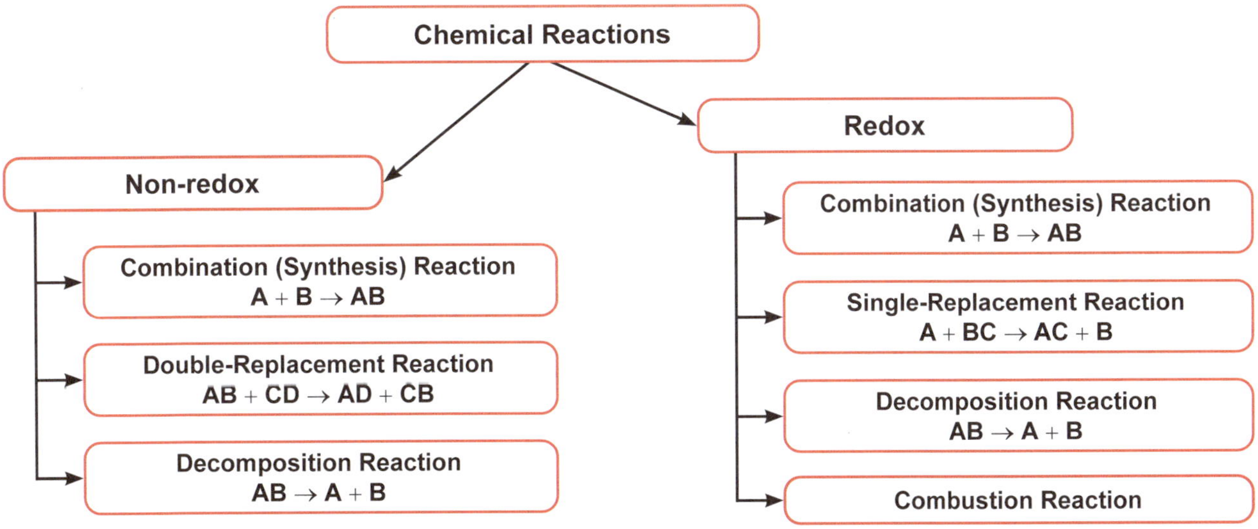

Note: Any reaction that does not involve the transfer of electrons (= change in oxidation numbers) qualifies as a non-redox reaction. Combination reactions qualify as non-redox reactions when all reactants and products are compounds and the oxidation numbers do not change. Decomposition reactions qualify as non-redox reactions when all reactants and products are compounds and the oxidation numbers do not change.

CHAPTER 3: Bonding

3.3 Partial Ionic Character: Polar Covalent Bonds

- This polar bond will also have a dipole moment given by:

$$D = q \cdot d$$

where q is the charge and d is the distance between these two atoms.

3.4 Lewis Acids and Lewis Bases

- The Lewis acid BF_3 and the Lewis base NH_3. Notice that the green arrows follow the flow of electron pairs. {Mnemonic: lEwis Acids: Electron pair Acceptors}

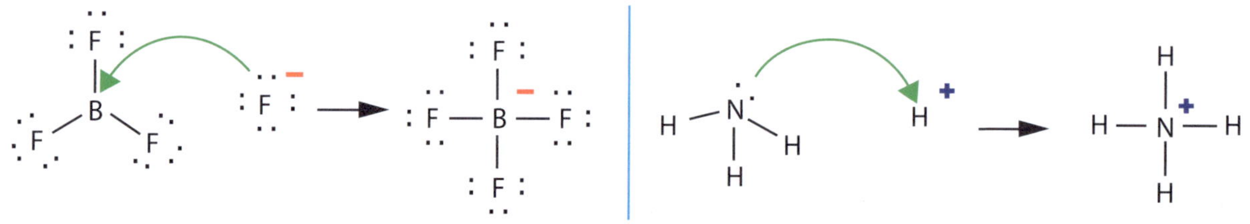

3.5 Valence Shell Electron Pair Repulsions (VSEPR Models)

- Geometry of simple molecules in which the central atom A has one or more lone pairs of electrons (= e⁻)

Total number of e⁻ pairs	Number of lone pairs	Number of bonding pairs	Electron Geometry, Arrangement of e⁻ pairs	Molecular Geometry (Hybridisation State)	Examples
3	1	2	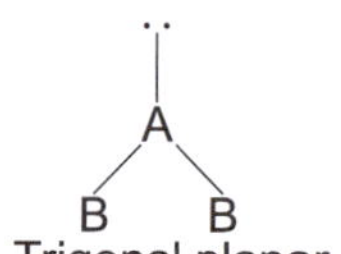 Trigonal planar	Bent (sp^2)	SO_2
4	1	3	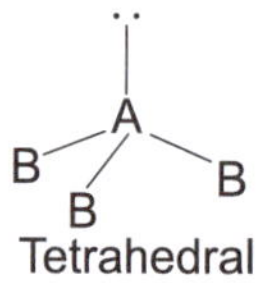 Tetrahedral	Trigonal pyramidal (sp^3)	NH_3
4	2	2	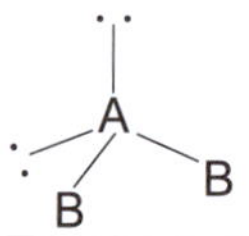 Tetrahedral	Bent (sp^3)	H_2O

5	1	4	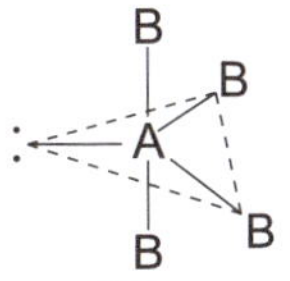 Trigonal bipyramidal	Seesaw (sp^3d)	SF_4
5	2	3	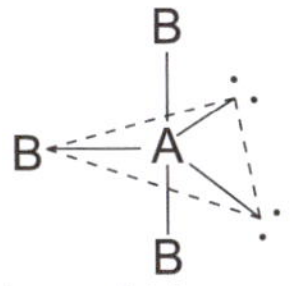 Trigonal bipyramidal	T-shaped (sp^3d)	ClF_3

Note: dotted lines only represent the overall molecular shape and not molecular bonds. In brackets under "Molecular Geometry" is the hybridisation.

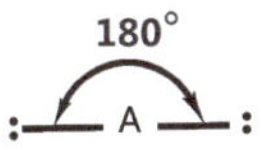

linear arrangement
of 2 electron pairs
around central atom A

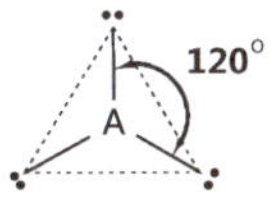

trigonal planar arrangement
of 3 electron pairs
around central atom A

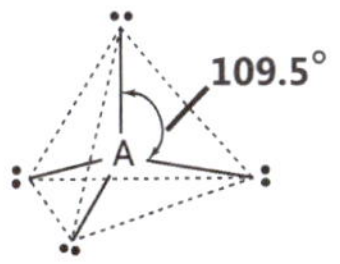

tetrahedral arrangement
of 4 electron pairs
around central atom A

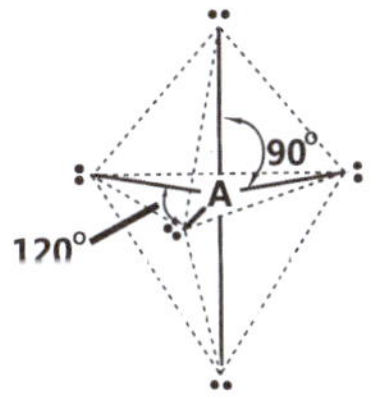

trigonal bipyramidal arrangement
of 5 electron pairs
around central atom A

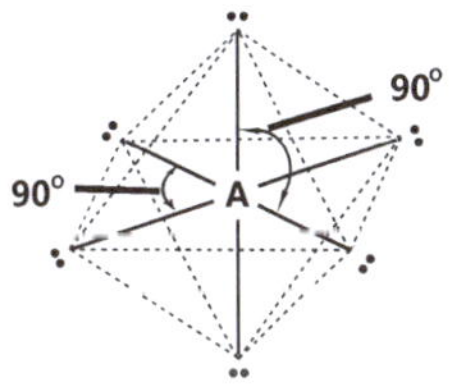

octahedral arrangement
of 6 electron pairs
around central atom A

Molecular arrangement of electron pairs around a central atom A. Dotted lines only represent the overall molecular shape and not molecular bonds.

CHAPTER 4: Phases and Phase Equilibria

4.1.1 Standard Temperature and Pressure, Standard Molar Volume

- 0 °C (273.15 K) and 1.00 atm (101.33 kPa = 760 mmHg = 760 torr); these conditions are known as the standard temperature and pressure (STP). {Note: the SI unit of pressure is the pascal (Pa).}
- The volume occupied by one mole of any gas at STP is referred to as the standard molar volume and is equal to 22.4 L.

4.1.2 Kinetic Molecular Theory of Gases (A Model for Gases)

- The average kinetic energy of the particles ($KE = 1/2\ mv^2$) increases in direct proportion to the temperature of the gas ($KE = 3/2\ kT$) when the temperature is measured on an absolute scale (i.e. the Kelvin scale) and k is a constant (the Boltzmann constant).

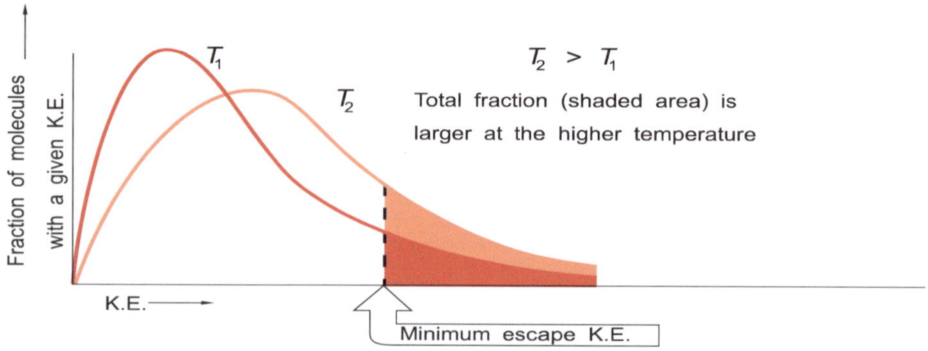

The Maxwell Distribution Plot

4.1.3 Graham's Law (Diffusion and Effusion of Gases)

$$\frac{Rate_1}{Rate_2} = \sqrt{\frac{M_2}{M_1}}$$

4.1.4 Charles' Law

$$V = \text{Constant} \times T \quad \text{or} \quad V_1/V_2 = T_1/T_2$$
$$\text{or} \quad V_1/T_1 = V_2/T_2$$

4.1.5 Boyle's Law

$$V = \text{Constant} \times 1/P \quad \text{or} \quad P_1V_1 = P_2V_2$$

4.1.6 Avogadro's Law

$$V/n = \text{Constant} \quad \text{or} \quad V_1/n_1 = V_2/n_2$$

4.1.7 Combined Gas Law

$$\frac{P_1V_1}{T_1} = k = \frac{P_2V_2}{T_2} \quad \text{(at constant mass)}$$

4.1.8 Ideal Gas Law

$$PV = nRT$$

since m/V is the density (d) of the gas:

$$P = \frac{dRT}{M}$$

4.1.9 Partial Pressure and Dalton's Law

$$P_T = P_1 + P_2 + \ldots + P_i$$

Of course, the sum of all mole fractions in a mixture must equal one:

$$\Sigma X_1 = 1$$

The partial pressure (P_i) of a component of a gas mixture is equal to:

$$P_i = X_i P_T$$

4.2 Liquid Phase (Intermolecular Forces)

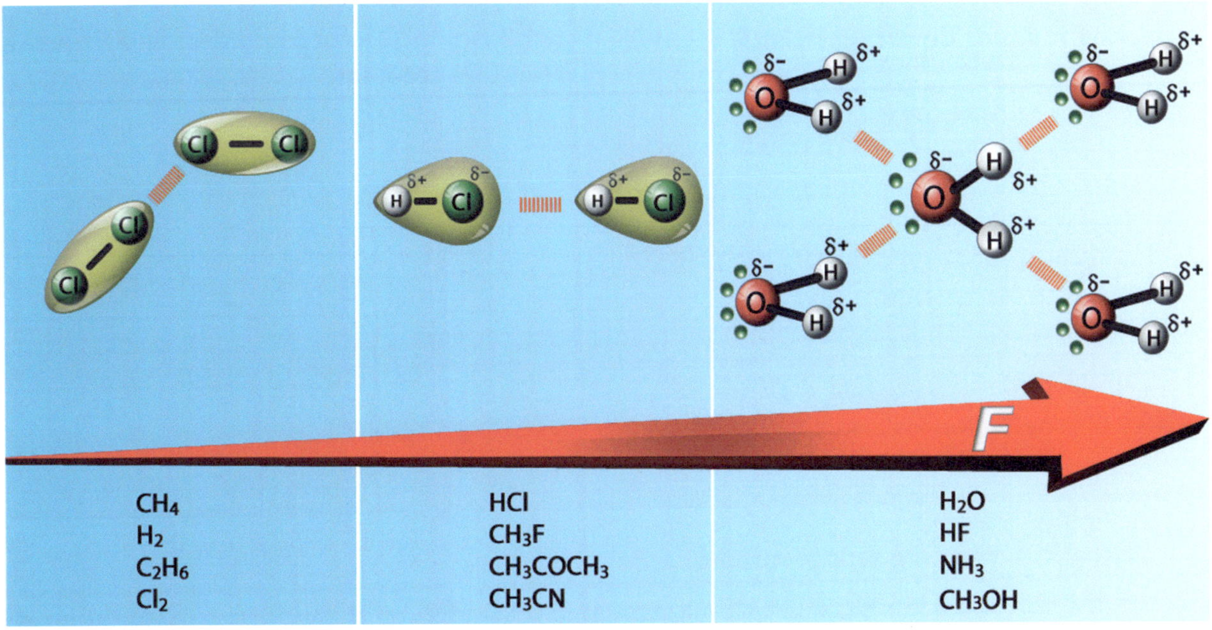

Intermolecular (*between different molecules*) bonding: Van Der Waal's forces (weak) and hydrogen bonding (strong). London forces between Cl_2 molecules, dipole-dipole forces between HCl molecules and H-bonding between H_2O molecules. Note that a partial negative charge on an atom is indicated by δ^- (delta negative), while a partial positive charge is indicated by δ^+ (delta positive). Notice that one H_2O molecule can potentially form 4 H-bonds with surrounding molecules which is highly efficient. The preceding is one key reason that the boiling point of water is higher than that of ammonia, hydrogen fluoride or methanol.

4.4.1 Phase Changes

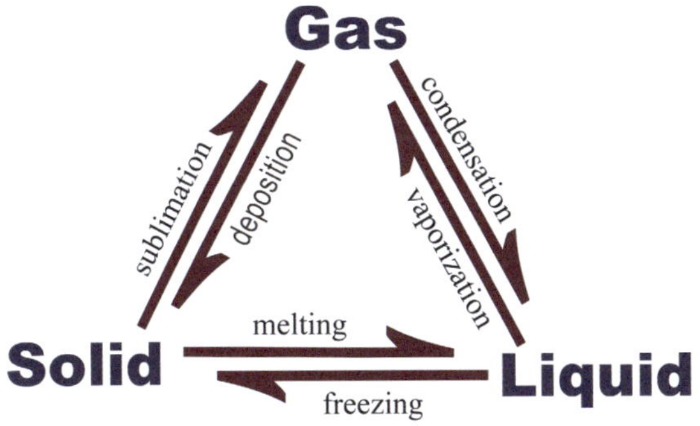

4.4.3 Phase Diagrams

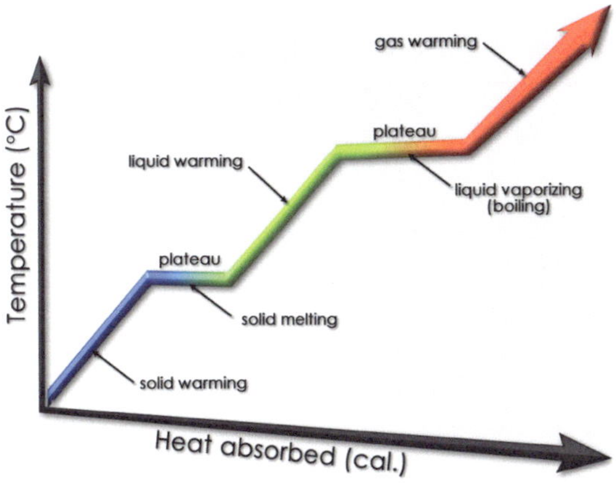

CHAPTER 5: Solution Chemistry

5.1.1 Vapor-Pressure Lowering (Raoult's Law)

$$P = P^{\circ}X_{solvent}$$

where P = vapor pressure of solution
P° = vapor pressure of pure solvent (at the same temperature as P)

5.1.2 Boiling-Point Elevation and Freezing-Point Depression

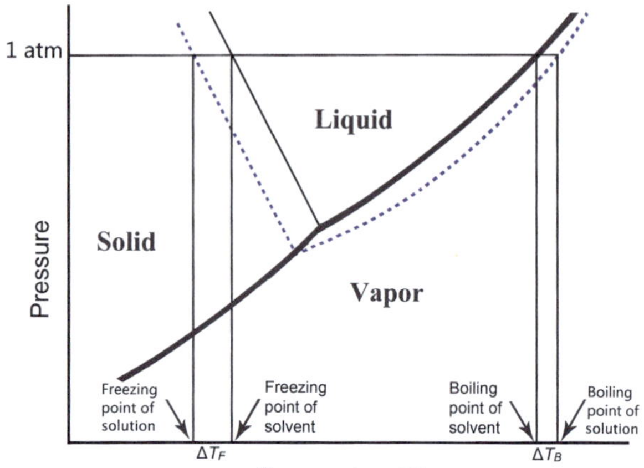

Phase diagram of water demonstrating the effect of the addition of a solute
$\Delta T_B = iK_b m$
$\Delta T_F = iK_F m$

5.1.3 Osmotic Pressure

$$\Pi = i\,MRT$$

where R = gas constant per mole
T = temperature in degrees K and
M = concentration of solute (mole/litre)
i = Van't Hoff factor

5.2 Ions in Solution

- Ions that are positively charged = cations; ions that are negatively charged = anions
- *Mnemonic: anions are negative ions*
- The word "aqueous" simply means containing or dissolved in water

Common Anions					
F^-	Fluoride	OH^-	Hydroxide	ClO^-	Hypochlorite
Cl^-	Chloride	NO_3^-	Nitrate	ClO_2^-	Chlorite
Br^-	Bromide	NO_2^-	Nitrite	ClO_3^-	Chlorate
I^-	Iodide	CO_3^{2-}	Carbonate	ClO_4^-	Perchlorate
O^{2-}	Oxide	SO_4^{2-}	Sulfate	SO_3^{2-}	Sulfite
S^{2-}	Sulfide	PO_4^{3-}	Phosphate	CN^-	Cyanide
N^{3-}	Nitride	$CH_3CO_2^-$	Acetate	MnO_4^-	Permanganate

Common Cations			
Na^+	Sodium	H^+	Hydrogen
Li^+	Lithium	Ca^{2+}	Calcium
K^+	Potassium	Mg^{2+}	Magnesium
NH_4^+	Ammonium	Fe^{2+}	Iron (II)
H_3O^+	Hydronium	Fe^{3+}	Iron (III)

5.3.1 Units of Concentration

- Molarity (M): moles of solute/litre of solution (solution = solute + solvent)
- Normality (N): one equivalent per litre
- Molality (m): one mole/1000g of solvent
- Molal concentrations are not temperature-dependent as molar and normal concentrations are
- Density (ρ): Mass per unit volume at the specified temperature
- Osmole (Osm): The number of moles of particles (molecules or ions) that contribute to the osmotic pressure of a solution
- Osmolarity: osmoles/litre of solution
- Osmolality: osmoles/kilogram of solution
- Mole Fraction: amount of solute (in moles) divided by the total amount of solvent and solute (in moles)
- Dilution: $M_iV_i = M_fV_f$

5.3.2 Solubility Product Constant, the Equilibrium Expression

$$AgCl\ (s) \rightleftharpoons Ag^+\ (aq) + Cl^-\ (aq)$$

$$K_{sp} = [Ag^+][Cl^-]$$

Because the K_{sp} product always holds, precipitation will not take place unless the product of $[Ag^+]$ and $[Cl^-]$ exceeds the K_{sp}.

5.3.5 Solubility Rules

1. All salts of alkali metals are soluble.
2. All salts of the ammonium ion are soluble.
3. All chlorides, bromides and iodides are water soluble, with the exception of Ag^+, Pb^{2+}, and Hg_2^{2+}.
4. All salts of the sulfate ion (SO_4^{2-}) are water soluble with the exception of Ca^{2+}, Sr^{2+}, Ba^{2+}, and Pb^{2+}.

5. All metal oxides are insoluble with the exception of the alkali metals and CaO, SrO and BaO.
6. All hydroxides are insoluble with the exception of the alkali metals and Ca^{2+}, Sr^{2+}, Ba^{2+}.
7. All carbonates (CO_3^{2-}), phosphates (PO_4^{3-}), sulfides (S^{2-}) and sulfites (SO_3^{2-}) are insoluble, with the exception of the alkali metals and ammonium.

CHAPTER 6: Acids and Bases

6.1 Acids

$$K_a = [H^+][A^-]/[HA]$$

STRONG	WEAK
Perchloric $HClO_4$	Hydrocyanic HCN
Chloric $HClO_3$	Hypochlorous HClO
Nitric HNO_3	Nitrous HNO_2
Hydrochloric HCl	Hydrofluoric HF
Sulfuric H_2SO_4	Sulfurous H_2SO_3
Hydrobromic HBr	Hydrogen Sulfide H_2S
Hydriodic HI	Phosphoric H_3PO_4
Hydronium Ion H_3O^+	Benzoic, Acetic and other Carboxylic Acids

6.2 Bases

$$K_b = [HB^+][OH^-]/[B]$$

- Strong bases include any hydroxide of the group 1A metals
- The most common weak bases are ammonia and any organic amine.

6.3 Conjugate Acid-Base Pairs

- The acid, HA, and the base produced when it ionises, A-, are called a conjugate acid-base pair.

6.4 Water Dissociation

$$K_w = [H^+][OH^-] = 1.0 \times 10^{-14}$$

6.5 The pH Scale

$$pH = -\log_{10}[H^+]$$

$$pOH = -\log_{10}[OH^-]$$

at 25°C, pH + pOH = 14.0

6.5.1 Properties of Logarithms

1. $\log_a a = 1$
2. $\log_a M^k = k \log_a M$
3. $\log_a(MN) = \log_a M + \log_a N$
4. $\log_a(M/N) = \log_a M - \log_a N$
5. $10^{\log_{10}(M)} = M$

6.7 Salts of Weak Acids and Bases

$$K_a \times K_b = K_w$$

6.8 Buffers

$$pH = pK_a + \log([salt]/[acid])$$

$$pOH = pK_b + \log([salt]/[base])$$

CHAPTER 7: Thermodynamics

7.2 The First Law of Thermodynamics

$$\Delta E = Q - W$$

- heat absorbed by the system: Q > 0
- heat released by the system: Q < 0
- work done by the system on its surroundings: W > 0
- work done by the surroundings on the system: W < 0

7.4 Temperature Scales

$$0\ K = -273\ °C.$$

7.6 State Functions

- W can be determined experimentally by calculating the area under a pressure-volume curve

	Work	Heat	Changes in internal energy
1st tranf.	w	0	$-w$
2nd transf.	$W = w + q$	q	$-w$

CHAPTER 8: Enthalpy and Thermochemistry

8.2 Heat of Reaction: Basic Principles

- A reaction during which heat is released is said to be exothermic (ΔH is negative).
- If a reaction requires the supply of a certain amount of heat it is endothermic (ΔH is positive).

$$\Delta H_{OVERALL} = \Delta H_1 + \Delta H_2$$

$$\Delta H°_{reaction} = \Sigma\Delta H_f°{}_{(products)} - \Sigma\Delta H_f°{}_{(reactants)}$$

8.6 Bond Dissociation Energies and Heats of Formation

$$\Delta H^\circ_{(reaction)} = \Sigma\Delta H_{(bonds\ broken)} + \Sigma\Delta H_{(bonds\ formed)}$$
$$= \Sigma BE_{(reactants)} - \Sigma BE_{(products)}$$

8.7 Calorimetry

$$Q = mC(T_2 - T_1)$$

$$Q = mL$$

8.8 The Second Law of Thermodynamics

- For any spontaneous process, the entropy of the universe increases which results in a greater dispersal or randomisation of the energy ($\Delta S > 0$).

8.9 Entropy

$$\Delta S^\circ_{reaction} = \Delta S^\circ_{products} - \Delta S^\circ_{reactants}$$

8.10 Free Energy

$$\Delta G = \Delta H - T\Delta S$$

- A reaction carried out at constant pressure is spontaneous if: $\Delta G < 0$
- It is not spontaneous if: $\Delta G > 0$
- It is in a state of equilibrium (reaction spontaneous in both directions) if: $\Delta G = 0$

CHAPTER 9: Rate Processes in Chemical Reactions

9.2 Dependence of Reaction Rates on Concentration of Reactants

$$\text{rate} = k\,[A]^m\,[B]^n$$

- [ ] is the concentration of the corresponding reactant in moles per litre
- k is referred to as the rate constant
- m is the order of the reaction with respect to A
- n is the order of the reaction with respect to B
- m+n is the overall reaction order

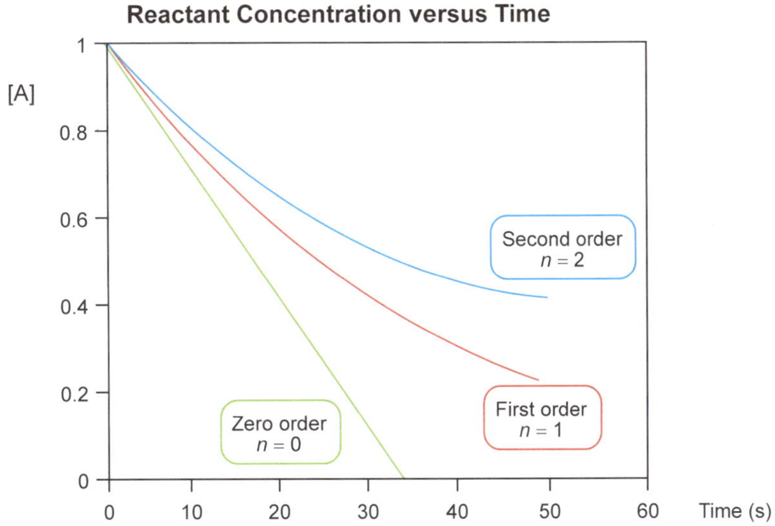

9.2.1 Differential Rate Law vs. Integrated Rate Law

Rate Law Summary					
Reaction Order	**Rate Law**	**Units of k**	**Integrated Rate Law**	**Straight-Line Plot**	**Half-Life Equation**
0	Rate $= k[A]^0$	$M \cdot s^{-1}$	$[A]_t = -kt + [A]_0$	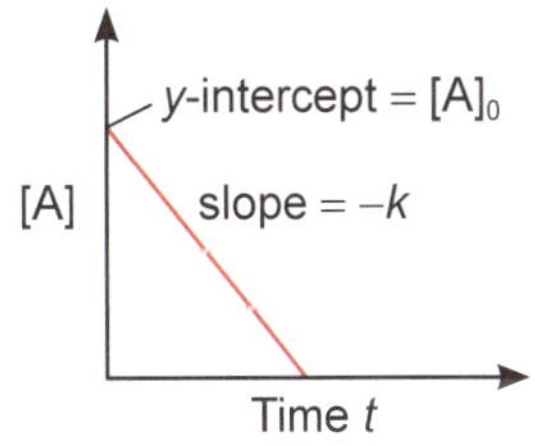	$t_{1/2} = \frac{[A]_0}{2k} = \frac{1}{k}\frac{[A]_0}{2}$
1	Rate $= k[A]^1$	s^{-1}	$\ln[A]_t = -kt + \ln[A]_0$ $\ln\frac{[A]_t}{[A]_0} = -kt$	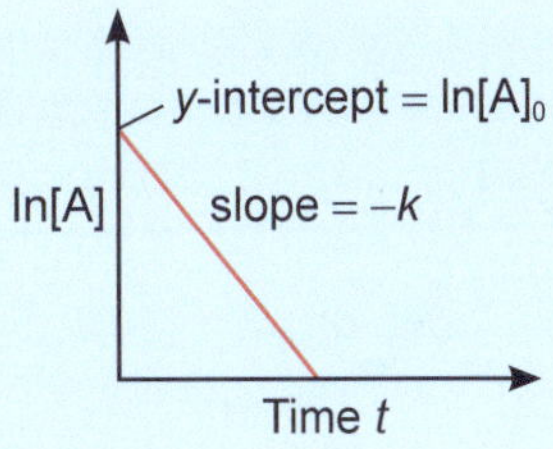	$t_{1/2} = \frac{0.693}{k} = \frac{1}{k}(0.693)$
2	Rate $= k[A]^2$	$M^{-1} \cdot s^{-1}$	$\frac{1}{[A]_t} = kt + \frac{1}{[A]_0}$	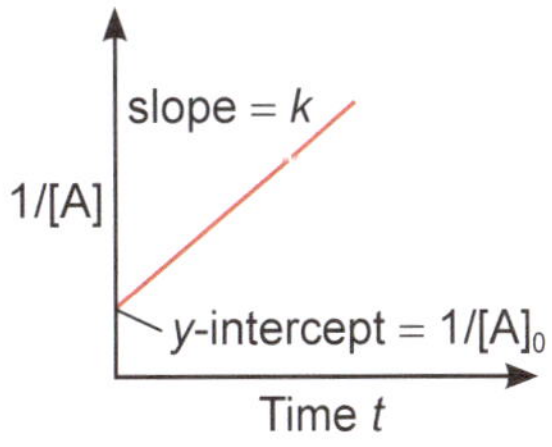	$t_{1/2} = \frac{1}{k[A]_0} = \frac{1}{k}\frac{1}{[A]_0}$

The 3 graphs in the table do not need to be memorised but you may be expected to match any Integrated Rate Law equation with its graph since they follow the simple standard of y = mx + b (CHM 9.2.1; GM 3.4.4, 3.5.1).

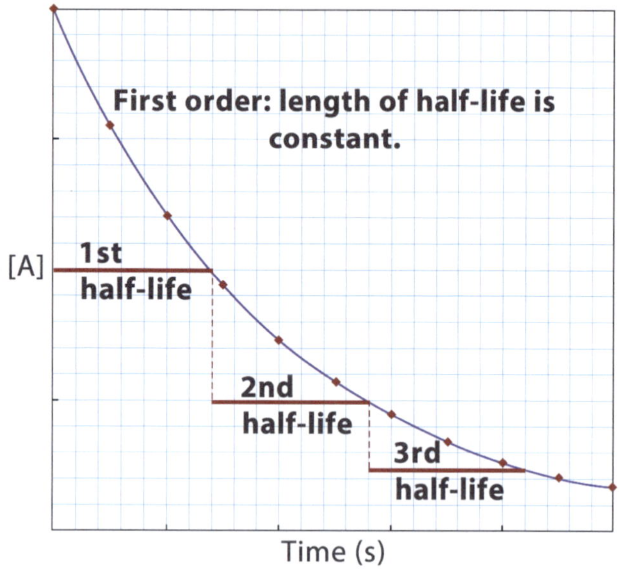

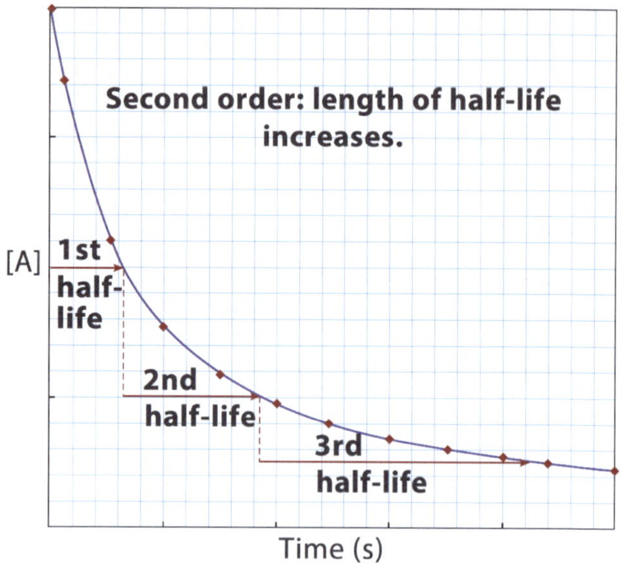

9.5 Dependence of Reaction Rates upon Temperature

$$k = A\,e^{-Ea/RT}$$

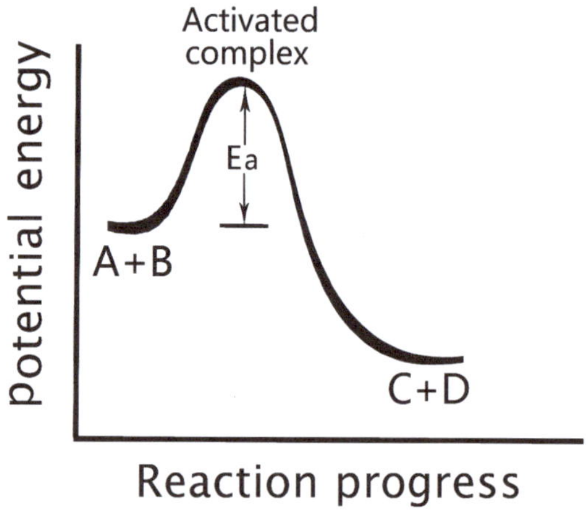

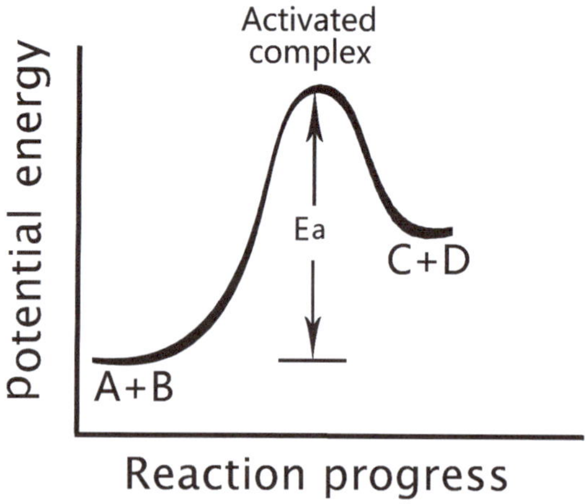

Potential Energy Diagrams: Exothermic vs. Endothermic Reactions

9.7 Catalysis

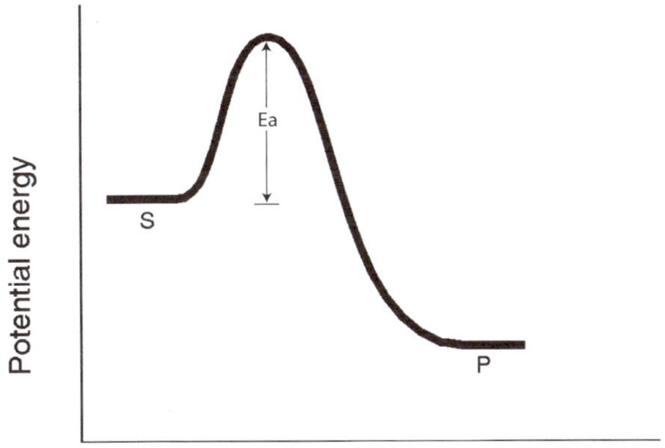

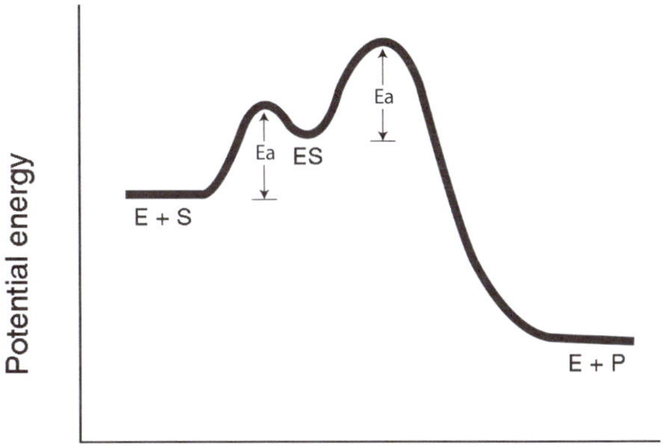

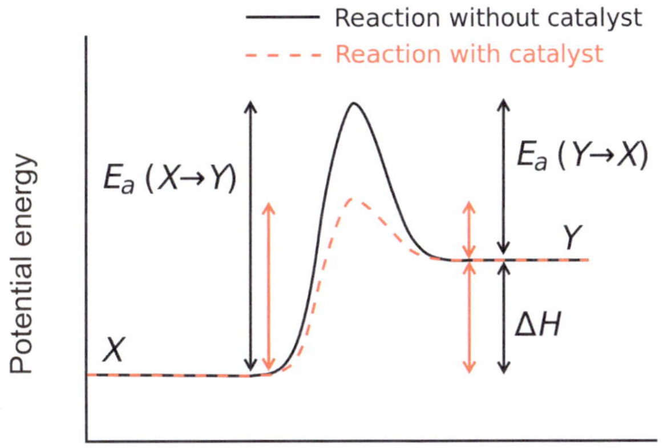

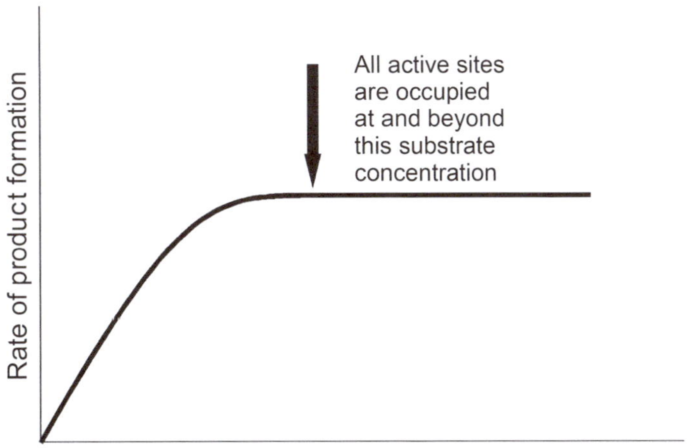

Saturation Kinetics

9.8 Equilibrium in Reversible Chemical Reactions

$$aA + bB \rightleftharpoons cC + dD$$

$$K_{eq} = \frac{[C]^c [D]^d}{[A]^a [B]^b}$$

- {Note: Catalysts speed up the rate of reaction without affecting K_{eq}}

9.9 Le Chatelier's Principle

- Le Chatelier's principle states that whenever a perturbation is applied to a system at equilibrium, the system evolves in such a way as to compensate for the applied perturbation.

9.10 Relationship between the Equilibrium Constant and the Change in the Gibbs Free Energy

$$\Delta G^\circ = -R\,T\,ln\,K_{eq}$$

CHAPTER 10: Electrochemistry

10.0.1 Oxidation Numbers, Redox Reactions, Oxidising vs. Reducing Agents

- Here are the general rules:
  - In elementary substances, the oxidation number of an uncombined element is zero
  - In monatomic ions the oxidation number of the elements that make up this ion is equal to the charge of the ion
  - In a neutral molecule the sum of the oxidation numbers of all the elements that make up the molecule is zero
- Some useful oxidation numbers to memorise
  - For H: +1, except in metal hydrides where it is equal to -1
  - For O: -2 in most compounds; In peroxides (e.g. in H_2O_2) the oxidation number for O is -1, it is +2 in OF_2 and -1/2 in superoxides
  - For alkali metals: +1
  - For alkaline earth metals: +2
  - Aluminium always has an oxidation number of +3 in all its compounds

10.1 Redox Reactions and Half-cell Potentials

- The more positive the E° value, the more likely the reaction will occur spontaneously as written.
- The strongest reducing agents have large negative E° values.
- The strongest oxidising agents have large positive E° values.
- The oxidising agent is reduced; the reducing agent is oxidised.

10.2 Galvanic Cells

- Mnemonic: LEO is A GERC
    - Lose Electrons Oxidation is Anode
    - Gain Electrons Reduction at Cathode

10.5 Faraday's Law

- Faraday's law relates the amount of elements deposited or gas liberated at an electrode due to current.
- One mole (= Avogadro's number) of electrons is called a faraday ($\mathfrak{F}$).
- A coulomb is the amount of electricity that is transferred when a current of one ampere flows for one second (1C = 1A · s).